Smart Nanovesicles for Drug Targeting and Delivery

Smart Nanovesicles for Drug Targeting and Delivery

Special Issue Editors

Maria Carafa
Carlotta Marianecci

MDPI • Basel • Beijing • Wuhan • Barcelona • Belgrade

MDPI

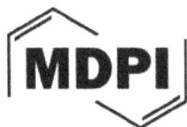

Special Issue Editors

Maria Carafa
Department Chimica e Tecnologie del
Farmaco Sapienza Università di Roma
Italy

Carlotta Marianecci
Department Chimica e Tecnologie del
Farmaco Sapienza Università di Roma
Italy

Editorial Office
MDPI
St. Alban-Anlage 66
4052 Basel, Switzerland

This is a reprint of articles from the Special Issue published online in the open access journal *Pharmaceutics* (ISSN 1999-4923) from 2018 to 2019 (available at: https://www.mdpi.com/journal/pharmaceutics/special_issues/nanovesicles).

For citation purposes, cite each article independently as indicated on the article page online and as indicated below:

LastName, A.A.; LastName, B.B.; LastName, C.C. Article Title. *Journal Name* **Year**, *Article Number*, Page Range.

ISBN 978-3-03897-894-7 (Pbk)
ISBN 978-3-03897-895-4 (PDF)

Contents

About the Special Issue Editors

Maria Carafa is an Associate Professor of Pharmaceutical Technology at the Faculty of Pharmacy and Medicine, University of Rome "Sapienza". She obtained her PhD in Pharmaceutical Sciences at the University of Rome "Sapienza" in 1992. She started her scientific carrier working in the field of pharmaceutical technology, on the development of prolonged/controlled drug delivery systems based on natural polysaccharides. In recent years, she has focused her research on the preparation and characterization of vesicular systems. Phospholipid and surfactant vesicles and pH-sensitive vesicles have been studied as drug delivery systems for several pharmaceutical applications: Topical, ophthalmic, diagnostic, pulmonary, oral, drug delivery in CNS disorders and cellular targeting. Recently, she has focused on the deep physical–chemical characterization of vesicular formulations as drug delivery systems, preparation of mixed systems polymer/vesicles, nanoemulsions, and nanobubbles for different therapeutic and diagnostic applications. She has published 85 journal articles and about 200 oral and poster presentations; she has served as a peer reviewer for about 20 journals focused on nanotechnology and drug delivery (e.g., *J. Control. Release*, *Pharmceutics*, *Int. J. Pharm.*, *Colloids Surf. B*, *Colloids Surf. A*, *BBA: Biomembranes*). She is the coauthor of 3 book chapters and 4 patents. Associate Editor: Recent Pat. Drug Deliv. Formul.—ISSN: 2212-4039 (Online)—ISSN: 1872-2113 (Print); Editorial Board: Int. J. Med. Nano Res.; Pharma. Front.

Carlotta Marianecci, Associate Professor at the Faculty of Pharmacy and Medicine, Department of Drug Chemistry and Technologies, "Sapienza" University of Rome. Her research activity is mainly focused on pharmaceutical technology, and in particular on: Preparation and characterization of phospholipid (liposomes), non-phospholipid (niosomes), pH-sensitive and not vesicular systems, surfactant stabilized nanoemulsions, surfactant and phospholipid nanobubbles; studies on their cell internalization pathways in different cell lines; application of niosomes for topical, pulmonary, and brain delivery of drugs; study on l-dopa delivery and DNA delivery by different liposomal formulations; deep chemical–physical characterization studies on vesicular nanocarriers and preparation and characterization of theranostic nanocarriers. She is the author of about 65 national and international research papers, 3 patents, 3 book chapters, and about 70 oral and poster presentations, as well as a referee for 10 international journals focused on nanotechnology and drug delivery and a member of the Editorial Board of the *Recent Pat. Drug Deliv. Formul.*.

pharmaceutics

MDPI

Editorial

Smart Nanovesicles for Drug Targeting and Delivery

Carlotta Marianecci * and Maria Carafa *

Dipartimento di Chimica e Tecnologie del Farmaco, Sapienza University of Rome, 00185 Rome, Italy
* Correspondence: carlotta.marianecci@uniroma1.it (C.M.); maria.carafa@uniroma1.it (M.C.);
  Tel.: +39-06-49913970 (C.M.); +39-06-49913603 (M.C.)

Received: 27 March 2019; Accepted: 27 March 2019; Published: 29 March 2019

This special issue is dedicated to our teacher, mentor and friend Prof. Eleonora Santucci to celebrate her 80-years birthday.

Nanovesicles are highly-promising and versatile systems for the delivery and/or targeting of drugs, biomolecules and contrast agents. Despite the fact that initial studies in this area were performed on phospholipid vesicles, there is an ever-increasing interest in the use of other molecules to obtain smart vesicular carriers focusing on strategies for targeted delivery. This special issue aims to highlight and capture the contemporary progress and current landscape of smart nanovesicles applied in drug targeting and delivery.

A series of research articles and one review are present in this special issue and offer a summary of the different researches by different countries' teams, thus making meaningful and significant contributions to the field.

Asprea et al. investigated the possibility to obtain monodisperse and stable nanocochleates from Natural Soy Lecithin Liposomes, using two different phospholipids, phosphatidylcholine and phosphatidylserine, loaded with a typical small hydrophobic natural product, andrographolide (AG). AG from the Asiatic medicinal plant *Andrographis paniculata* shows numerous potential activities ranging from anti-inflammatory to neuroprotection, antidiabetic to anti-obesity properties, and antitumor activity to hepatoprotective activity. It has poor water solubility which deeply limits its biodistribution and localization, resulting in low bioavailability and additionally, is unstable in gastrointestinal media and has a very short biological half-life ($t_{\frac{1}{2}}$ = 1.33 h) after a single oral dose. The stability of developed nanocochleates after lyophilisation and in simulated gastrointestinal fluids was investigated. In addition, the studied nanocarriers show high EE%, and suitable drug release properties for oral delivery, but with possible uses in other routes of administration [1].

In a second study Piazzini et al. evaluated the possibility of using liposomes to enhance the penetration into the brain of AG. The AG-loaded liposomes showed protection against damage induced by amyloid-oligomers in vitro, reduction of amyloid levels and tau phosphorylation in mice, modulation of the formation of amyloid plaques and recovery of spatial memory functions in Alzheimer's disease transgenic mouse model. Liposomal surface was modified by adding Tween 80 alone or in combination with Didecyldimethylammonium bromide to confer cationic surface charge. Liposomes were evaluated for various formulation parameters (size, polydispersity, ζ-potential, morphology, chemical and physical stability, in vitro release) and the optimized formulations were studied and characterized with in vitro tests. Both formulations enhanced solubility and cellular permeability of AG, as in vitro tests with PAMPA and hCMEC/D3 cells and increase the permeation of AG into the cell without alterations in cell viability and monolayer integrity. The presence of positive charge elevated the cellular internalization of liposomes [2].

Another interesting study on a natural compound is the one by Santos-Rebelo and colleagues. In this research study, Parvifloron D was efficiently extracted and isolated from *P. ecklonii* and it showed more selectivity to human pancreatic tumor cells than healthy cells or breast cancer cells, but Parvifloron D is affected by low water-solubility, thus, small and spherical albumin nanoparticles (water soluble particles) have been formulated with high encapsulation efficiency to enhance drug solubility and targeted delivery. Those nanoparticles led to a controlled release of the drug, which was stable, and therefore, they can be considered a suitable and promising carrier to deliver the drug to the tumor site, improving the treatment of pancreatic cancer [3].

The great interest around natural compound delivery was confirmed by the study reported by Di Sotto and colleagues. They performed a deep physical-chemical characterization of soybean phosphatidylcholine (SPC) liposomes used to improve the dissolution of the natural sesquiterpene-caryophyllene (CRY) in biological fluids and its cellular uptake. Both unilamellar (ULV) and multilamellar (MLV) formulations were studied. The lipid composition, lamellarity, the manufacturing process and drug incorporation can all influence the physicochemical properties of a liposomal formulation, including the drug release performance. In particular, the influence of the drug–lipid ratio on the arrangement of the nonpolar region of the vesicles' membrane must be considered to design a carrier able to entrap and then release the loaded drug to obtain the therapeutic effect. The antiproliferative activity of CRY-loaded SPC ULV and MLV with respect to that of CRY alone was also studied in liver cancer HepG2 cells and MDA-MB-468 [4].

In the research study carried out by Coccè and colleagues, the application of extracellular vesicles in the paclitaxel delivery was evaluated. In particular, the anticancer activity of secretomes from both untreated and paclitaxel (PTX)-primed GinPaMSCs, by demonstrating that both PTX-loaded GinPaMSCs and the corresponding extracellular vesicles (EVs/PTX) were active against cancer cells. This research study provides a strong proof of concept, suggesting a possible application of the procedure to collect PTX-associated EVs from drug-primed GinPaMSC working as "natural anticancer liposomes" [5].

The study of Palchetti and colleagues focused on an important aspect related to liposomal administration: the understanding that the limited success of liposomal drugs in clinical practice is due to our poor knowledge of the nano–bio interactions experienced by liposomes in vivo. In this study, a library of 10 liposomal formulations with systematic changes in lipid composition were prepared and exposed to human plasma. Size, zeta-potential, and corona composition of the resulting liposome–protein complexes were thoroughly characterized. According to the recent literature, enrichment in protein corona fingerprints (PCFs) was used to predict the targeting ability of synthesized liposomal formulations. In this study, the predicted targeting capability of liposome–protein complexes was clearly correlated with cellular uptake in pancreatic adenocarcinoma (PANC-1) and insulinoma (INS-1) cells. The cellular uptake of the liposomal formulation with the highest abundance of PCFs was found to be much larger than that of Onivyde®, an Irinotecan liposomal drug approved by the Food and Drug Administration in 2015 for the treatment of metastatic pancreatic ductal adenocarcinoma [6].

An example of a pH sensitive targeting by using non-ionic surfactant vesicles is represented by the research study by Marzoli and colleagues. The anti-inflammatory and analgesic activity in acute and chronic models of pain of ibuprofen loaded pH sensitive vesicles was evaluated. These niosomes, with increased affinity for an acidic pH microenvironment, can take advantage of pathological conditions (ischemia, infection, inflammation, and cancer where extracellular pH values range from 5.5 to 7.0) for selective targeting. In particular pH-Tw20Gly niosomes loaded with ibuprofen were compared to free ibuprofen in animal models of acute and chronic pain. pH sensitive niosomal formulations increase Ibuprofen's analgesic activity, promoting a longer duration of action of this drug [7].

In the study of Rodrigues et al., multifunctional liposomes containing manganese ferrite/gold core/shell nanoparticles were developed in order to obtain simultaneous chemotherapy and phototherapy. In order to develop applications in cancer therapy, the prepared nanoparticles were entrapped in liposomes (aqueous magnetoliposomes, AMLs) or covered with a lipid bilayer (solid magnetoliposomes, SMLs). These new nanosystems were tested in this scenario as nanocarriers for a potential anticancer drug, especially active against melanoma, breast adenocarcinoma, and non-small cell lung cancer. The local heating capability of the developed systems was also monitored [8].

An alternative route of administration by means of a nanotechnological strategy was proposed by Touitou and colleagues for buspirone delivery. In particular, the nasal administration of buspirone incorporated in a new nanovesicular delivery system (NDS) to be tested in a hot flushes animal model was studied. The role of the carrier in the design of an efficient nasal product is fundamental, so to this aim, in this work, buspirone NDS was appropriately designed and extensively characterized, then the pharmacodynamic effect in an ovariectomized (OVX) animal model for hot flushes, and the drug levels in brain and plasma were evaluated. The safety of the local application of the nanovesicular system on the animal nasal cavity was also examined [9].

Finally, the review by Narayan and colleagues reported an overview on mesoporous silica nanoparticles (MSNs), a material with high thermal, chemical and mechanical properties, that have garnered immense attention as drug carriers owing to their distinctive features over the others [10].

All the articles presented in the special issue represent a small cross-section of a great research interest in the field of nanovesicular system applications in drug delivery.

From the overall presented results, several interesting potentialities of these systems have been highlighted together with their high versatility and excellent biocompatibility. These qualities make them attractive and we hope that they will soon be able to represent an evolution in products available on the market.

Conflicts of Interest: The authors declare no conflict of interest.

References

1. Asprea, M.; Tatini, F.; Piazzini, V.; Rossi, F.; Bergonzi, M.C.; Bilia, A.R. Stable, Monodisperse, and Highly Cell-Permeating Nanocochleates from Natural Soy Lecithin Liposomes. *Pharmaceutics* **2019**, *11*, 34. [CrossRef] [PubMed]
2. Piazzini, V.; Landucci, E.; Graverini, G.; Pellegrini-Giampietro, D.E.; Bilia, A.R.; Bergonzi, M.C. Stealth and Cationic Nanoliposomes as Drug Delivery Systems to Increase Andrographolide BBB Permeability. *Pharmaceutics* **2018**, *10*, 128. [CrossRef] [PubMed]
3. Santos-Rebelo, A.; Garcia, C.; Eleutério, C.; Bastos, A.; Castro Coelho, S.; Coelho, M.A.N.; Molpeceres, J.; Viana, A.S.; Ascensão, L.; Pinto, J.F.; et al. Development of Parvifloron D-Loaded Smart Nanoparticles to Target Pancreatic Cancer. *Pharmaceutics* **2018**, *10*, 216. [CrossRef] [PubMed]
4. Di Sotto, A.; Paolicelli, P.; Nardoni, M.; Abete, L.; Garzoli, S.; Di Giacomo, S.; Mazzanti, G.; Casadei, M.A.; Petralito, S. SPC Liposomes as Possible Delivery Systems for Improving Bioavailability of the Natural Sesquiterpene β-Caryophyllene: Lamellarity and Drug-Loading as Key Features for a Rational Drug Delivery Design. *Pharmaceutics* **2018**, *10*, 274. [CrossRef] [PubMed]
5. Coccè, V.; Franzè, S.; Brini, A.T.; Giannì, A.B.; Pascucci, L.; Ciusani, E.; Alessandri, G.; Farronato, G.; Cavicchini, L.; Sordi, V.; et al. In Vitro Anticancer Activity of Extracellular Vesicles (EVs) Secreted by Gingival Mesenchymal Stromal Cells Primed with Paclitaxel. *Pharmaceutics* **2019**, *11*, 61. [CrossRef] [PubMed]
6. Palchetti, S.; Caputo, D.; Digiacomo, L.; Capriotti, A.L.; Coppola, R.; Pozzi, D.; Caracciolo, G. Protein Corona Fingerprints of Liposomes: New Opportunities for Targeted Drug Delivery and Early Detection in Pancreatic Cancer. *Pharmaceutics* **2019**, *11*, 31. [CrossRef] [PubMed]
7. Marzoli, F.; Marianecci, C.; Rinaldi, F.; Passeri, D.; Rossi, M.; Minosi, P.; Carafa, M.; Pieretti, S. Long-Lasting, Antinociceptive Effects of pH-Sensitive Niosomes Loaded with Ibuprofen in Acute and Chronic Models of Pain. *Pharmaceutics* **2019**, *11*, 62. [CrossRef] [PubMed]
8. Rodrigues, A.R.O.; Matos, J.O.G.; Nova Dias, A.M.; Almeida, B.G.; Pires, A.; Pereira, A.M.; Araújo, J.P.; Queiroz, M.-J.R.P.; Castanheira, E.M.S.; Coutinho, P.J.G. Development of Multifunctional Liposomes Containing Magnetic/Plasmonic MnFe$_2$O$_4$/Au Core/Shell Nanoparticles. *Pharmaceutics* **2019**, *11*, 10. [CrossRef] [PubMed]
9. Touitou, E.; Natsheh, H.; Duchi, S. Buspirone Nanovesicular Nasal System for Non-Hormonal Hot Flushes Treatment. *Pharmaceutics* **2018**, *10*, 82. [CrossRef] [PubMed]

10. Narayan, R.; Nayak, U.Y.; Raichur, A.M.; Garg, S. Mesoporous Silica Nanoparticles: A Comprehensive Review on Synthesis and Recent Advances. *Pharmaceutics* **2018**, *10*, 118. [CrossRef] [PubMed]

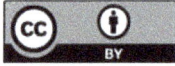

pharmaceutics

MDPI

Article

Stable, Monodisperse, and Highly Cell-Permeating Nanocochleates from Natural Soy Lecithin Liposomes

Martina Asprea [1], Francesca Tatini [2], Vieri Piazzini [1], Francesca Rossi [2],
Maria Camilla Bergonzi [1] and Anna Rita Bilia [1,*]

[1] Department of Chemistry, University of Florence, Via U. Schiff 6, 50019 Sesto Fiorentino, Florence, Italy;
aspreamartina@gmail.com (M.A.); vieri.piazzini@unifi.it (V.P.); mc.bergonzi@unifi.it (M.C.B.)
[2] Institute of Applied Physics "N. Carrara" (IFAC-CNR), Via Madonna del Piano 10, 50019 Sesto Fiorentino,
Italy; f.tatini@ifac.cnr.it (F.T.); f.rossi@ifac.cnr.it (F.R.)
* Correspondence: ar.bilia@unifi.it; Tel.: +39-055-4573708

Received: 13 November 2018; Accepted: 8 January 2019; Published: 16 January 2019

Abstract: (1) Background: Andrographolide (AN), the main diterpenoid constituent of *Andrographis paniculata*, has a wide spectrum of biological activities. The aim of this study was the development of nanocochleates (NCs) loaded with AN and based on phosphatidylserine (PS) or phosphatidylcholine (PC), cholesterol and calcium ions in order to overcome AN low water solubility, its instability under alkaline conditions and its rapid metabolism in the intestine. (2) Methods: The AN-loaded NCs (AN–NCs) were physically and chemically characterised. The in vitro gastrointestinal stability and biocompatibility of AN–NCs in J77A.1 macrophage and 3T3 fibroblasts cell lines were also investigated. Finally, the uptake of nanocarriers in macrophage cells was studied. (3) Results: AN–NCs obtained from PC nanoliposomes were suitable nanocarriers in terms of size and homogeneity. They had an extraordinary stability after lyophilisation without the use of lyoprotectants and after storage at room temperature. The encapsulation efficiency was 71%, while approximately 95% of AN was released in PBS after 24 h, with kinetics according to the Hixson–Crowell model. The in vitro gastrointestinal stability and safety of NCs, both in macrophages and 3T3 fibroblasts, were also assessed. Additionally, NCs had extraordinary uptake properties in macrophages. (4) Conclusions: NCs developed in this study could be suitable for both AN oral and parental administration, amplifying its therapeutic value

Keywords: soy lecithin liposomes; nanocochleates; andrographolide; freeze-drying; gastrointestinal stability; uptake and safety

1. Introduction

The design and production of appropriate drug delivery systems, in particular, nanosized ones, offer an advanced approach to optimised bioavailability and/or the stability of drugs, to control drug delivery and to maintain drug stability during transport to the site of action. A successful drug carrier system should possess a long shelf life, optimal drug loading and release properties, and exert a much higher therapeutic efficacy as well as have low side effects [1,2].

Phospholipids are the main amphiphilic components of the cell membrane and currently represent the main constituents of nanovectors because they can self-assembly in aqueous milieu, generating different supramolecular structures such as micelles and vesicles [1,3]. Typically, their variation in head groups, aliphatic chains and alcohols leads to a wide variety of phospholipids, generally classified as glycerophospholipids and sphingomyelins. The most common natural glycerophospholipids are phosphatidylcholine (PC), phosphatidylinositol, phosphatidylserine (PS), phosphatidylglycerol and phosphatidic acid, having diverse acyl moieties, principally myristoyl, palmitoyl, oleoyl and stearoyl.

In particular, glycerophospholipids are the specific constituents of liposomes, which are widely used as drug vectors because of their high biocompatibility, non-toxicity, complete biodegradability, and non-immunogenic effects after both systemic and non-systemic routes of administration [4]. Conversely, the therapeutic use of vesicles has some limitations, principally poor stability and availability under the harsh conditions typically presented in the gastrointestinal tract [1,2,5,6]. A very limited number of studies report on the use of cochleates as an alternative platform to vesicles in order to overcome these limitations. Cochleates were first observed by Verkleij et al. [7] using phosphatidylglycerol liposomes and later by Papahadjopoulos et al. [8], using phosphatidylserine liposomes in the presence of divalent metal cations (Me^{2+}), i.e., Ca^{2+}, Ba^{2+}, Fe^{2+}, Mg^{2+} and Zn^{2+}. Cochleates can be produced as nano- and microstructures and they are extremely biocompatible, with excellent stability due to their unique compact structure. They present an elongated shape and a carpet roll-like morphology always accompanied by narrowly packed bilayers, through the interaction with Me^{2+} as bridging agents between the bilayers (Figure 1). During this arrangement, the close approach of bilayers is dependent on dehydration of the head group of the phospholipid. They roll-up in order to minimise their interaction with water and, consequently, cochleates possess little or no aqueous phase. The relevant differences between cochleates and different liposomes, i.e., small unilamellar vesicle (SUV), large unilamellar vesicle (LUV), multilamellar vesicle (MLV) and multivesicle vesicle (MVV), are reported in Figure 1.

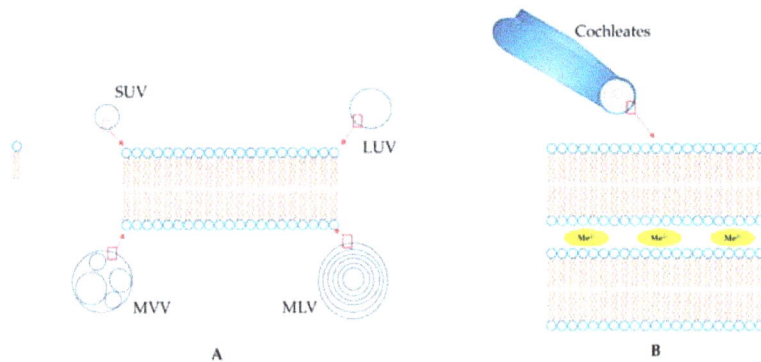

Figure 1. Schematic representation of the structures of liposomes (**A**) and nanocochleates (**B**).

The bilayers in a cochleate are organised very precisely at a very close repeating distance of 54 Angstrom [9] with a water-free interior, which is a rigid, stable, rod-shaped structure. Due to this unique structure, cochleates can be easily lyophilised to a free-flowing powder that can be incorporated in capsules for oral administration or re-dispersed in water for parental administration. Yet what remains very unclear is their mechanism of permeation throughout the biological membranes. It is reported that after oral administration, cochleates cross the epithelium, delivering the loaded drug into the blood vessel [10]. There are two current hypotheses to explain the mechanism of permeation. According to the first assumption, the contact of the calcium-rich membrane of the cochleate with a cell can cause a perturbation and the reordering of the cell membrane. Subsequently, there is fusion between the outer layer of the cochleate and the cell membrane [10]. An alternative hypothesis for the delivery mechanism of cochleates is phagocytosis. In both cases, once within the interior of a cell, a low calcium concentration results in the opening of the cochleate crystal and the release of the entrapped drug [11–13].

Currently, cochleates represent difficult drug delivery systems for clinical use, principally due to the numerous difficulties in producing monodisperse systems because of a tendency to form stable and huge aggregates, which represent a serious drawback at the industrial level. Diverse patents and publications have reported different strategies to overcome these limitations [11], in particular, the use of methylcellulose, casein, or albumin, but proteins may decrease stability and safety due to the change of pharmacokinetic parameters. Methylcellulose is able only in part to disrupt the formed aggregates.

Other natural polysaccharides (including celluloses, gums, and starches) have been recommended as inhibitors of the aggregation processes, but their efficiency still remains ambiguous [11,12]. In recent times, the ability of citric acid to remove Ca^{2+} ions from the external surface of cochleates, leading to the dispersion of the aggregates, has been investigated [13]. Furthermore, a recent approach compared a novel microfluidics-based strategy with the conventional cochleate production methods; however, the formation of aggregates was still present in the samples [14].

The aim of this study was the production of monodisperse and stable nanocochleates (NCs) using two different phospholipids, PC and PS, loaded with a typical small hydrophobic natural product, andrographolide (AN) from the Asiatic medicinal plant *Andrographis paniculata*. Besides the numerous potential activities ranging from anti-inflammatory to neuroprotection, antidiabetic to anti-obesity properties, and antitumor activity to hepatoprotective activity [15], AN has poor water solubility (3.29 ± 0.73 µg at 25 °C) [16], which deeply limits its biodistribution and localisation, resulting in low bioavailability [17]. Additionally, AN is unstable in gastrointestinal media and has a very short biological half-life ($t^{1/2} = 1.33$ h) after a single oral dose [18]. The stability of developed nanocochleates after lyophilisation and in simulated gastrointestinal fluids was investigated. In addition, the possible hazards and the cellular effects of NCs were determined using J774a.1 murine macrophages and 3T3 fibroblasts. Lastly, studies on uptake using a confocal microscope were carried out in the macrophages cell line.

2. Materials and Methods

2.1. Materials

The phospholipon 90G (soy phosphatidylcholine, PC) was sourced from the Italian agent AVG srl (Milan, Italy) of Lipoid AG (Cologne, Germany). The dioleoyl phosphatidylserine (PS) was a kind gift from Lipoid AG (Cologne, Germany). The following reagents were from Sigma-Aldrich (Milan, Italy): pepsin from porcine gastric mucosa, bile salts, andrographolide (AN), fluorescein isothiocyanate (FITC, purity ≥ 90%, HPLC), lipase from porcin pancreas, sodium hydroxide (NaOH), calcium chloride ($CaCl_2$), cholesterol, phosphate buffered saline (PBS) bioperformance certified, paraformaldehyde (PFA), Dulbecco's Modified Eagle Medium (DMEM), fetal bovine serum (FBS), l-glutamine, penicillin–streptomycin solution, WST-8 kit, acetonitrile (HPLC grade), methanol (HPLC grade), formic acid (analytical grade), hydrochloric acid (HCl) (analytical grade) and dichloromethane (CH_2Cl_2). The water used was from the Milli-Q$_{plus}$ system from Millipore (Milford, CT, USA). The phosphotungstic acid (PTA) was from Electron Microscopy Sciences (Hatfield, PA, USA). The dialysis kit was from Spectrum Laboratories, Inc. (Breda, The Netherlands). The J774a.1 murine macrophages and the 3T3 fibroblasts were purchased from the American Type Culture Collection (ATCC® TIB-67™, Manassas, VA, USA). A LT-4000 reader from Labtech was used to read the absorbance (Bergamo, Italy).

2.2. Preparation of PC- and PS-based Liposomes and NCs

The NCs were obtained from nano-sized liposomes (LPs), which were prepared according to the film hydration method [19]. The liposomes were formulated as follows: the required amounts of phospholipids (60 mg) and cholesterol (20 mg) were dissolved in a dichloromethane/methanol mixture (20 mL of a mixture, 3:2 *v/v*). The obtained organic solution was evaporated under vacuum and the lipid film was hydrated by the addition of PBS (10 mL) using a mechanical stirrer (RW20 digital, IKA, Staufen im Breisgau, Germany) for 30 min in a water bath at a constant temperature of 37 °C for PC and 60 °C for PS. The resulting formulations were optimised by ultrasonication (3 min, two cycles of 90 s) in an ice bath to prevent lipid degradation. Subsequently, a gentle centrifugation (1205× *g*, 1 min) was performed to remove possible metallic particles released during the ultrasonication. The NCs were prepared from the nanoliposomes according to the trapping method, described by Asprea et al. [20]. Briefly, a 0.1 M solution of $CaCl_2$ was added drop-by-drop to the liposomal suspension under magnetic stirring (150 rpm, room temperature) until the formulation appeared cloudy, indicating the formation of NCs. The molar ratio between PC and $CaCl_2$ was 1:1, while the molar ratio between PS and $CaCl_2$ was 1:4.

2.3. Characterisation of Nanocarriers: Size, Polydispersity Index and ζ-Potential

The Zsizer Nano series ZS90 (Malvern Instruments, Malvern, UK) outfitted with a JDS Uniphase 22 mW He-Ne laser operating at 632.8 nm, an optical fiber-based detector, a digital LV/LSE-5003 correlator and a temperature controller (Julabo water-bath) set at 25 °C was used for Dynamic Light Scattering (DLS) measurements, including for the particle size, polydispersity index (PdI) and ζ-potential. The cumulant method was used to analyse time correlation functions, obtaining the mean diameter of the nanocarriers (Z-average) and the size distribution using the ALV-60X0 software V.3.X provided by Malvern. The size characterisation technique for the nanoparticles in suspension, based on the measurement of their translational diffusion coefficient, related to the length, L, of their major axis is as

$$D = \frac{kBT}{3\pi\eta L} FD, \tag{1}$$

where η represents the viscosity of the solvent, kB represents the Boltzmann constant and T represents the sample temperature. FD is a geometrical coefficient depending on the shape, but not the size, of the particles [21,22]. In particular, for NCs, the expressions of FD corresponding to these particle shapes are

$$FD = \log\rho + 0.312 + 0.565/\rho - 0.1/\rho^2, \tag{2}$$

ζ-potential values were obtained from the electrophoretic mobility, using the Henry correction to Smoluchowski's equation. The samples were diluted in distilled water and an average of three measurements at the stationary level were taken. A Haake temperature controller kept the temperature constant at 25 °C.

2.4. Morphological and Size Characterisation by Transmission Electron Microscopy (TEM)

A transmission electron microscope (TEM, Jeol Jem 1010, Tokyo, Japan) was used to evaluate the morphology, shape and dimensions of NCs. The NCs dispersion was diluted 10-fold and placed on a carbon film-covered copper grid and stained with a phosphotungstic acid solution 1 g/100 mL in sterile water, before the TEM analysis. The samples were dried for 1 min and then examined under TEM and photographed at an accelerating voltage of 64 kV.

2.5. Stability Study of NCs after Lyophilisation

The lyophilisation process of NCs provides an extended storage period at room temperature and can be carried out without the use of lyoprotectants because of the very low water content. The samples were frozen by a freezer (−23 °C) overnight before lyophilisation. Then, the samples were moved to a freeze-drier. The temperature was set to −23 °C and the pressure was −1.0 bar. The drying time was 24 h. The pressure and the temperature remained unchanged during the process.

The stability of the lyophilised NCs was evaluated after reconstitution of the colloidal system to the original volume with distilled water, using a vortex mixer at room temperature. The samples were stored in sealed glass containers after being placed into a desiccator containing silica gel to absorb water vapor. The samples were also protected from light. The stability of the lyophilised NCs was assessed by checking the size, ζ-potential, polydispersity and morphology every week for 2 months.

2.6. Stability Study of NCs in Gastrointestinal Media

NCs could be used to protect the entrapped compound from the effects of the gastrointestinal fluids. Accordingly, NC formulations were tested for their stability using simulated gastrointestinal conditions. Simulated gastric fluid (SGF) was used to investigate the gastric stability of NCs, as previously reported [23,24]. Briefly, 5 mL of NCs was suspended in 5 mL of SGF (0.32% *w/v* pepsin, 2 g of sodium chloride and 7 mL HCl dissolved in 1 L water and pH adjusted to 1.8 using 1 M HCl) and incubated at 37 °C under shaking at a speed of 100 strokes/min. After 2 h, the sample was collected. The size and PdI were analysed by DLS, while the morphology of the colloidal systems was analysed by TEM.

The stability of the samples was also investigated in simulated intestinal fluid (SIF) containing an intestinal enzyme complex (lipase 0.4 mg/mL, bile salts 0.7 mg/mL and pancreatin 0.5 mg/mL) and 750 mM calcium chloride solution at 37 °C, under shaking, with a speed of 100 strokes/min. The pH of the mixture was adjusted to a value of 7.0 with NaOH 0.1 N. After 2 h, the sample was collected and its physical and morphological properties were assessed by size and PDI analysis by DLS and TEM.

2.7. Preparation of Nanocarriers Based on AN and FITC

NCs were obtained from nanoliposomes (SUVs), which were prepared using the film hydration method. The nanoliposomes were formulated as follows: phospholipids (60 mg), cholesterol (20 mg) and AN (20 mg) or FITC (5 mg) were dissolved in dichloromethane/methanol mixture (20 mL of a mixture 3:2 *v/v*). The obtained organic solution was evaporated under vacuum to obtain a lipid film, which was hydrated by the addition of PBS (10 mL) using a mechanical stirrer (RW20 digital, IKA, Staufen im Breisgau, Germany) for 30 min in a water bath at a constant temperature of 37 °C for PC and 60 °C for PS. The resulting formulations were reduced in size using an ultrasonication probe for 3 min (two cycles of 90 s). During the sonication, the samples were kept in an ice bath to prevent lipid degradation. After that, a gentle centrifugation (1205× *g*, 1 min) was performed to remove possible metallic particles released during the ultrasonication. The NCs were prepared by the trapping method, according to Asprea et al. [20]. A 0.1 M solution of CaCl₂ was added drop-by-drop to the liposomal suspension under magnetic stirring (150 rpm, at room temperature) until the formulation became cloudy, indicating the formation of NCs. The molar ratio between PC and CaCl₂ was 1:1, while the molar ratio between PS and CaCl₂ was 1:4.

2.8. Determination of Encapsulation Efficiency of AN–NCs by HPLC

After preparation of the NCs, free AN was removed by dialysis using bags with a pore size of 3.5–5 kD, and according to previous studies [25]. The dialysis bag was placed in 1 L of distilled water at room temperature for 1 h under stirring. The physical mixture was used as a control to validate the procedure. The AN-loaded content was quantified by HPLC–DAD analysis using a standard sample of AN, after the treatment of NCs with methanol to destroy the cochleates. HPLC–DAD analyses were performed with a HP 1200 Liquid Chromatograph (Agilent Technologies, Palo Alto, CA, USA), equipped with a Diode Array Detector (DAD), managed by a HP 9000 workstation (Agilent Technologies). The column was a Varian Polaris RP18 (250 mm × 4.6 mm i.d., particle size 5 μm) (Agilent Technologies) maintained at 27 °C. The chromatograms were acquired at 223 nm. The eluents were acetonitrile (A) and formic acid/water at pH 3.2 (B) at a flow rate of 1 mL/min. The following gradient profile was applied: 0–3 min, 10% A, and 90% B; 3–11 min, 10–38% A, and 90–62% B; 11–25 min, 38% A, and 62% B; 25–30 min, 38–50% A, and 62–50% B; and 30–34 min, 50–10% A, and 50–90% B. The post time was 10 min. The injected volume of the samples was 10–20 μL.

The calibration curve was obtained from a dilution series of the AN reference standard solubilised in MeOH, in the range between 56 and 0.56 ng/mL. Linear regression was used to establish the calibration curve. AN was quantified using the peak areas acquired at 223 nm. The correlation coefficient (R^2) was 0.9995. The data are expressed as the mean ± SD of the three experiments.

The encapsulation efficiency (EE%) for each preparation was calculated using the following equation:

$$EE\% = (Wt/Wi) \times 100\%, \tag{3}$$

where *Wt* is the total amount of the loaded AN and *Wi* is the total quantity of AN added initially during the preparation. The encapsulation efficiency was determined in triplicate.

2.9. Determination of Encapsulation Efficiency of FITC–NCs by HPLC

Free FITC was removed by means of dialysis, as previously described. The contents of FITC were determined by the same HPLC instrument used for AN quantification. The column was a Lichrosorb RP18 (4.6 mm × 100 mm i.d., 5 µm) (Agilent Technologies) maintained at 27 °C. The mobile phases were (A) acetonitrile and (B) formic acid/water pH 3.2, at a flow rate of 0.8 mL/min and an injection volume of 10 µL. The following gradient profile was used: 0–5 min, 10–40% A, and 90–60% B; 5–10 min, 40–50% A, and 60–50% B; 10–12 min 50–55% A, and 50–45% B; 12–15 min, 55% A, and 45% B; 15–18 min, 55–90% A, and 45–10% B; and 18–20 min, 10% A, and 90% B. The post time was 5 min. The chromatograms were acquired at 224 nm. The linearity range of responses of FITC dissolved in CH_3OH was determined on five concentration levels from 6.40 ng/mL to 520 ng/mL and the correlation coefficient (R^2) was 0.9994 [26].

The encapsulation efficiency was calculated using the equation described in the previous paragraph. In this case, Wt is the total amount of the loaded FITC and Wi is the total quantity of FITC added initially during the preparation.

2.10. In Vitro Release Study

The in vitro release of AN from the NCs was investigated using the dialysis bag method. In order to simulate the physiological conditions, PBS (pH 7.4) and enzyme-free SGF and SIF were used as dissolution media. A total of 2 mL of AN–NCs suspension was deposited into the dialysis membrane (pore size 3.5 kD) and placed in 200 mL of the release medium. The temperature was set at 37 °C and the system was stirred at 150 rpm. Release into the PBS was monitored for 24 h while in SGF and for 2 h while in SIF, corresponding to the theoretical transit through the gastrointestinal tract; aliquots of one millilitre were withdrawn in duplicate and replaced with fresh dissolution medium. The samples were analysed by HPLC for the quantification of released AN. The percentage of AN released was calculated as follows:

$$\%AN\ released = \left(\frac{AN_r}{AN_{tot}}\right) \times 100, \tag{4}$$

where AN_r is the amount of AN detected by HPLC analyses and AN_{tot} is the total quantity of AN deposited into the dialysis membrane.

Furthermore, to evaluate the kinetics of drug release from the NCs, different mathematical models were used, i.e., zero order and first order kinetics model, the Higuchi model, the Korsmeyer–Peppas model and the Hixson–Crowell model. The best fitting model was selected according to the best regression coefficient (R^2) value for the release data.

2.11. Cell Viability and Uptake Studies

The albino mouse embryonic 3T3 fibroblast cell line and the murine monocyte/macrophage cell line J774a.1 were used for cell viability and uptake studies [27,28]. The cell lines were maintained in Dulbecco's Modified Eagle's Medium (DMEM, Sigma-Aldrich) supplemented with foetal bovine serum, 100 units/mL penicillin, and 100 µg/mL streptomycin; for the 3T3 cell line, an additional glucose concentration (4.5 g/L) was used. The cells were maintained under standard culture conditions (37 °C, 5% CO_2, 95% air and 100% relative humidity).

The cells were inoculated into 96-well microplates and maintained under standard culture conditions for 24 h to test the cell viability. Thereafter, the medium was replaced with fresh medium containing different concentrations of NCs or LPs. After 24 h, a WST-8 test was performed following the kit protocol as indicated by the manufacturer and as described in [28]. Briefly, 100 µL of DMEM supplemented with 10% WST-8 reagent was incubated in each well for 2 h at 37 °C. The formazan concentration was quantified by an optical absorbance at 450 nm, with a reference wavelength of 630 nm and by subtracting blank values. The data were expressed as a percentage of the optical absorbance with respect to the controls.

The cells were inoculated into a 33-mm petri dish and maintained under standard culture conditions for 24 h for uptake experiments. Subsequently, the medium was replaced with fresh medium containing different concentrations of FITC loaded in NCs or SUVs. After 1 h, the medium was removed and the cells were fixed in 3.6% PFA in PBS for 10 min at room temperature, stained with DAPI and analysed by confocal imaging. Images were acquired by a Leica SP7 confocal microscope and underwent no subsequent manipulation. A minimum of five different fields was acquired from each sample and all samples were performed in triplicate.

3. Results

3.1. Preparation and Characterisation of NCs

The NCs were prepared according to the multi-step preparation reported in Figure 2.

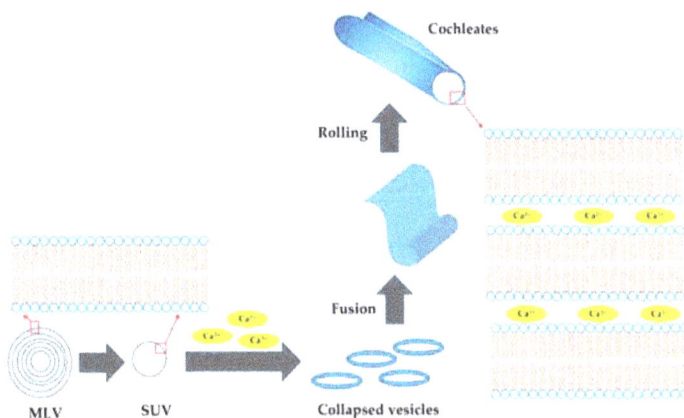

Figure 2. Multi-step preparation process of nanocochleates.

Briefly, as a first step, nanosized LPs were prepared according to the film hydration method using PC or PS and cholesterol, in the gravimetric ratio reported in the experimental part. The lipid film was dispersed in PBS to obtain MLVs. The formation of the SUVs was performed using an ultrasonication probe. In a further step, the SUVs collapsed after the addition of $CaCl_2$ solution when added in the molar ratio 1:1 to PC liposomes (PC–SUVs) and in the molar ratio 4:1 to PS liposomes (PS–SUVs). Then, the collapsed vesicles fused giving large sheets, which rolled-up to give NCs. The calcium ions were essential for the stability of the system, and the aqueous phase in the structure of NCs was very limited, as reported in Figure 2. Both the SUV and NC formulations were characterised in terms of size, homogeneity and ζ-potential by dynamic and electrophoretic light scattering (Table 1).

Table 1. Physical characterisation of empty liposomes and nanocochleates.

Sample	Size (nm)	PdI	ζ-Potential (mV)
PC–SUVs	150 ± 2	0.20 ± 0.02	−29.3 ± 0.9
PC–NCs	150 ± 2	0.24 ± 0.01	−21.6 ± 1.3
PS–SUVs	205 ± 37	0.25 ± 0.03	−37.2 ± 7.1
PS–NCs	207 ± 44	0.55 ± 0.05	−36.4 ± 1.4

PC–SUVs: liposomes made of phosphatidylcholine; PC–NCs: nanocochleates made of phosphatidylcholine; PS–SUVs: liposomes made of phosphatidylserine; PS–NCs nanocochleates made of phosphatidylserine. The data are displayed as the mean ± SD; *n* = 3.

Both PC–SUVs and PC–NCs had a narrow size of ca. 150 nm and they were highly homogeneous as evinced by the PdI (Table 1). Both the liposomes and the NCs based on PC were smaller than those prepared with PS. In particular, the PS–NCs were not homogeneous (Table 1). The dimension of the nanocarriers in the suspension was based on the measurement of their translational diffusion coefficient. This value is related to the length, L, of their major axis as described by Equation (1). The shape of the particles, but not the size, is linked by the geometrical coefficient, FD, which is 1 for spheres. However, it was determined for the NCs using a simplified geometry of long rods, according to Equation (2) [19,20]. All the nanovectors were negatively charged, and, as expected, the ζ-potential was a very low for the nanocarriers based on PS.

The morphological characterisation was completed by the observation of TEM pictures. The size and homogeneity of the liposomes based on PC and PS were confirmed (data not reported). The cigar-like shape of PC–NCs was strongly assessed (Figure 3a). PC–NCs dimensions were comparable with the dimensional distribution results obtained from the DLS analysis. The TEM images of PS–NCs confirmed the presence of polydisperse systems with structures different to NCs (Figure 3b).

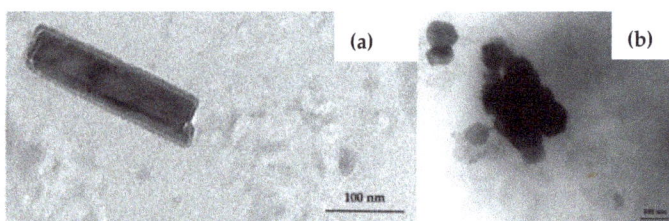

Figure 3. TEM images of PC–NCs (**a**) and PS–NCs (**b**) (scale 100 nm).

3.2. Stability Study of Empty NCs

Firstly, the stability of the NCs was assessed by measuring the changes in terms of the average dimensions, polydispersity and ζ-potential values after the lyophilisation process and resuspension at room temperature with distilled water. The analysis was performed immediately after the lyophilisation process, which did not affect the physical characteristics, when re-suspended in water, as reported in Table 2. All the samples were reconstituted and analysed by DLS, ELS and TEM every week. It was only the PC–NCs that did not experience considerable modification in size, homogeneity and ζ-potential values (Table 2).

Table 2. The particle size, polydispersity index (PdI) and ζ-potential of PC–NCs and PS–NCs as a lyophilised product after two-month storage at 25 °C.

PC–NCs	t_0	After 30 Days	After 60 Days
Size (nm)	150 ± 2	166 ± 5	172 ± 3
PdI	0.24 ± 0.01	0.25 ± 0.02	0.25 ± 0.01
ζ-Potential (mV)	−21.6 ± 1.3	−19.4 ± 1.1	−18.5 ± 1.0
PS–NCs	t_0	After 30 days	After 60 days
Size (nm)	207 ± 44	292 ± 22	280 ± 25
PdI	0.55 ± 0.05	0.53 ± 0.04	0.55 ± 0.05
ζ-Potential (mV)	−36.4 ± 1.4	−31.4 ± 2.1	−27.2 ± 1.1

PC–NCs: nanocochleates made of phosphatidylcholine; PS–NCs nanocochleates made of phosphatidylserine. The data are displayed as the mean ± SD; n = 3.

TEM analyses confirmed the dimensional data obtained by DLS concerning PC–NCs (Figure 4). Instantly after the preparation, PC–NCs had a dimension of 150 nm, while in the following 60 days their size increased by about 20 nm, while their ζ-potential values remained almost constant during this stability study. By contrast, the PS–NCs were not stable and their size increased by about 80 nm during storage. The TEM pictures showed the presence of aggregates (data not reported), confirming the results reported in Table 2.

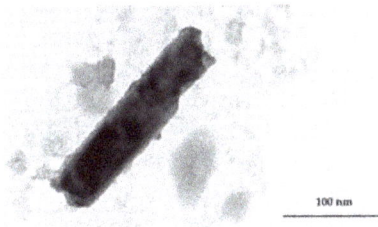

Figure 4. TEM image of PC–NCs re-suspended with distilled water after two months of storage at room temperature in the lyophilised state (scale 100 nm).

3.3. AN–NCs and FITC–NCs Production

As a result of the stability testing of the two NC formulations, PC–NCs were selected as drug delivery systems to be investigated in the present study. AN or FITC was added to the lipid phase and their preparation was carried out using the same scheme reported in Figure 2.

FITC–LPs and FITC–NCs had a good size and homogeneity to test their performance for uptake in the macrophage J774a.1 cell line (Table 3). The average FITC-entrapment efficiency in the SUVs and NCs obtained by HPLC–DAD analyses was 87.5 ± 1.0 and 87.2 ± 0.1%, respectively.

Table 3. Physical and chemical characterisation of AN- and FITC-loaded LPs and NCs.

Sample	Size (nm)	PdI	ζ-Potential (mV)	EE (%)
AN–SUVs	148 ± 2	0.13 ± 0.01	−27.5 ± 2.9	71.1 ± 2.3
AN–NCs	140 ± 1	0.22 ± 0.05	−22.3 ± 3.1	70.6 ± 5.9
FITC–SUVs	180 ± 2	0.20 ± 0.05	−29.2 ± 0.9	87.5 ± 1.0
FITC–NCs	177 ± 1	0.13 ± 0.02	−20.4 ± 2.3	87.2 ± 0.1

AN–SUVs: andrographolide-loaded liposomes; AN–NCs: andrographolide-loaded nanocochleates; FITC–SUVs: fluorescein isothiocyanate-loaded liposomes; FITC–NCs: fluorescein isothiocyanate-loaded nanocochleates. The data are displayed as the mean ± SD; $n = 3$.

The dimensions of the AN–NCs was ca. 150 nm, with a very low PdI, which resulted in suitability for all routes of administration, not only oral [29]. These data were also reflected by the TEM which exhibited NCs as tubular rod structures (Figure 5). The structure of the NCs is not modified in terms of size by AN loading, which means that AN does not interfere with the cohesion and packing of the apolar chains of the cochleate membrane. This is typical of small terpenes, which are able to decrease the size of lipid nanocarriers by forcing the PC structure to increase its surface curvature [30].

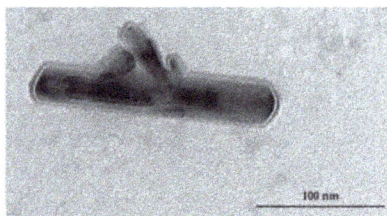

Figure 5. TEM image of AN–NCs (scale 100 nm).

The average AN-entrapment efficiency in both SUVs and NCs was obtained by HPLC–DAD; the results were 71.1 ± 2.3 and 70.6 ± 5.9%, respectively (Table 3).

3.4. Stability of AN–NCs in Gastrointestinal Fluids

It is known that AN is not stable in the presence of gastrointestinal enzymes. Accordingly, one of the aims of this study was the development of a formulation able to protect the incorporated compound from degradation in gastrointestinal fluids. The gastrointestinal fluids may have an influence on the integrity of NCs. The physical stability of AN–NCs was assessed in SGF (pH 2) and in SIF (pH 7). These media did not affect their structure after two hours of incubation. The DLS analyses revealed that the mean diameter of the NCs was not affected by these conditions: after incubation in both gastro-enteric media, their mean size was 143 ± 1 nm with PdI 0.25 ± 0.02.

3.5. In Vitro Release Studies

After demonstrating the physical stability of NCs in gastrointestinal conditions, the in vitro release of AN from NCs was investigated by the dialysis bag diffusion technique. The test was carried out in both SGF (pH 2) and SIF (pH 7) for two hours and in physiological pH conditions (PBS, pH 7.4) for 24 h.

The percentage of AN released in SGF was only 2.31 ± 0.02%, while in SIF, it was 14.75 ± 1.14%. These results suggest that NCs may prevent AN burst release in the gastrointestinal tract, since about 85% of the compound remained entrapped in the NCs.

In PBS, the release of AN from NCs was not immediate, but gradual, unlike in the case of free-AN, indicating that the formulation results in a more prolonged effect (Figure 6).

The AN release from NCs can be described as a biphasic process and the mathematical model of the drug release data was found to best fit the Hixson–Crowell release model: $W_0^{\frac{1}{3}} - W_t^{\frac{1}{3}} = K_s t$; where W_0 is the initial amount of the drug in the pharmaceutical dosage form; W_t is the remaining amount of the drug in the pharmaceutical dosage form, at time t; and K_s is a constant, incorporating the surface–volume relation. The R^2 was 0.9961. This model has been frequently used to describe drug release from several dosage forms with modified release. According to this model, the drug release is described by dissolution, characterised by the surface area and diameter of the particles. Consequently, based on the obtained results, it is possible to hypothesise that this behaviour may be due to the strong affinity of hydrophobic AN to the lipid structure of NCs.

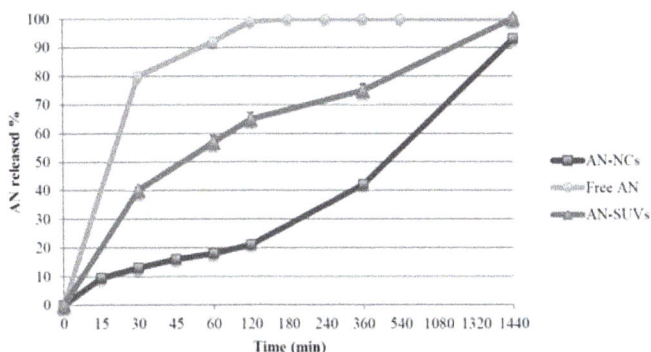

Figure 6. In vitro release profiles of free AN, AN–NCs and AN–SUVs in PBS. AN solution and AN–SUVs were tested to evidence the superiority of AN–NCs on the gradual release of AN. The data are displayed as the mean ± SD; $n = 3$.

3.6. Biocompatibility Studies

The biocompatibility of NCs was tested using two cell lines: macrophage J774a.1 and fibroblasts 3T3. SUVs were used as comparable reference nanovesicles. As a colorimetric, non-radioactive assay, the WST-8 test was selected for assessing cell viability and proliferation because it indicates the mitochondrial activity and hence reflects the cell viability. WST-8, a highly water-soluble tetrazolium salt, is reduced to a soluble purple formazan derivative by trans-plasma membrane electron transport from NADH via an electron mediator. The concentration of formazan was quantified by optical absorbance at 450 nm, with a reference wavelength of 630 nm and by subtracting blank values. The mean value and the standard deviation are the results of nine measurements: the test was performed in three independent experiments and in each experiment, the samples were tested in triplicate. The data were expressed as the percent of optical absorbance with respect to the controls. As indicated in Figure 7, both SUVs and NCs showed no cytotoxicity at the concentration needed for massive uptake, namely, with a dilution of 1:40. Higher concentrations showed a decrease in cell viability, validating the dose–response curve. By contrast, it is remarkable that lower concentrations of the nanovesicles increased the cell metabolism rates, which was probably due to the active uptake process.

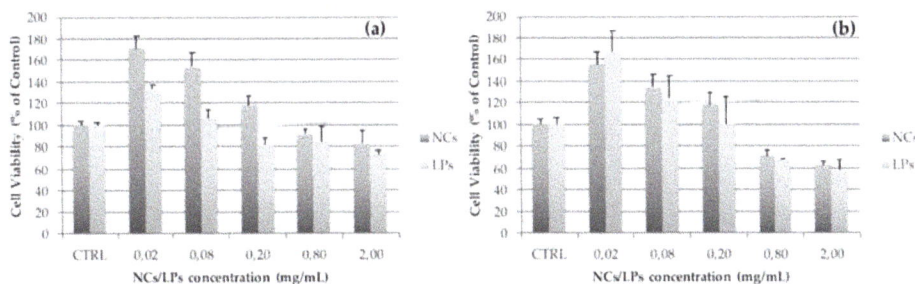

Figure 7. Cell viability after 24 h of exposition to NCs or LPs. The concentrations are expressed in mg/mL. The data represent the percentage of control ± SD. The J774a.1 (**a**) is a monocytes/macrophages cell line; the 3T3 (**b**) is a fibroblasts cell line.

3.7. Cellular Uptake Studies

In Figure 8, the uptake of both NCs and SUVs by macrophage J774a.1 cell line, using nanoparticles loaded with FITC (FITC–NCs and FITC–SUVs), is reported. The uptake was tracked by the green fluorescence of FITC using a confocal microscope (Figure 8).

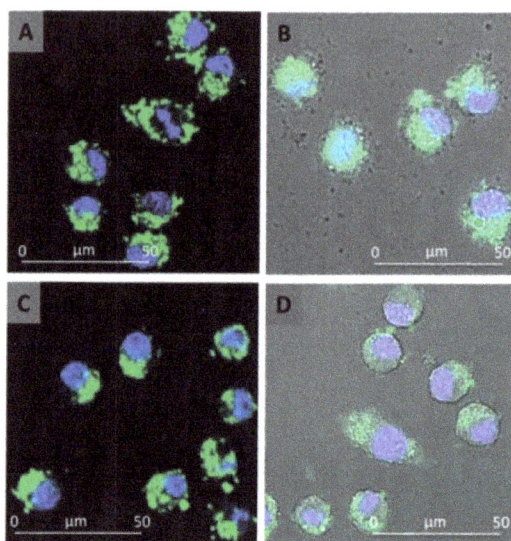

Figure 8. Confocal images of the macrophage uptake of NCs (**a**) and SUVs (**c**). Following nuclear staining with DAPI and FITC encapsulation into NCs and SUVs, the cell nuclei appear in blue and the NCs/SUVs appear in green. The confocal images are also superimposed to Bright Field acquisition (**b,d** for NCs and SUVs, respectively) to show the unaltered morphology of the cells and the localisation of intracellular nanocarriers.

As reported in Figure 8, massive uptake takes place but the fluorescence is typically in the cytoplasm without entering the cell nuclei. NCs and SUVs exhibit very similar uptake capability.

4. Discussion

In the present study, the potential of NCs is explored for the delivery of AN, a very promising active natural constituent with various potential therapeutic benefits, but due to the low bioavailability and instability in gastrointestinal media when administered with conventional dosage forms, it has never reached a milestone therapeutic potential. Accordingly, the development of suitable delivery systems for AN represents an urgent issue to formulate effective therapeutic approaches. Lipid-based delivery systems, especially vesicles, have attracted huge efforts as high bio-compatible and biodegradable nanocarriers crossing membrane delivery systems because of their resemblance to the cell membrane. One of the main drawbacks of conventional liposomes for oral administration is their poor stability in the gastrointestinal environment. By contrast, NCs can easily be lyophilised to obtain solid, stable, biocompatible and biodegradable nanovectors [1,2,5,6].

The NCs were simply developed from nanoliposomes (Figure 2), selecting both PS and PC and cholesterol as lipid phases due to their close resemblance to natural membranes and their high compatibility for human use. Ca^{2+} was selected among the diverse divalent cations to generate NCs because it can enhance membrane fusion and phagocytosis. It is well documented that calcium ions induce perturbations of the contact region and thereby promote the membrane fusion [11,31]. Astonishingly, in our studies, only PC and cholesterol generated monodisperse NCs with a tightly packed structure after the addition of Ca^{2+}. As previously reported, PS-based NCs are not stable, producing systems with elevated polydispersity because of a tendency to form stable and huge aggregates, which represents a serious drawback at the industrial level [15]. By contrast, developed PC-based NCs were stable after lyophilisation and re-suspension in distilled water, and after incubation in simulated gastric and intestinal media. In vitro dissolution studies explained an extended release, making AN available over a prolonged period after administration. The PC-based NCs were biocompatible. Even at high concentrations, the cell morphology and vitality were not affected by internalisation. Moreover, high cellular uptake of PC-based NCs was found in macrophages using fluorescent nanovectors. After treatment of the cells with NCs, a bright fluorescent color of the cytoplasm arose due to the FITC and it was clearly distinguished from the nucleus stained with DAPI. Due to the similar uptake performances of SUVs and NCs, it is plausible that the developed NCs fuse with the cell membrane due to the interaction of calcium ions with the membrane containing negatively charged lipids, entering into the cells as nanovesicles [11]. A distinctive geometry, together with peculiar internal interactions, makes NCs ideal as pharmaceutical carriers, which may provide unparalleled protection for the molecular species in order to be carried harmlessly toward its destination. Developed NCs are inexpensive, stable, monodisperse, highly safe, biocompatible, and cell-permeating delivery systems. Moreover, they have high EE%, and suitable drug release properties for oral delivery, but with possible uses in other routes of administration. NCs are characterised by a series of solid-lipid bilayers; the components within the interior of this structure remain intact, even though the outer layers of NCs may be exposed to harsh external environmental conditions or enzymes. This interior structure of NCs is essentially free of water and resistant to penetration by oxygen, which leads to an increased shelf-life of the formulation. NCs can be stored at room temperature or 4 °C, and can be lyophilised to a powder form. Thus, NCs can be used to formulate capsules, pills, tablets, granules, suspensions or emulsions. Due to the ease of the internalisation process, this system could be exploited by employing future in vivo experiments and could be of interest in various therapeutic options.

Author Contributions: The design of the study, A.R.B., M.A. and F.T.; the experimental part, M.A., V.P. and F.T.; data curation, F.T., V.P., M.C.B.; resources, A.R.B., F.R., M.C.B.; writing—original draft preparation, A.R.B., F.T., V.P.; writing—review and editing, A.R.B., F.R.

Funding: This research received no external funding.

Acknowledgments: Maria Cristina Salvatici, Electron Microscopy Centre "Laura Bonzi" (Ce.M.E.), ICCOM, CNR, Sesto Fiorentino, Florence, Italy.

Conflicts of Interest: The authors declare no conflict of interest.

References

1. Bilia, A.R.; Piazzini, V.; Guccione, C.; Risaliti, L.; Asprea, M.; Capecchi, G.; Bergonzi, M.C. Improving on Nature: The Role of Nanomedicine in the Development of Clinical Natural Drugs. *Planta Med.* **2017**, *83*, 366–381. [CrossRef]
2. Bilia, A.R.; Piazzini, V.; Risaliti, L.; Vanti, G.; Casamonti, M.; Wang, M.; Bergonzi, M.C. Nanocarriers: A Successful Tool to Increase Solubility, Stability and Optimise Bioefficacy of Natural Constituents. *Curr. Med. Chem.* **2018**. [CrossRef]
3. Sinico, C.; Caddeo, C.; Valenti, D.; Fadda, A.M.; Bilia, A.R.; Vincieri, F.F. Liposomes as carriers for verbascoside: Stability and skin permeation studies. *J. Liposome Res.* **2008**, *18*, 83–90. [CrossRef]
4. Bozzuto, G.; Molinari, A. Liposomes as nanomedical devices. *Int. J. Nanomed.* **2015**, *10*, 975–999. [CrossRef]
5. Nguyen, T.X.; Huang, L.; Gauthier, M.; Yang, G.; Wang, Q. Recent advances in liposome surface modification for oral drug delivery. *Nanomedicine* **2016**, *11*, 1169–1185. [CrossRef]
6. Sankar, V.R.; Reddy, Y.D. Nanocochleate—A new approach in lipid drug delivery. *Int. J. Pharm. Pharm. Sci.* **2010**, *2*, 220–223.
7. Verkleij, A.J.; De Kruyff, B.; Verversgaert, P.H.J.T.; Tocanne, J.F.; Van Deenen, L.L.M. The influence of pH, Ca²⁺ and protein on the thermotropic behaviour of the negatively charged phospholipid, phosphatidylglycerol. *Biochim. Biophys. Acta Biomembr.* **1974**, *339*, 432–437. [CrossRef]
8. Papahadjopoulos, D.; Vail, W.J.; Jacobson, K.; Poste, G. Cochleate lipid cylinders: Formation by fusion of unilamellar lipid vesicles. *Biochim. Biophys. Acta* **1975**, *394*, 483–491. [CrossRef]
9. Zarif, L. Elongated supramolecular assemblies in drug delivery. *J. Control. Release* **2002**, *81*, 7–23. [CrossRef]
10. Syed, U.M.; Woo, A.F.; Plakogiannis, F.; Jin, T.; Zhu, H. Cochleates bridged by drug molecules. *Int. J. Pharm.* **2008**, *363*, 118–125. [CrossRef]

11. Panwar, V.; Mahajan, V.; Panwar, A.S.; Darwhekar, G.N.; Jain, D.K. Nanocochleate as drug delivery vehicle. *Int. J. Pharm. Biol. Sci.* **2011**, *1*, 31–36.

12. Mannino, R.J.; Gould-Fogerite, S.; Krause-Elsmore, S.L.; Delmarre, D.; Lu, R. Novel Encochleation Methods, Cochleates and Methods of Use. U.S. Patent 8,642,073 B2, 4 February 2014.

13. Bozó, T.; Wacha, A.; Mihály, J.; Bóta, A.; Kellermayer, M.S.Z. Dispersion and stabilization of cochleate nanoparticles. *Eur. J. Pharm. Biopharm.* **2017**, *117*, 270–275. [CrossRef] [PubMed]

14. Nagarsekar, K.; Ashtikar, M.; Steiniger, F.; Thamm, J.; Schacher, F.H.; Fahr, A. Micro-spherical cochleate composites: Method development for monodispersed cochleate system. *J. Liposome Res.* **2017**, *27*, 32–40. [CrossRef] [PubMed]

15. Dai, Y.; Chen, S.R.; Chai, L.; Zhao, J.; Wang, Y.; Wang, Y. Overview of Pharmacological Activities of Andrographis paniculata and its Major Compound Andrographolide. *Crit. Rev. Food Sci. Nutr.* **2018**. [CrossRef] [PubMed]

16. Bothiraja, C.; Shinde, M.B.; Rajalakshmi, S.; Pawar, A.P. Evaluation of molecular pharmaceutical and in-vivo properties of spray-dried isolated andrographolide—PVP. *J. Pharm. Pharmacol.* **2009**, *61*, 1465–1472. [CrossRef]

17. Guccione, C.; Oufir, M.; Piazzini, V.; Eigenmann, D.E.; Jähne, E.A.; Zabela, V.; Faleschini, M.T.; Bergonzi, M.C.; Smiesko, M.; Hamburger, M.; et al. Andrographolide-loaded nanoparticles for brain delivery: Formulation, characterisation and in vitro permeability using hCMEC/D3 cell line. *Eur. J. Pharm. Biopharm.* **2017**, *119*, 253–263. [CrossRef] [PubMed]

18. Chellampillai, B.; Pawar, A.P. Improved bioavailability of orally administered andrographolide from pH-sensitive nanoparticles. *Eur. Drug Metab. Pharmacokinet.* **2011**, *35*, 123–129. [CrossRef]

19. Righeschi, C.; Coronnello, M.; Mastrantoni, A.; Isacchi, B.; Bergonzi, M.C.; Mini, E.; Bilia, A.R. Strategy to provide a useful solution to effective delivery of dihydroartemisinin: Development, characterization and in vitro studies of liposomal formulations. *Colloids Surf. B Biointerfaces* **2014**, *116*, 121–127. [CrossRef]

20. Asprea, M.; Leto, I.; Bergonzi, M.C.; Bilia, A.R. Thyme essential oil loaded in nanocochleates: Encapsulation efficiency, in vitro release study and antioxidant activity. *LWT* **2017**, *77*, 497–502. [CrossRef]

21. Arenas-Guerrero, P.; Delgado, A.V.; Donovan, K.J.; Scott, K.; Bellini, T.; Mantegazza, F.; Jiménez, M.A. Determination of the size distribution of non-spherical nanoparticles by electric birefringence-based methods. *Sci. Rep.* **2018**, *8*, 9502–9508. [CrossRef]

22. Tirado, M.; Martınez, C.; de la Torre, J. Comparison of theories for the translational and rotational diffusion coefficients of rod-like macromolecules. Application to short DNA fragments. *J. Chem. Phys.* **1984**, *81*, 2047–2052. [CrossRef]

23. Piazzini, V.; Rosseti, C.; Bigagli, E.; Luceri, C.; Bilia, A.R.; Bergonzi, M.C. Prediction of Permeation and Cellular Transport of *Silybum marianum* Extract Formulated in a Nanoemulsion by Using PAMPA and Caco-2 Cell Models. *Planta Med.* **2017**, *83*, 1184–1193. [CrossRef] [PubMed]

24. Aditya, N.P.; Shim, M.; Lee, I.; Lee, Y.; Im, M.H.; Ko, S. Curcumin and genistein coloaded nanostructured lipid carriers: In vitro digestion and antiprostate cancer activity. *J. Agric. Food Chem.* **2013**, *61*, 1878–1883. [CrossRef] [PubMed]

25. Piazzini, V.; Landucci, E.; Graverini, G.; Pellegrini-Giampietro, D.; Bilia, A.; Bergonzi, M. Stealth and cationic nanoliposomes as drug delivery systems to increase andrographolide BBB permeability. *Pharmaceutics* **2018**, *10*, 128. [CrossRef] [PubMed]

26. Graverini, G.; Piazzini, V.; Landucci, E.; Pantano, D.; Nardiello, P.; Casamenti, F.; Pellegrini-Giampietro, D.E.; Bilia, A.R.; Bergonzi, M.C. Solid lipid nanoparticles for delivery of andrographolide across the blood-brain barrier: In vitro and in vivo evaluation. *Colloids Surf. B Biointerfaces* **2018**, *161*, 302–313. [CrossRef]

27. Borri, C.; Centi, S.; Ratto, F.; Pini, R. Polylysine as a functional biopolymer to couple gold nanorods to tumor-tropic cells. *J. Nanobiotechnol.* **2018**, *16*, 50–58. [CrossRef] [PubMed]

28. Ralph, P.; Nakoinz, I. Phagocytosis and cytolysis by a macrophage tumour and its cloned cell line. *Nature* **1975**, *257*, 393–394. [CrossRef] [PubMed]

29. Bhosale, R.R.; Ghodake, P.P.; Mane, A.N.; Ghadge, A.A. Nanocochleates: A novel carrier for drug transfer. *J. Sci. Ind. Res.* **2013**, *2*, 964–969.

30. Turina, A.V.; Nolan, M.V.; Zygadlo, J.A.; Perillo, M.A. Natural terpenes: Self-assembly and membrane partitioning. *Biophys. Chem.* **2006**, *122*, 101–113. [CrossRef]
31. Papahadjopoulos, D.; Portis, A.; Pangborn, W. Calcium induced lipid phase transitions and membrane fusion. *Ann. N. Y. Acad. Sci.* **1978**, *308*, 50–66. [CrossRef]

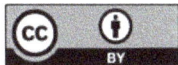

pharmaceutics

MDPI

Article

Stealth and Cationic Nanoliposomes as Drug Delivery Systems to Increase Andrographolide BBB Permeability

Vieri Piazzini [1] , Elisa Landucci [2], Giulia Graverini [1], Domenico E. Pellegrini-Giampietro [2], Anna Rita Bilia [1] and Maria Camilla Bergonzi [1,*]

[1] Department of Chemistry, University of Florence, Via Ugo Schiff 6, Sesto Fiorentino, 50019 Florence, Italy; vieri.piazzini@unifi.it (V.P.); giulia.graverini@stud.unifi.it (G.G.); ar.bilia@unifi.it (A.R.B.)
[2] Department of Health Sciences, Section of Clinical Pharmacology and Oncology, University of Florence, Viale Pieraccini 6, 50139 Florence, Italy; elisa.landucci@unifi.it (E.L.); domenico.pellegrini@unifi.it (D.E.P.-G.)
*   Correspondence: mc.bergonzi@unifi.it; Tel.: +39-055-457-3678

Received: 22 June 2018; Accepted: 8 August 2018; Published: 13 August 2018

Abstract: (1) Background: Andrographolide (AG) is a natural compound effective for the treatment of inflammation-mediated neurodegenerative disorders. The aim of this investigation was the preparation of liposomes to enhance the penetration into the brain of AG, by modifying the surface of the liposomes by adding Tween 80 (LPs-AG) alone or in combination with Didecyldimethylammonium bromide (DDAB) (CLPs-AG). (2) Methods: LPs-AG and CLPs-AG were physically and chemically characterized. The ability of liposomes to increase the permeability of AG was evaluated by artificial membranes (PAMPA) and hCMEC/D3 cells. (3) Results: Based on obtained results in terms of size, homogeneity, ζ-potential and EE%. both liposomes are suitable for parenteral administration. The systems showed excellent stability during a month of storage as suspensions or freeze-dried products. Glucose resulted the best cryoprotectant agent. PAMPA and hCMEC/D3 transport studies revealed that LPs-AG and CLPs-AG increased the permeability of AG, about an order of magnitude, compared to free AG without alterations in cell viability. The caveolae-mediated endocytosis resulted the main mechanism of up-take for both formulations. The presence of positive charge increased the cellular internalization of nanoparticles. (4) Conclusions: This study shows that developed liposomes might be ideal candidates for brain delivery of AG.

Keywords: liposomes; brain delivery; surfactant; cationic liposomes; andrographolide; PAMPA; hCMEC/D3 cells

1. Introduction

The major hindrance in the treatment of brain disorders is the blood–brain barrier (BBB), which prevents the transfer of most drugs, peptides and large molecules across the endothelial cell lining to protect the brain from undesirable side effects. To overcome such problems various approaches are used.

The liposomes offer a promising tool to resolve the low permeability and high selectivity of the BBB.

Liposomes are non-toxic, biocompatible and biodegradable drug carrier systems. Their structure which is composed of phospholipids with an aqueous reservoir allows the encapsulation of a wide variety of hydrophilic and hydrophobic agents [1–4]. Their phospholipid bilayer structure, similar to physiological membranes, makes them more compatible with the lipoid layer of BBB and increase the permeability of the drug.

Liposomes allow relatively higher intracellular uptake than other particulate systems, due to their sub-cellular size. They are highly studied for the treatment of central nervous system's pathologies such as infections, cerebral ischemia, brain tumors and neurodegenerative diseases, for instance Parkinson's and Alzheimer's [5,6]. Several studies have reported an increased transport across the BBB of encapsulated drugs both through intracerebral and intravenous administration [7].

The surface can be modified with functional ligands to enhance the brain targeting. The functionalized nanoparticles with structures able to interact with targets on the surface of the BBB represents a tool of enormous potentiality to ameliorate the bioavailability and to reduce side effects. Several studies on animal models of Alzheimer's disease demonstrated the efficacy of functionalized liposomes to cross BBB and ameliorate impaired cognitions [8–10].

In a previous research studies, the authors developed solid lipid nanoparticles [11] and polymeric nanoparticles [12] to deliver the andrographolide (AG), a natural compound, through the central nervous system and ameliorate its biopharmaceutical characteristics.

AG is one of the characteristic diterpenoids from *Andrographis paniculata* with a wide spectrum of biological activities, being anti-inflammatory, anticancer, hepatoprotective and antihyperlipidemic. AG is involved in oxidative stress-related pathways implicated in stroke pathogenesis and it protects against ischemic stroke [13]. Furthermore, it has shown protection against damage induced by amyloid-β oligomers in vitro, it reduces amyloid-β levels and tau phosphorylation in mice, it modulates the formation of amyloid plaques and it retrieves spatial memory functions in Alzheimer's disease transgenic mouse model [14]. The high lipid solubility of AG would permit its penetration of the BBB but its poor water solubility and stability reduces its bioavailability: indeed, these factors are the greatest drawbacks for clinical application [15,16].

In recent years, surfactants such as Tween 80 have been studied for the application in liposomal formulations. The sterically stabilized liposomes exhibited a superior entrapment stability compared with surfactant-free liposomes [17]. The surfactant during preparation of liposomes helps in efficient emulsification resulting in decreasing the size of vesicles and promotes the flexibility of the vesicle to penetrate the biological cell membranes. Tween 80 was also able to enhance liposomes half-life [18] and, in addition, has interesting properties including the formation of a superficial coating on liposomes that can produce "stealth" nanocarriers. Tween 80 can adsorb ApoE, which subsequently binds to its specific LDL receptor by increasing carrier endocytosis at the level of cerebral endothelial cells [4,19–22]. Finally, this surfactant is also an inhibitor of the P-gp effluent pump [23].

Another approach is the use of the cationic liposomes, able to cross the BBB via absorption-mediated transcytosis [24]. Several studies have shown that these cationic nanocarriers are more efficient vehicles for drug delivery to the brain than conventional, neutral, or anionic liposomes, possibly due to the electrostatic interactions between the cationic liposomes and the negatively charged cell membranes, enhancing nanoparticle uptake. In particular, this kind of liposome interacts with the endothelial cells of microvessels rich in lecithin, which binds positively charged material and induces its cell internalization process through endocytosis [6,24]. Furthermore, the cationic liposomes very easily fuse with cells.

The aim of the present study was the formulation of nano-sized liposomes of AG for brain targeting. Tween 80 alone or in combination with Didecyldimethylammonium bromide (DDAB) were considered to investigate the effects, on chemical and physical aspects, stability, release characteristics, in vitro uptake and permeability of the AG liposomes and to ameliorate the loading and the solubility of AG.

Liposomes were evaluated for various formulation parameters (size, polydispersity, ζ-potential, morphology, chemical and physical stability, in vitro release) and the optimized formulations were studied and characterized with in vitro tests. The ability of liposomes to increase the permeability of AG was evaluated by a Parallel Artificial Membrane Permeability Assay (PAMPA) [25]. Furthermore, the uptake of liposomes as well as their permeability across hCMEC/D3 monolayer cells, as an in vitro BBB model [11,26,27], were considered. Cell viability and cytotoxicity studies were also conducted.

2. Materials and Methods

2.1. Materials

Egg phosphatidylcholine (Phospholipon 90G) was purchased from Lipoid AG, Cologne, Germany with the support of its Italian agent AVG srl, Milan, Italy. Andrographolide, Cholesterol ≥95%, Didecyldimethylammonium bromide (DDAB, 98%), Coumarin-6 (6C), Fluorescein sodium salt (NaF), Human Serum Albumin (HSA), Phosphate Buffered Saline (PBS 0.01 M) powder (29 mM NaCl, 2.5 mM KCl, 7.4 mM $Na_2HPO_4 \cdot 7H_2O$, 1.3 mM KH_2PO_4) pH 7.4 and Tween 80 were from Sigma Aldrich, Milan, Italy. Glucose anhydrous and sucrose came from Merck, Darmstadt, Germany. 96-well Multi-Screen PAMPA filter plate (pore size 0.45 μm) were purchased from Millipore Corporation, Tullagreen, Carrigtwohill, County Cork, Ireland. Porcine polar brain lipid was obtained from Avanti Polar Lipids, Inc., Alabaster, AL, USA. All the solvents used (acetonitrile, dichloromethane, dodecane, ethanol, formic acid, methanol) were HPLC grade from Sigma Aldrich, Milan, Italy. Water was purified by Millipore, Milford, MA, USA, Milli-Qplus system. Phosphotungstic acid (PTA) was from Electron Microscopy Sciences, Hatfield, PA, USA.

2.2. Preparation of Liposomal Carriers

Stealth liposomes containing Tween 80 (LPs) and cationic liposomes (CLPs) with Tween 80 and DDAB were prepared according to the thin layer evaporation method [28]. For LPs, 160 mg of egg phosphatidylcholine (P90G) and 10 mg of cholesterol (CHOL) were dissolved in dichloromethane. The organic solvent was vacuum evaporated, and the dry lipid film was hydrated by adding 10 mL PBS containing Tween 80 at a concentration of 3% *w/v*. The aqueous dispersion was shaken with a mechanical stirrer for 30 min in a water bath at the constant temperature of 37 °C. In order to obtain small unilamellar vesicles from multilamellar vesicles, an ultrasonication probe was used for 10 min (with pulsed duty cycles of $\frac{1}{2}$ s on and $\frac{1}{2}$ s off, amplitude 50%) with the sample in an ice bath to prevent lipid degradation [29]. Finally, a gentle centrifugation of 1 min at $1205 \times g$ was performed to remove possible metallic particles released by the ultrasonic probe inside the liposomal dispersion [30].

In addition, for CLPs, 10 mg of DDAB were weighted together with P90G and CHOL and then vesicles were prepared by hydrating the dry lipid film with 10 mL PBS containing 3% of Tween 80 [31].

AG-loaded LPs (LPs-AG) and AG-loaded CLPs (CLPs-AG) were prepared with the same method described above, adding 8.5 mg of AG (0.85 mg/mL, corresponding to 5% of the weight of the lipid component) together with P90G, CHOL, DDAB in the case of CLPs-AG and 1–2 mL of methanol with dichloromethane to completely dissolve AG.

Coumarin-6-loaded liposomes (LPs-6C and CLPs-6C) were prepared using the same method, adding 5 mg of the probe (λ_{max} = 444, λ_{ex} = 420 nm, λ_{em} = 505 nm, green), corresponding to 3% of the weight of the lipid component, to the organic phase.

2.3. Physical and Morphological Characterization

Liposomes' hydrodynamic diameter, size distribution and ζ-potential were measured by Light Scattering (LS), using a Zsizer Nano series ZS90 (Malvern Instruments, Malvern, UK) outfitted with a JDS Uniphase 22 mW He-Ne laser operating at 632.8 nm, an optical fiber-based detector, a digital LV/LSE-5003 correlator and a temperature controller (Julabo water-bath) set at 25 °C. Time correlation functions were analyzed by the Cumulant method, to obtain the hydrodynamic diameter of the vesicles ($Z_{average}$) and the particle size distribution (polydispersity index, PdI) using the ALV-60 × 0 software V.3.X provided by Malvern. ζ-potential, instead, was calculated from the electrophoretic mobility, using the Henry correction to Smoluchowski's equation. The samples were diluted 100-fold in distilled water and an average of three measurements at stationary level was taken. A Haake temperature controller kept the temperature constant at 25 °C.

Liposomes were also analyzed in terms of morphology, shape, and dimensions by the transmission electron microscopy (TEM). The aqueous dispersion was diluted 10-fold in PBS and 5 μL were applied to a carbon film-covered copper grid. Most of the sample was blotted from the grid with filter paper to form a thin film. After the adhesion of liposomes, 5 µL of phosphotungstic acid solution (1% *w/v* in sterile water) were dropped onto the grid as a staining medium and the excess solution was removed with filter paper. Samples were dried for 3 min, after which they were examined with a JEOL 1010 electron microscope and then photographed at an accelerating voltage of 64 kV.

2.4. Chemical Characterization of Formulations

The percentage of the AG or 6C entrapped into liposomes in respect to the amount of substances initially used in the liposomal preparation was expressed as encapsulation efficiency (EE%) and calculated using the direct method. Free AG or 6C was removed by means of dialysis. 2 mL of liposomal suspensions were transferred in a dialysis bag (cut-off 3500–5000 Dalton), which was stirred in 1 L of water at room temperature for 1 h [29]. The content of AG or 6C entrapped within liposomes was quantified by HPLC-DAD analysis, respectively after disruption with methanol of purified liposomes (placed in the ultrasonic bath for 30 min) and ultracentrifugation for 10 min at $11,330 \times g$.

LC% for liposomal formulations was calculated using the following Equation (1):

$$LC\% = \frac{\text{Total amount of determined drug}}{\text{Weight of liposomes}} \times 100 \qquad (1)$$

The Recovery% was carried out with the same procedure but without initial dialysis and was calculated using the following Formula (2):

$$\text{Recovery}\% = \frac{\text{Total amount of determined drug}}{\text{Initial amount of drug loading}} \times 100 \qquad (2)$$

2.5. HPLC-DAD and HPLC-FLD Methods

An HP 1100 liquid chromatograph equipped with a DAD detector was used to carry out the quali-quantitative determinations of AG. A 150 mm × 4.6 mm i.d., 5 µm Zorbax Eclipse XDB, RP18 column (Agilent Technologies, Santa Clara, CA, USA) was employed. The mobile phases were (A) CH_3CN and (B) formic acid/water pH 3.2. Flow rate was 0.8 mL/min and temperature were set to 27 °C. The following gradient profile was utilized: 0–2 min, 5–15% A, 95–85% B; 2–5 min, 15% A, 85% B; 5–7 min 15–50% A, 85 50% B; 7–12 min, 50% A, 50% B; 12–15 min, 50–30% A, 50–70% B; 15–20 min, 30% A, 70% B; 20–25 min, 30–5% A, 70–95% B with equilibration time of 5 min. Injection volume was 10 µL. The UV/vis spectra were recorded in the range 200–800 nm and the chromatograms were acquired at 223 nm.

6C characterization was performed using an HP 1200 liquid chromatograph with Luna RP18 column (4.6 mm × 250 mm i.d., 5 µm) maintained at 25 °C. The mobile phase was composed of (A) CH_3CN and (B) formic acid/water pH 3.2 with a flow rate of 1 mL/min. The gradient profile was: 0–2 min, 30% A, 70% B; 2–26 min 30–100% A, 70–0% B; 26–29 min 100% A, 0% B; 29–35 min 100–30% A, 0–70% B with post-time of 5 min. Chromatograms were acquired at 444 nm.

An HP 1200 liquid chromatograph equipped with a FLD detector was used for the quantification of NaF probe (λ_{ex} = 460 nm, λ_{em} = 515 nm, green). The column was a Kinetex C18 (4.6 mm × 150 mm i.d., 5 µm) maintained at 27 °C. The mobile phases were (A) CH_3CN and (B) formic acid/water pH 3.2. Flow rate was 0.8 mL/min and the injection volume was 10 µL. The following gradient profile was utilized: 0–3 min, 20% A, 80% B; 3–23 min, 20–80% A, 80–20% B; 23–25 min 80–100% A, 20–0% B; 25–27 min, 100–20% A, 0–80% B with equilibration time of 5 min.

Diluting stock solutions in CH_3OH (0.5 mg/mL for AG and 0.1 mg/mL for 6C) and in H_2O (0.1 mg/mL for NaF), standard solutions were freshly prepared. To quantify each compound, an external standard method was applied using a regression curve and analyses were performed in triplicate. Results were expressed as the mean ± SD of the 3 experiments.

All the compounds showed a linear response: AG from 0.05 to 25 µg/mL, NaF from 0.05 to 46 µg/mL and 6C from 0.515 to 51.5 µg/mL. All the curves had coefficients of linear correlation $R^2 \geq 0.999$.

Progressive dilutions of standard solutions were used to calculate the limit of detection LOD $(S/N \geq 3)$ and the limit of quantification LOQ $(S/N \geq 10)$. LOD and LOQ for AG were 2.6 ng and 5.3 ng, respectively.

2.6. Stability Studies

The stability of empty and AG-loaded liposomes was studied for one month. Aqueous dispersions were kept at 4 °C and, at fixed time intervals, their physical and chemical stabilities were assayed: physical stability was checked by monitoring sizes, polydispersity index and ζ-potential, while chemical stability was determined by quantification of encapsulated drug by HPLC-DAD analysis.

The freeze-drying process in the absence of cryoprotectant and in the presence of 1% *w/v* of glucose or sucrose was also considered. Afterwards, lyophilization physical stability was checked for one month at 25 °C.

200 µL of LPs and CLPs dispersions were incubated at body temperature with a solution of human serum albumin (HSA, 40 mg/mL in PBS) for two hours under magnetic stirring to mimic in vivo conditions [32,33]. Physical stability of the formulations was evaluated using Dynamic Light Scattering, by controlling liposomes sizes at regular intervals.

The yield of the preparation of freeze-dried LPs-AG and CLPs-AG was calculated as the weight of the product obtained after the freeze-drying, compared to the weight of the components used in the reaction (3):

$$\text{Yield\%} = \frac{\text{real weight (mg)}}{\text{teoric weight (mg)}} \times 100 \tag{3}$$

2.7. In Vitro Release

AG in vitro release from liposomes was performed using a dialysis membrane (cut-off 3000–5000 Dalton) in PBS at 37 °C. Two mL of AG solution (0.85 mg/mL in methanol), LPs and CLPs suspensions were filled in pre-soaked dialysis tubes and placed in 200 mL of release medium using a magnetic stirrer. An aliquot of 1 mL of release medium was removed at pre-determined time intervals and replaced with 1 mL of fresh PBS maintained at 37 °C [34]. AG concentration at different times was calculated using HPLC analyses: the mean of triplicate drug release and standard deviation (mean ± SD, $n = 3$) was used to draw the drug release profiles.

The following Formula (4) was applied to calculate the percentage of AG released in the medium at pH 7.4 at each time interval (0, 30, 60, 120, 240, 360 and 1440 min):

$$\text{\% drug released} = \frac{\text{drug(t) (mg)}}{\text{total drug (mg)}} \times 100 \tag{4}$$

To evaluate the kinetics and mechanism of drug release from the liposomes, the Korsmeyer–Peppas model, Hixson Crowell model, Higuchi model, first order and zero order mathematical models were used and the best fitted model was selected based on high regression coefficient (R^2) value for the release data.

2.8. PAMPA Studies

PAMPA studies for LPs-AG and CLPs-AG were carried out using the method previously published [11]. A solution (2% *w/v*) of Porcine Polar Brain Lipid (PBL) in n-dodecane was prepped and the mixture was sonicated. PBL solution (5 µL) was added to each donor plate well [16]. Right after the application of the artificial membrane, 250 µL of formulation were added to each donor compartment, whilst the acceptor compartment was filled with PBS/Ethanol solution. Then the drug-filled donor compartment was installed into the acceptor plate. After incubation for 18 h, the donor and acceptor plate samples were withdrawn and analyzed by HPLC-DAD analyses for quantification of AG concentration: 150 μL were taken from both compartments, later diluted with methanol, placed in the ultrasonic bath for 30 min and finally ultra-centrifuged for 10 min at $11,330 \times g$ (4 °C). The permeability of AG was calculated using the following Formula (5) [35]:

$$P_e = -\ln\left[1 - C_A(t)/C_{equilibrium}\right]/A \times (1/V_D + 1/V_A) \times t \tag{5}$$

where P_e is permeability in the unit of cm/s, effective filter area (A) = f $\times$ 0.3 cm^2, where f = apparent porosity of the filter, $C_A(t)$ = compound concentration in receptor well at time t, V_D = donor well volume (mL), V_A = receptor well volume (mL), t = incubation time (s), $C_D(t)$ = compound concentration in donor well at time t, and (6)

$$C_{equilibrium} = [C_D(t) \times V_D + C_A(t) \times V_A]/(V_D + V_A) \tag{6}$$

The experiments were performed in triplicate.

2.9. hCMEC/D3 Cell Culture

This cell line (Millipore Cat. # SCC066) derives from human temporal lobe micro-vessels isolated from tissue excised during surgery for epilepsy control. Cells were seeded in a concentration of 2.5×10^4 cells/cm^2 and grown at 37 °C in an atmosphere of 5% CO_2 in 25 cm^2 rat tail collagen type I coated culture flasks. EndoGRO^{TM}-MV Complete Media Kit (Cat. # SCME004) supplemented with 1 ng/mL FGF-2 (Cat. #GF003) was changed every three days and cells were grown until they were 90% confluent. Cells were passaged at least twice before use. Confluent hCMEC/D3 cells were split by Accumax^{TM} Cell Counting Solution in DPBS.

2.10. 3-(4,5-Dimethylthiazol-2-yl)-2,5-diphenyltetrazolium Bromide (MTT) Assay

To assess cell viability after AG and LPs-AG and CLPs-AG exposure, an MTT assay was performed [36,37]. Cells were seeded in a 24-well plate (6×10^4 cells/cm^2) pre-coated with Collagen Type I, Rat Tail (Cat. #08–115) and grown at 37 °C in an atmosphere of 5% CO_2 in EndoGRO^{TM} Basal Medium (EBM-2). When the cells were approximately 70–80% confluent they were incubated with different concentrations of AG (10 and 100 μM), LPs-AG (0.085 and 0.0085 mg/mL) and CLPs-AG (0.085 and 0.0085 mg/mL), obtained by dilution (1:10 and 1:100) of the formulation in EBM-2 for 2, 4 and 24 h. The liposome formulations were previously filtered through 0.4 μm sterile filter units. The medium of each well was separated from the cells and stored for lactate dehydrogenase (LDH) assay, and cells were treated with 1 mg/mL of MTT for 1 h at 37 °C and 5% CO_2. Finally, DMSO was added to dissolve MTT formation and absorbance was measured at 550 and 690 nm. Cell viability was expressed as a percentage compared to the cells incubated only with EBM-2 (positive control). Triton X-100 was used in the MTT assay as the negative control since its detergent action disrupts the cells.

2.11. LDH Assay

Cytotoxicity after AG and liposomes exposure was verified with LDH assay. The medium resulting from incubation of AG and liposomes with cells was centrifuged ($250 \times g$, 10 min at RT) and the supernatant separated from the deposited cells in each well. This centrifugation process allowed us to remove any waste and cellular debris as well as AG and liposomes. The release of LDH into culture supernatants was detected by adding catalyst and dye solutions of a Cytotoxicity Detection Kit (LDH) (Roche Diagnostics, Indianapolis, IN, USA). The absorbance values were recorded at 490 nm and 690 nm. Cytotoxicity was expressed as a percentage compared to the maximum LDH release in the presence of triton X-100 (positive control). EBM-2 was used as negative control since no cytotoxicity was detected in such conditions.

2.12. hCMEC/D3 Cell Culture for Transwell Permeability Studies

High density pore (2×10^6 pores/cm^2) transparent PET membrane filter inserts (0.4 µm, 23.1 mm diameter, Falcon, Corning BV, Amsterdam, Netherlands) were used in 6-well cell culture plates (Falcon, Corning, Amsterdam, Netherlands) for all transcytosis assays. The transparent PET membrane filter inserts were coated with rat tail collagen type I at a concentration of 0.1 mg/mL and incubated at 37 °C for 1 h prior to cell barrier coating. Inserts were subsequently washed with PBS and incubated for 1 h, after which PBS was removed and replaced with the assay medium. The inserts were calibrated for at least 1 h with assay medium at 37 °C. Optimum media volumes were calculated to be 1 mL and 1.2 mL respectively for apical and basolateral chambers. The transwell inserts were calibrated with assay medium for 1 h, then the medium was removed and hCMEC/D3 cells were seeded onto the apical side of the inserts at a density of 6×10^4 cells/cm^2 in 1 mL assay media. 1.2 mL of fresh medium was added to the basolateral chamber. The assay medium was changed every 3 days following transwell apical insert seeding with hCMEC/D3. For seven days, cells were grown to confluence. hCMEC/D3 monolayers were used as a permeability assay for AG and AG-loaded liposomes. Fluorescein sodium salt (NaF) was considered at a concentration of 10 µg/mL as an integrity control marker with a known permeability coefficient (P_{app}) for this cell line [19]. The integrity of monolayer cells was confirmed also by observation of cultures under phase-contrast microscopy or under bright-field optics using of transparent membranes. The image was observed using an inverted microscope (Olympus IX-50; Solent Scientific, Segensworth, Fareham, UK) with a low-power objective (20X). The images were digitized using a video image obtained with a CCD camera (Diagnostic Instruments Inc., Sterling Heights, MI, USA) controlled by software (InCyt Im1TM; Intracellular Imaging Inc., Cincinnati, OH, USA).

For permeability studies, AG (10, and 100 µM), LPs-AG and CLPs-AG (0.085 mg/mL, corresponding to AG 240 µM) obtained by dilution 1:10 of the formulation in EBM-2 were tested and incubated for 1, 2, 3 and 4 h in the apical donor compartment. At the end of the incubation, the amount of NaF and AG were quantified both in apical and basolateral compartments by HPLC-FLD or HPLC-DAD method. In the case of the formulation, EBM-2 was diluted with methanol and placed in the ultrasonic bath for 30 min and then ultra-centrifuged for 1 h at $11,330 \times g$ (4 °C). The apparent permeability coefficients (P_{app}) of free AG and AG encapsulated in LPS and CLPs were calculated according to the Equation (7):

$$P_{app} \text{ (cm/s)} = V_D/(A \cdot M_D) \times (\Delta M_R/\Delta t) \tag{7}$$

where: V_D = apical (donor) volume (cm^3), M_D = apical (donor) amount (mol), $\Delta M_R/\Delta t$ = change in amount (mol) of compound in receiver compartment over time.

The recovery for AG and NaF was calculated according to the Equation (8) [19]:

$$\text{Recovery (\%)} = C_{Df} \cdot V_D + C_{Rf} \cdot V_R/(C_{D0} \cdot V_D) \times 100 \tag{8}$$

where C_{Df} and C_{Rf} are the final compound concentrations in the donor and receiver compartments, C_{D0} is the initial concentration in the donor compartment and V_D and V_R are the volumes in the donor and receiver compartments, respectively. All experiments were performed at least in triplicate.

2.13. Cellular Uptake of LPs-6C and CLPs-6C

For the evaluation of the intracellular content of 6-Coumarin, hCMEC/D3 cells (1×10^4) were exposed for 2 h to the LPs-6C and CLPs-6C loaded with 0.5 mg/mL of 6C and diluted 1:100 into EBM-2, and to a saturated solution of fluorescent probe. To elucidate the endocytic uptake mechanisms, these experiments were carried out in presence/absence of endocytic inhibitors. Control cells were exposed to liposomal formulations without any agent pre-treatment and their uptake was assumed to be 100%. A second group of cells was pre-treated with 15 μM chlorpromazine for 30 min followed by incubation with liposomes. A third group of cells was pre-treated with 25 μM of indomethacin for 30 min; and, finally, a fourth group of cells was maintained at 4 °C during the LPs-6C and CLPs-6C exposure to observe the effect of low temperature, a general metabolic inhibitor.

At the end of the treatments, the amount of 6C was quantified on cellular lysate by HPLC. For control cells and cells maintained at 4 °C during exposure, a morphological evaluation of cellular uptake was also performed: hCMEC/D3 cells were cultured on histological slides, treated as described above, fixed in 4% formaldehyde in 0.1 mol/L phosphate buffer, pH 7.4, for 10 min then stained with Fluoro scheld with DAPI (Sigma, Milan, Italy) to display the nucleus and observed by fluorescence microscopy (Labophot-2 Nikon, Tokyo, Japan). Ten photomicrographs were randomly taken for each sample.

Cellular uptake was investigated by confocal microscopy Nikon Eclipse Ti using liposomes labeled with 6C, with S Fluor 20x, NA = 0.75 high pressure Hg vapor lamp (Intensilight, Nikon, Tokyo, Japan).

Filter set: excitation 365 nm emission 400 nm hi-pass DAPI, excitation 485 nm emission 524 nm 6Co and CCD camera: Coolsnap HQ^2, Princeton instruments, Trenton, NJ, USA, 1392 × 1040, 6.45 um square pixels.

2.14. Statistical Analysis

The experiments were repeated three times and results expressed as a mean ± standard deviation. Statistical significance of hCMEC/D cell viability and cellular uptake was analyzed using one-way ANOVA followed by the post hoc Tukey's w-test for multiple comparisons. All statistical calculations were performed using GRAPH-PAD PRISM v. 5 for Windows (GraphPad Software, San Diego, CA, USA). A probability value (*p*) of <0.05 was considered significant.

3. Results and Discussion

3.1. Preparation and Characterization of Liposomes

LPs were prepared by using P90G, CHOL and Tween 80. This compound was selected as a coating agent to increase the stability of the formulation, to produce "stealth" nanovesicles and to promote endocytosis of the carrier at the level of cerebral endothelial cells [23]. Various ratios of the two lipid constituents were tested to obtain small sizes, good polydispersity and favorable ζ-potential. In particular, the ratios P90G:CHOL 18:1, 16:1, 14:1, 12:1, and 10:1 were considered. The best ratio resulted to be 16:1, corresponding to 160 mg of P90G and 10 mg of CHOL. Then, 3% *w/v* of Tween 80 was added (LPs). Furthermore, different sonication times were tested to optimize LPs physical characteristics. The selected conditions consisted in two cycles of 5 min of sonication, each including 0.5 s of sonication alternating with 0.5 s of pause, as reported in the materials and methods section. LPs were nanosized unilamellar vesicles, with a PdI less than 0.25 and a ζ-potential, around −20 mV (Table 1), confirming a homogeneous and stable dispersion. LC% was 2.28% ± 0.22. The mean vesicle sizes and the width of the particle distribution are important parameters as they govern physical stability and permeation through BBB [38]. Moreover, the vesicles sizes highly affected the interaction of the liposomes with the hCMEC/D3 cellular model [39,40].

AG does not influence the stability of the formulation (Table 1); when LPs were loaded with AG, LPs-AG showed the same physical parameters as LPs. The electron microscope analysis confirmed the liposomal structure; the results evidenced the presence of spherical vesicles, with a defined phospholipid bilayer, well separated, due to the presence of the surfactant that prevents agglomeration, and with dimensions around 100 nm, confirming the DLS results (Figure 1a).

Next, LPs were functionalized with positive surface charges by using DDAB (cationic liposomes, CLPs) in the same amount of CHOL (10 mg in the total formulation). In this case, ζ-potential resulted positive, indicating the presence of positive charges on the surface of the carrier.

Then, CLPs loaded with 8.5 mg of AG (corresponding to 5% of the weight of the lipid component) were prepared (CLPs-AG); the presence of DDAB and AG did not modify the physical characteristics of the formulation (Table 1). LC% was 3.08% ± 0.21. TEM analysis showed well separated spherical shape vesicles, with a distinct phospholipid bilayer (Figure 1b).

The compound 6-Coumarin (6C), a lipophilic fluorescent dye, was incorporated into liposomes to investigate the ability of nanoparticles to penetrate into hCMEC/D3 cells, as BBB-model, and to elucidate trans-endothelial transport in vitro. The preparation of fluorescent liposomes was performed as reported for LPs and CLPs, by adding 6C (0.5 mg/mL) to the organic phase. Their physical and chemical parameters are shown in Table 1. The same dimensions of the two types of liposomes, was very important to interact with the HCMEC/D3 equally [39]. LPs-6C and CLPs-6C resulted larger but useful for a parenteral administration. AG and 6C are lipophilic compounds and there are inserted in the bilayer, but the effect on the sizes of nanoparticles is different due to their unlike chemical structure. The high ζ-potential of all formulations is indicative of their stability, as also supported by stability studies.

Table 1. Physical characterization of empty, andrographolide (AG) and coumarin-6 (6C) loaded liposomes.

Sample	Size (nm)	PdI	ζ-Potential	EE%	Recovery%
LPs	80.2 ± 3.6	0.22 ± 0.03	−20.4 ± 4.1	-	-
CLPs	84.6 ± 8.1	0.23 ± 0.02	20.7 ± 4.7	-	-
LPs-AG	96.4 ± 9.5	0.23 ± 0.03	−22.8 ± 1.2	44.7 ± 3.2	91.1 ± 5.3
CLPs-AG	82.1 ± 9.3	0.25 ± 0.01	20.3 ± 3.7	47.5 ± 3.3	94.9 ± 4.7
LPs-6C	193.1 ± 3.0	0.21 ± 0.02	−27.4 ± 0.4	46.0 ± 1.4	71.2 ± 4.2
CLPs-6C	197.1 ± 1.4	0.27 ± 0.03	31.1 ± 0.6	63.1 ± 0.1	80.6 ± 5.0

LPs: liposomes with Tween 80, CLPs: liposomes with Tween 80 and DDAB. Data displayed as mean ± SD; *n* = 3.

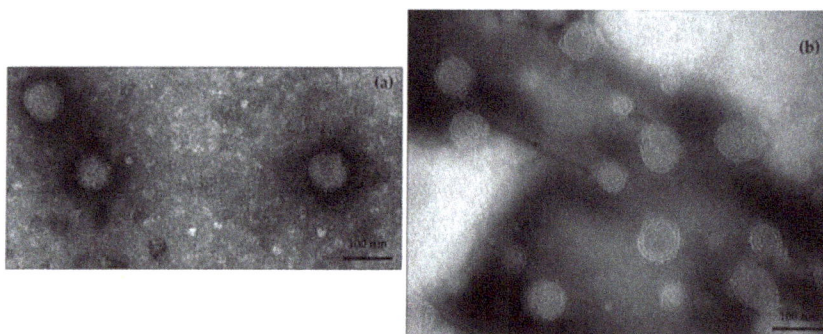

Figure 1. TEM images of LPs-AG (**a**) and CLPs-AG (**b**) (scale 100 nm).

3.2. Stability Studies

Liposomes stability was evaluated both as a colloidal dispersion and in the freeze-dried form. The ability of the aqueous dispersions to maintain their physicochemical properties in terms of particle size, PdI, surface charge and drug entrapment was assessed after 1-month storage at 4 °C and the Light Scattering analyses were performed to control the stability over time. No significant changes were observed in physical parameters of empty or LPs-AG and CLPs-AG dispersions (Figure 2). The presence of non-ionic surfactant is expected to reduce the agglomeration between liposomes via steric repulsion. Also, the presence of DDAB on the surface of liposomes prevented the aggregation and the precipitation of the vesicles and increased the systems stability. In addition, the entrapment efficiency remained constant, around 45%.

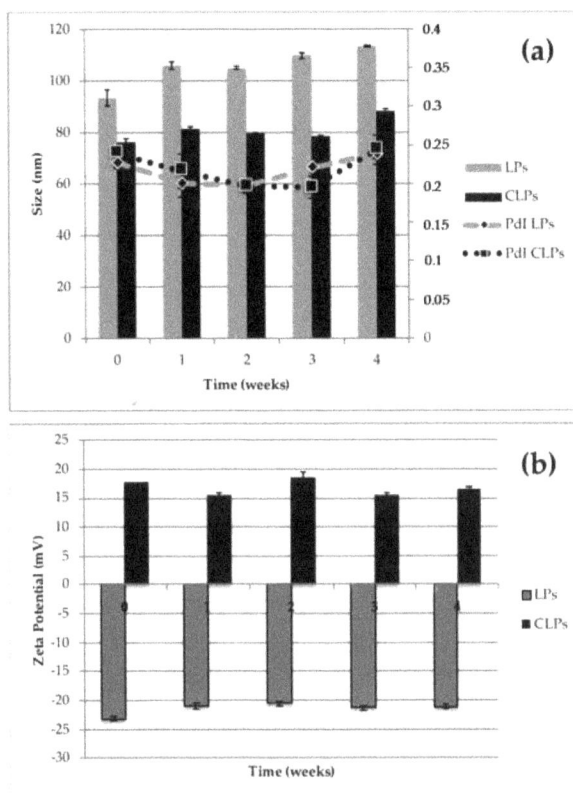

Figure 2. Particle size, polydispersity index (PdI) (**a**) and zeta-potential (**b**) of LPs-AG and CLPs-AG as dispersion after one-month storage at 4 °C. (Data displayed as mean ± SD; *n* = 3).

The major limitation to liposomes use is due to their physical and chemical instability, when the aqueous suspension is stored for an extended period. The poor stability in an aqueous medium forms a real obstacle against the clinical application of nanoparticles.

To improve the physical and chemical stability, water needs to be removed. Freeze-drying is a good technique to enhance the chemical and physical stability of formulations over prolonged periods.

The stability of LPs-AG and CLPs-AG with time was evaluated also in the freeze-dried form. However, the freezing process of the sample might cause problems of possible structural and/or functional damages of the system, and/or subsequent difficulties in sample re-solubilization, due to particle aggregation phenomena. The addition of cryoprotectants improves the quality of the dehydrated product, decreases particle aggregation phenomena and allows to obtain an easier re-dispersion of the freeze-dried product.

Therefore, to estimate the effect of the presence and type of cryoprotectant, empty, LPs-AG and CLPs-AG formulations were freeze-dried with and without sucrose or glucose (1% *w*/*v*). After the lyophilization process, all formulations were dispersed in PBS and analyzed by DLS and ELS (Table 2). As shown in Table 2, the drying process produced an increase in terms of size and PdI, respect to the values reported before the freeze-drying process (Table 1). However, all liposomes maintained characteristics suitable for parenteral administration. The best freeze-drying process was obtained in the presence of glucose both for LPs-AG and CLPs-AG. The EE% remained almost constant around 43%. The yield % of the preparation process was also calculated, in this case without addition of the cryoprotectant, and resulted 69.5% ± 0.1 for LPs and 71.2% ± 0.1 for CLPs (mean ± SD; $n = 3$). After a month of storage at 25 °C the freeze-dried product retained the starting characteristics.

Table 2. Physical parameters of andrographolide loaded liposomes, after the freeze-drying process with and without cryoprotectant, 1% w/v of sucrose or glucose.

LPs-AG	No Cryoprotector	Glucose	Sucrose
Size (nm)	148.8 ± 1.4	135.0 ± 0.9	147.5 ± 1.2
PdI	0.32 ± 0.03	0.25 ± 0.02	0.35 ± 0.01
ζ (mV)	−21.3 ± 0.9	−19.4 ± 1.1	−18.5 ± 1.0
CLPs-AG			
Size (nm)	144.6 ± 2.2	131.3 ± 5.1	149.3 ± 1.2
PdI	0.38 ± 0.02	0.28 ± 0.01	0.29 ± 0.01
ζ (mV)	+28.6 ± 0.9	+27.0 ± 0.8	+26.5 ± 0.9

LPs-AG: liposomes with Tween 80 loaded with AG, CLPs-AG: liposomes with Tween 80 and DDAB loaded with AG. Data displayed as mean ± SD; $n = 3$.

A drawback to the use of nanocarriers, in particular cationic nanocarriers, for brain delivery is their binding to serum proteins that attenuates their surface charge. Therefore, the stability of LPs-AG and CLPs-AG in presence of human serum albumin (HSA) at physiological concentration was also tested. After 2 h of incubation, DLS analyses confirmed that sizes were not affected by the presence of HSA and therefore revealed coexistence of free serum proteins and optimized nanocarrier without any protein corona effect (Table 3).

Table 3. Physical stability of LPs-AG and CLPs-AG in presence of human serum albumin.

	LPs-AG		CLPs-AG	
Time	Size (nm)	Pd	Size (nm)	Pd
0	94.8 ± 2.4	0.23 ± 0.02	76.4 ± 1.2	0.24 ± 0.01
30′	103.8 ± 2.0	0.39 ± 0.01	82.9 ± 0.5	0.41 ± 0.02
1 h	97.2 ± 3.2	0.39 ± 0.02	83.5 ± 4.8	0.40 ± 0.01
2 h	99.1 ± 5.1	0.39 ± 0.01	81.9 ± 3.4	0.43 ± 0.02

LPs-AG: liposomes with Tween 80 loaded with AG, CLPs-AG: liposomes with Tween 80 and DDAB loaded with AG. Data displayed as mean ± SD; $n = 3$.

3.3. In Vitro Release

AG in vitro release at 37 °C from LPs-AG and CLPs-AG was evaluated for 24 h by using a dialysis bag and PBS as receptor medium to mimic sink conditions. The release profiles of AG from AG solution, LPs-AG and CLPs-AG were reported in Figure 3. The result indicated that the release of AG from methanol solution through the dialysis membrane was much faster, with a fast release during the first 2 h and approximately 100% of the drug released within 6 h. In contrast, the immediate release of the drug (burst effect) does not occur in the case of LPs-AG and CLPs-AG. The percentages of AG released from LPs and CLPs were gradual: only 56.8% and 69.7% of drug was released within 6 h, respectively. The percentages rose to 83.5% and 77.4%, after 24 h, respectively. The almost linear and gradual trend of the release indicated that the liposomal systems can release AG for prolonged periods and in greater quantities compared to the saturated aqueous solution, were the solubility of AG resulted very low (0.05 mg/mL). Optimized liposomal formulations are able to solubilize 0.85 mg/mL of drug.

Different theoretical models were considered to examine the nature of release. The drug release mechanism was defined by fitting AG release data with various kinetics models. By comparing the regression coefficient values, the Higuchi model ($R^2 = 0.8366$ and 0.9264, respectively, Table 4) resulted as the best to describe the kinetics of these two types of liposomes. Thus, the liposomal membrane disruption controlled the release mechanism [41].

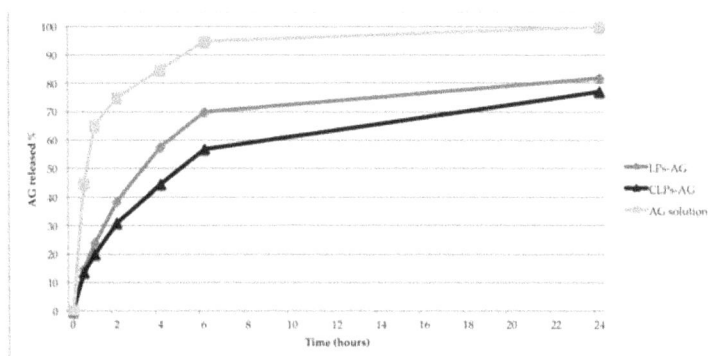

Figure 3. In vitro release profiles of LPs-AG and CLPs-AG in PBS. (each data point represents the average of three samples).

Table 4. Regression coefficient (R^2) obtained in different kinetics models for AG release from LPs-AG and CLPs-AG.

Release Kinetics	LPs-AG	CLPs-AG
Zero order	0.5722	0.7079
First order	0.7685	0.8816
Korsmeyer-Peppas	0.4552	0.4980
Hixson	0.7033	0.8292
Higuchi	0.8366	0.9264

LPs-AG: liposomes with Tween 80 loaded with AG, CLPs-AG: liposomes with Tween 80 and DDAB loaded with AG.

Due to the very low solubility of AG in water and the related problems of bioavailability, both the liposomal formulations allow the administration of a high amount of solubilized molecule according to the requirements for parenteral preparations.

3.4. PAMPA Study

Parallel Artificial Membrane Permeability Assay (PAMPA) was performed to estimate passive transcellular permeability. It is a non-cell-based permeability model because it lacks transporter- and pore-mediated permeability, but is considered robust, reproducible and it results in a helpful complement to the cellular permeability model for its speed, low cost and versatility, and readily provides information about passive transport permeability.

AG is a molecule with low BBB permeability (effective permeability, P_e value of $0.49 \pm 0.16 \times 10^{-6}$ cm/s [11] and therefore liposomal formulation could represent a useful tool to improve its permeation. P_e of AG-loaded liposomes resulted as increased, in particular $3.94 \pm 0.60 \times 10^{-6}$ cm/s for LPs-AG and $3.87 \pm 0.36 \times 10^{-6}$ cm/s for CLPs-AG. These values confirmed that LPs-AG and CLPs-AG increased the permeability of the drug, of about an order of magnitude, compared to the aqueous solution.

Though this test does not discriminate the different behavior of the two systems because the artificial membrane fails to mimic all properties of a cell, a mechanism of permeation through the artificial membrane was hypothesized. An interaction between the phospholipid bilayer, which is a flexible system, with the lipid that covers the artificial membrane, similar to one of mechanisms of liposome-cell interaction.

3.5. MTT and LDH Assays

MTT and LDH assays were performed in the hCMEC/D3 cell line to evaluate the effect of AG and LPs-AG and CLPs-AG in cell viability and cytotoxicity, and permeability studies were also conducted in transwell devices using the same cell line. The in vitro cytotoxicity of the developed LPs-AG and CLPs-AG and AG was assessed by cell viability determination and membrane integrity evaluation using the hCMEC/D3 cell line in MTT and LDH assays, respectively (Figure 4). When cells were exposed to different concentrations of AG (10 and 100 µM) and LPs-AG and CLPs-AG (0.0085 and 0.085 mg/mL) for 2 (Figure 4a) and 4 h (Figure 4b), no significant changes were observed in MTT metabolization, except for LPs-AG and CLPs-AG (0.085 mg/mL) or LDH release when compared to cells exposed to the EBM-2 medium alone, indicating that AG and LPs-AG and CLPs-AG affected neither the metabolic activity of the cells nor the membrane integrity at these time points. On the other hand, when the cells were incubated for 24 h with AG at a dose of 100 µM, LPs-AG (0.085 mg/mL) and CLPs-AG (0.0085 and 0.085 mg/mL) we observed a significant reduction of cell viability and an increase in cytotoxicity compared to the control (Figure 4c).

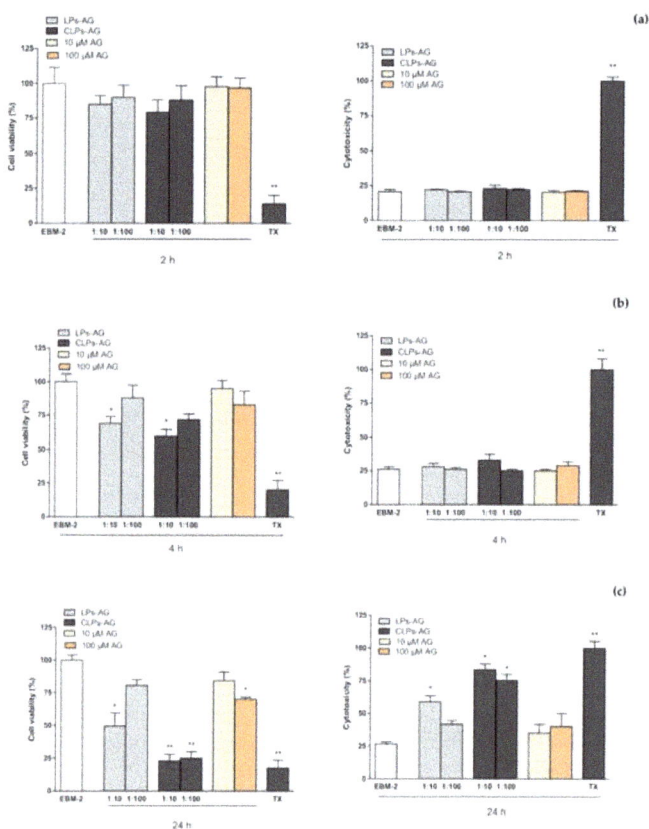

Figure 4. hCMEC/D3 cell viability evaluated by MTT assay (left panel) and cytotoxicity by LDH assay (right panel) when exposed for 2 h (**a**), 4 h (**b**) and 24 h (**c**) to AG (10 and 100 µM) or LPs-AG and CLPs-AG (0.0085 and 0.085 mg/mL). Data is expressed as percentage of control (EBM-2 medium) and Triton-X (TTX) which represent, respectively, the maximum cell viability and cell cytotoxicity. Values represent the mean ± SEM of at least three experiments performed in triplicate. * $p < 0.05$ and ** $p < 0.01$ vs. EBM-2 alone.

3.6. BBB Permeability Studies

hCMEC/D3 brain microvascular endothelial cell line is a model of human BBB utilized to study the drug transport mechanisms [18,42]. The cells retain the expression of most transporters and receptors expressed in vivo in the human BBB. hCMEC/D3 apparent permeability coefficient (P_{app}) correlates well with in vivo permeability data, and therefore permeability studies were performed to predict the permeability of free AG and LPs-AG and CLPs-AG across the BBB. NaF was used as the negative control and its P_{app} was determined during all transport experiments to monitor the integrity of the cell layer. This aspect was also been checked by phase-contrast microscopy [11].

P_{app} of NaF was $8.27 \pm 1.81 \times 10^{-6}$ cm/s, in agreement with the literature values [11,12,19]. This value remained constant during the permeability assay, and demonstrates the confluence of the monolayer and assesses the tight junction integrity. P_{app} of LPs-AG and CLPs-AG were only slightly higher than the P_{app} values of the free AG for the first 3 h. However, at 4 h, the P_{app} value for both LPs-AG and CLPs-AG was significantly higher (about double) than that of the free AG (P_{app} of AG: $8.67 \pm 0.95 \times 10^{-6}$ cm/s; P_{app} LPs-AG: $16.8 \pm 1.70 \times 10^{-6}$ cm/s; P_{app} CLPs-AG: $17.2 \pm 1.43 \times 10^{-6}$ cm/s). The amount of AG that permeated when loaded into liposomes increased about 200 times in respect to the free molecule, as confirmed by the increase of the P_{app} values during the time reported in Figure 5. AG transport across the cell was in a time-dependent manner. The obtained P_{app} data are useful for in vitro prediction, as confirmed by the recovery value, which was above 80% in all experiments. The data agrees with PAMPA results.

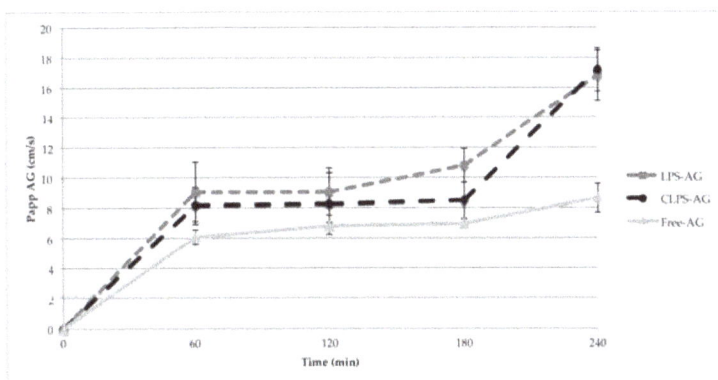

Figure 5. The apparent permeable coefficient of different liposomal formulations for different treatment time in the in vitro BBB model. (Data represent means $\pm$ S.D, $n = 3$).

A combination assay of PAMPA and unidirectional (apical to basal) hCMEC/D3 permeability model can synergistically provide invaluable permeability/absorption assessment of AG. The P_{app} values are greater than those of P_e, due to the presence of an active endocytic mechanism in addition to a passive one, as seen by following uptake studies.

3.7. Liposome Uptake by hCMEC/D3 Cells

Figure 6 shows the fluorescence images of hCMEC/D3 cells treated with LPs-6C and CLPs-6C after 2 h of incubation. The images revealed that the probe was internalized and LPs-6C and CLPs-6C were punctually concentrated in intracellular vesicles (endosomes or lysosomes) which can be related to their endocytic mechanism of uptake [42]. Besides their cytoplasmic location, green fluorescence indicates that nanoparticles were also transported to the perinuclear area. This is an important finding for pharmaceutical drug delivery research, since the nucleus is the target site for several drugs [43].

Nuclei   6C-loaded LPs   Overlay

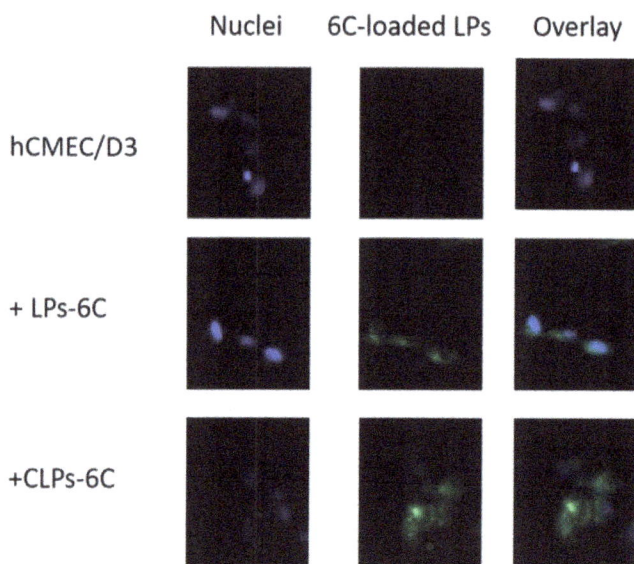

Figure 6. Cellular uptake of LPs-6C and CLPs-6C by hCMEC/D3 cells after 2 h incubation at 37 °C. Images of nuclei stained with DAPI (blue), 6-Coumarin (green) and their overlay. Scale bar: 20 μm.

Concerning the uptake of liposomes by hCMEC/D3 cells, it was different for both liposomes LPs-6C and CLPs-6C: 6.4% and 14.0%, respectively. The result proves that the internalization ability of liposomes increases in the presence of positive charge on the bilayer that improves the binding affinity between carrier and cellular membrane [31].

Furthermore, a group of cells was maintained at 4 °C in the presence of LPs-6C and CLPs-6C, to observe the effect of low temperature, a general metabolic inhibitor. The fluorescence of cells incubated with 6C loaded liposomes in the absence of any inhibitor was considered as 100%, while the fluorescence after incubation in the presence of inhibitors was expressed as a relative percentage compared to the cells without inhibitor. As shown in Figure 7, a significant reduction (about 80%) in hCMEC/D3 cell uptake efficiency was observed at 4 °C for all two formulations as compared with that at physiological temperature, suggesting that their uptake relied on an energy-dependent pathway and it was mediated by endocytosis [44].

To elucidate the endocytic uptake mechanisms, the experiments were also carried out in the presence of endocytic inhibitors, such as chlorpromazine, a clathrin blocker, and indomethacin, a caveolin-dependent endocytosis inhibitor.

Liposomes could be internalized into cells by different mechanisms, according to the type of cell, composition, surface charge, and size of the liposome [45–47]. In our study, the cellular association of the liposomes was significantly influenced by indomethacin, with a reduction in cellular association of about 44% and 63% for LPs-6C and CLPs-6C, respectively (Figure 7). Caveolae-mediated endocytosis is involved in the uptake of liposomes. However, it did not completely inhibit active uptake of the nanoparticles when compared with the results at 4 °C, confirming that cellular uptake of liposomes involved more that on an energy-dependent pathway. In fact, as evidenced in the Figure 7, an uptake reduction of 15% for LPs-6C and 20% for CLPs-6C was observed in the presence of chlorpromazine, even if less pronounced than with indomethacin. This indicates that clathrin-mediated endocytosis is also a mechanism involved in the uptake.

Therefore, the preferential mechanism of the liposomes uptake by hCMEC/D3 cells was found to be caveolae-mediated endocytosis, with a greater effect of inhibitors in the case of CLPs-6C.

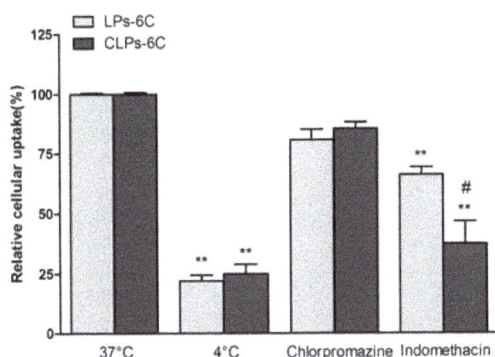

Figure 7. Effect of the temperature (4 °C) and different inhibitors on hCMEC/D3 cell internalization pathways of LPs-6C and CLPs-6C after 2 h incubation at 37 °C. (Data represent the mean ± standard deviation (n = 3). Bars represent the mean ± SD of at least 6 experiments ** $p < 0.01$ vs. corresponding liposome at 37 °C; # $p < 0.05$ CLPs-6C vs. LPs-6C. (ANOVA + Tukey's test).

4. Conclusions

Based on the obtained results in terms of size, homogeneity, ζ-potential and EE%, both optimized liposomal formulations of AG are suitable for parenteral administration. The systems showed excellent chemical and physical stability during a month of storage as suspensions or freeze-dried products. The optimized liposomes enhanced solubility and cellular permeability of AG, as demonstrated by in vitro tests with PAMPA and hCMEC/D3 cells. Both carriers increase the permeation of AG into the cell without alterations in cell viability and monolayer integrity. The presence of positive charge elevated the cellular internalization of liposomes. Uptake experiments suggest an energy-dependent pathway as a possible transport mechanism across the hCMEC/D3 monolayer, with caveolae-mediated endocytosis, in particular, being the main mechanism.

Author Contributions: V.P., E.L. and M.C.B. conceived and designed the experiments; V.P., E.L. and G.G. performed the experiments; V.P., E.L., G.G. and M.C.B. analyzed the data; M.C.B., E.L. and V.P. wrote the paper; M.C.B., A.R.B. and D.E.P.-G. provided materials and equipment for the experiments; A.R.B. and D.E.P.-G. reviewed and revised the paper.

Funding: This research received no external funding.

Acknowledgments: Maria Cristina Salvatici, Electron Microscopy Centre "Laura Bonzi" (Ce.M.E.), ICCOM, CNR, Sesto Fiorentino, Florence, Italy and Alessio Gnerucci Department of Experimental and Clinical Biomedical Sciences, University of Florence, Florence, Italy

Conflicts of Interest: The authors declare no conflict of interest.

References

1. Saenz del Burgo, L.; Hernández, R.M.; Orive, G.; Pedraz, J.L. Nanotherapeutic approaches for brain cancer management. *Nanomed. NBM* **2014**, *10*, e905–e919. [CrossRef] [PubMed]
2. Pattni, B.S.; Chupin, V.V.; Torchilin, V.P. New developments in liposomal drug delivery. *Chem. Rev.* **2015**, *115*, 10938–10966. [CrossRef] [PubMed]
3. Bilia, A.R.; Bergonzi, M.C.; Guccione, C.; Manconi, M.; Fadda, A.M.; Sinico, C. Vesicles and micelles: Two versatile vectors for the delivery of natural products. *J. Drug Deliv. Sc. Technol.* **2016**, *32*, 241–255. [CrossRef]
4. Grossi, C.; Guccione, C.; Isacchi, B.; Bergonzi, M.C.; Luccarini, I.; Casamenti, F.; Bilia, A.R. Development of blood–brain barrier permeable nanoparticles as potential carriers for salvianolic acid B to CNS. *Planta Med.* **2017**, *83*, 382–391. [CrossRef] [PubMed]

5. Conti, E.; Gregori, M.; Radice, I.; Da Re, F.; Grana, D.; Re, F.; Salvati, E.; Masserini, M.; Ferrarese, C.; Zola, C.P.; et al. Multifunctional liposomes interact with Abeta in human biological fluids: Therapeutic implications for Alzheimer's disease. *Neurochem. Int.* **2017**, *108*, 60–65. [CrossRef] [PubMed]

6. Agrawal, M.; Tripathi, A.D.K.; Saraf, S.; Saraf, S.; Antimisiaris, S.G.; Mourtas, S.; Margareta, H.-U.; Alexander, A. Recent advancements in liposomes targeting strategies to cross blood-brain barrier (BBB) for the treatment of Alzheimer's disease. *J. Control. Release* **2017**, *260*, 61–77. [CrossRef] [PubMed]

7. Garcia-Garcia, E.; Andrieux, K.; Gil, S.; Couvreur, P. Colloidal carriers and blood–brain barrier (BBB) translocation: A way to deliver drugs to the brain? *Int. J. Pharm.* **2005**, *298*, 274–292. [CrossRef] [PubMed]

8. Balducci, C.; Mancini, S.; Minniti, S.; La Vitola, P.; Zotti, M.; Sancini, G.; Mauri, M.; Cagnotto, A. Multifunctional liposomes reduce brain β-amyloid burden and ameliorate memory impairment in Alzheimer's disease mouse models. *J. Neurosci.* **2014**, *34*, 14022–14031. [CrossRef] [PubMed]

9. Ordóñez-Gutiérrez, L.; Re, F.; Bereczki, E.; Ioja, E.; Gregori, M.; Andersen, A.J.; Antón, M.; Moghimi, S.M.; Pei, J.J.; Masserini, M.; et al. Repeated intraperitoneal injections of liposomes containing phosphatidic acid and cardiolipin reduce amyloid-β levels in APP/PS1 transgenic mice. *Nanomedicine* **2015**, *11*, 421–430. [CrossRef] [PubMed]

10. Mancini, S.; Minniti, S.; Gregori, M.; Sancini, G.; Cagnotto, A.; Couraud, P.O.; Ordóñez-Gutiérrez, L.; Wandosell, F.; Salmona, M.; Re, F. The hunt for brain Aβ oligomers by peripherally circulating multi-functional nanoparticles: Potential therapeutic approach for Alzheimer disease. *Nanomedicine* **2016**, *12*, 43–52. [CrossRef] [PubMed]

11. Graverini, G.; Piazzini, V.; Landucci, E.; Casamenti, F.; Pantano, D.; Pellegrini-Giampietro, D.; Bilia, A.R.; Bergonzi, M.C. Solid lipid nanoparticles for delivery of andrographolide across the blood-brain barrier: In vitro and in vivo evaluation. *Colloid. Surf. B Biointerfaces* **2018**, *161*, 302–313. [CrossRef] [PubMed]

12. Guccione, C.; Oufir, M.; Piazzini, V.; Eigenmann, D.E.; Jähne, E.A.; Zabela, V.; Faleschini, M.T.; Bergonzi, M.C.; Smiesko, M.; Hamburger, M.; et al. Andrographolide-loaded nanoparticles for brain delivery: Formulation, characterisation and in vitro permeability using hCMEC/D3 cell line. *Eur. J. Pharm. Biopharm.* **2017**, *119*, 253–263. [CrossRef] [PubMed]

13. Yen, T.L.; Chen, R.J.; Jayakumar, T.; Lu, W.J.; Hsieh, C.Y.; Hsu, M.J.; Yang, C.H.; Chang, C.C.; Lin, Y.K.; Lin, K.H. Andrographolide stimulates p38 mitogen-activated protein kinase-nuclear factor erythroid-2-related factor2-heme oxygenase 1 signaling in primary cerebral endothelial cells for definite protection against ischemic stroke in rats. *Transl. Res.* **2016**, *170*, 57–72. [CrossRef] [PubMed]

14. Serrano, F.G.; Tapia-Rojas, C.; Carvajal, F.J.; Hancke, J.; Cerpa, W.; Inestrosa, N.C. Andrographolide reduces cognitive impairment in young and mature AβPPswe/PS-1 mice. *Mol. Neurodegener.* **2014**, *9*, 61. [CrossRef] [PubMed]

15. Yu, B.T.; Zhang, Z.R.; Liu, W.S.; Yang, P.W.; Wang, P. Study on stability in vitro of andrographolide. *Chin. Tradit. Pat. Med.* **2002**, *24*, 33133.

16. Wang, M.; Ren, X.L.; Gao, X.M.; Vincieri, F.F.; Bilia, A.R. Stability of active ingredients of traditional Chinese medicine (TCM). *Nat. Prod. Commun.* **2009**, *4*, 1761–1776.

17. Crosasso, P.; Ceruti, M.; Brusa, P.; Arpicco, S.; Dosio, F.; Cattel, L. Preparation characterization and properties of sterically stabilized paclitaxel-containing liposome. *J. Control. Release* **2000**, *63*, 19–30. [CrossRef]

18. Bucke, W.E.; Leitzke, S.; Diederichs, J.E.; Muller, RH. Surface-modified amikacin-liposomes: Organ distribution and interaction with plasma proteins. *J. Drug Target.* **1998**, *5*, 99–108. [CrossRef] [PubMed]

19. Gulyaev, A.E.; Gelperina, S.E.; Skidan, I.N.; Antropov, A.S.; Kivman, G.Y.; Kreuter, J. Significant transport of doxorubicin into the brain with polysorbate 80-coated nanoparticles. *Pharm. Res.* **1999**, *16*, 1564–1569. [CrossRef] [PubMed]

20. Kreuter, J.; Shamenkov, D.; Petrov, V.; Ramge, P.; Cychutek, K.; Koch-Brandt, C.; Alyautdin, R. Apolipoprotein-mediated transport of nanoparticle-bound drugs across the blood-brain barrier. *J. Drug Target.* **2002**, *10*, 317–325. [CrossRef] [PubMed]

21. Wohlfart, S.; Gelperina, S.; Kreuter, J. Transport of drugs across the blood–brain barrier by nanoparticles. *J. Control. Release* **2012**, *161*, 264–273. [CrossRef] [PubMed]

22. Kreuter, J. Mechanism of polymeric nanoparticle-based drug transport across the blood-brain barrier (BBB). *J. Microencapsul.* **2013**, *30*, 49–54. [CrossRef] [PubMed]

23. Gastaldi, L.; Battaglia, L.; Peira, E.; Chirio, D.; Muntoni, E.; Solazzi, I.; Gallarate, M.; Dosio, F. Solid lipid nanoparticles as vehicles of drugs to the brain: Current state of the art. *Eur. J. Pharm. Biopharm.* **2014**, *87*, 433–444. [CrossRef] [PubMed]

24. Wong, H.L.; Wu, X.Y.; Bendayan, R. Nanotechnological advances for the delivery of CNS therapeutics. *Adv. Drug Deliv. Rev.* **2012**, *64*, 686–700. [CrossRef] [PubMed]

25. Di, L.; Kerns, E.H.; Fan, K.; McConnell, O.J.; Carter, G.T. High throughput artificial membrane permeability assay for blood–brain barrier. *Eur. J. Med. Chem.* **2003**, *38*, 223–232. [CrossRef]

26. Weksler, B.; Romero, I.A.; Couraud, P.O. The hCMEC/D3 cell line as a model of the human blood brain barrier. *Fluids Barriers CNS* **2013**, *10*, 16. [CrossRef] [PubMed]

27. Eigenmann, D.E.; Xue, G.; Kim, K.S.; Moses, A.V.; Hamburger, M.; Oufir, M. Comparative study of four immortalized human brain capillary endothelial cell lines, hCMEC/D3, hBMEC, TY10, and BB19, and optimization of culture conditions, for an in vitro blood–brain barrier model for drug permeability studies. *Fluids Barriers CNS* **2013**, *10*, 33. [CrossRef] [PubMed]

28. Bangham, A.D.; Hill, M.W.; Miller, N.G.A. Preparation and use of liposomes as models of biological membranes. In *Methods in Membrane Biology*; Springer: Boston, MA, USA, 1974; pp. 61–68. [CrossRef]

29. Righeschi, C.; Coronnello, M.; Mastrantoni, A.; Isacchi, B.; Bergonzi, M.C.; Mini, E.; Bilia, A.R. Strategy to provide a useful solution to effective delivery of dihydroartemisinin: Development, characterization and in vitro studies of liposomal formulations. *Colloids Surf. B Biointerfaces* **2014**, *116*, 121–127. [CrossRef] [PubMed]

30. Dua, J.S.; Rana, A.C.; Bhandari, A.K. Liposome: Methods of preparation and applications. *Int. J. Pharm. Stud. Res.* **2012**, *3*, 14–20.

31. Saengkrit, N.; Saesoo, S.; Srinuanchai, W.; Phunpee, S.; Ruktanonchai, U.R. Influence of curcumin-loaded cationic liposome on anticancer activity for cervical cancer therapy. *Colloids Surf. B Biointerfaces* **2014**, *114*, 349–356. [CrossRef] [PubMed]

32. Gualbert, J.; Shahgaldian, P.; Coleman, A.W. Interactions of amphiphilic calix [4] arene-based solid lipid nanoparticles with bovine serum albumin. *Int. J. Pharm.* **2003**, *257*, 69–73. [CrossRef]

33. Koziara, J.M.; Lockman, P.R.; Allen, D.D.; Mumper, R.J. Paclitaxel nanoparticles for the potential treatment of brain tumors. *J. Control. Release* **2004**, *99*, 259–269. [CrossRef] [PubMed]

34. Righeschi, C.; Bergonzi, M.C.; Isacchi, B.; Bazzicalupi, C.; Gratteri, P.; Bilia, A.R. Enhanced curcumin permeability by SLN formulation: The PAMPA approach. *LWT-Food Sci. Technol.* **2016**, *66*, 475–483. [CrossRef]

35. Wohnsland, F.; Faller, B. High-throughput permeability pH profile and high-throughput alkane/water log P with artificial membranes. *J. Med. Chem.* **2001**, *44*, 923–930. [CrossRef] [PubMed]

36. Conti, P.; Pinto, A.; Tamborini, L.; Madsen, U.; Nielsen, B.; Bräuner-Osborne, H.; Hansen, K.B.; Landucci, E.; Pellegrini-Giampietro, D.E.; De Sarro, G.; et al. Novel 3-carboxy-and 3-phosphonopyrazoline amino acids as potent and selective NMDA receptor antagonists: Design, synthesis, and pharmacological characterization. *ChemMedChem* **2010**, *5*, 1465–1475. [CrossRef] [PubMed]

37. Landucci, E.; Lattanzi, R.; Gerace, E.; Scartabelli, T.; Balboni, G.; Negri, L.; Pellegrini-Giampietro, D.E. Prokineticins are neuroprotective in models of cerebral ischemia and ischemic tolerance in vitro. *Neuropharmacology* **2016**, *108*, 39–48. [CrossRef] [PubMed]

38. Chavan, S.S.; Ingle, S.G.; Vavia, P.R. Preparation and characterization of solid lipid nanoparticle-based nasal spray of budesonide. *Drug Deliv. Transl. Res.* **2013**, *3*, 402–408. [CrossRef] [PubMed]

39. Papadia, K.; Markoutsa, E.; Antimisiaris, S.G. How do the physicochemical properties of nanoliposomes affect their interactions with the hCMEC/D3 cellular model of the BBB? *Int. J. Pharm.* **2016**, *509*, 431–438. [CrossRef] [PubMed]

40. Markoutsa, E.; Pampalakis, G.; Niarakis, A.; Romero, I.A.; Weksler, B.; Couraud, P.-O.; Antimisiaris, S.G. Uptake and permeability studies of BBB-targeting immunoliposomes using the hCMEC/D3 cell line. *Eur. J. Pharm. Biopharm.* **2011**, *77*, 265–274. [CrossRef] [PubMed]

41. Mohan, A.; Narayanan, S.; Balasubramanian, G.; Sethuraman, S.; Krishnan, U.M. Dual drug loaded nanoliposomal chemotherapy: A promising strategy for treatment of head and neck squamous cell carcinoma. *Eur. J. Pharm. Biopharm.* **2016**, *99*, 73–83. [CrossRef] [PubMed]

42. Benfer, M.; Kissel, T. Cellular uptake mechanism and knockdown activity of siRNA-loaded biodegradable DEAPA-PVAg-PLGA nanoparticles. *Eur. J. Pharm. Biopharm.* **2012**, *80*, 247–256. [CrossRef] [PubMed]

43. Poller, B.; Gutmann, H.; Krähenbühl, S.; Weksler, B.; Romero, I.; Couraud, P.O.; Tuffin, G.; Drewe, J.; Huwyler, J. The human brain endothelial cell line hCMEC/D3 as a human blood-brain barrier model for drug transport studies. *J. Neurochem.* **2008**, *107*, 1358–1368. [CrossRef] [PubMed]

44. Rajendran, L.; Knolker, H.J.; Simons, K. Subcellular targeting strategies for drug design and delivery. *Nat. Rev. Drug Discov.* **2010**, *9*, 29–42. [CrossRef] [PubMed]

45. Lin, K.H.; Hong, S.-T.; Wang, H.-T.; Lo, Y.-L.; Lin, A.M.-Y.; Yang, J.C.-H. Enhancing Anticancer Effect of Gefitinib across the Blood–Brain Barrier Model Using Liposomes Modified with One α-Helical Cell-Penetrating Peptide or Glutathione and Tween 80. *Int. J. Mol. Sci.* **2016**, *17*, 1998. [CrossRef] [PubMed]

46. Takeuchi, H.; Makhlof, A.; Fujimoto, S.; Tozuka, Y. In vitro and in vivo evaluation of WGA-carbopol modified liposomes as carriers for oral peptide delivery. *Eur. J. Pharm. Biopharm.* **2011**, *77*, 216–224. [CrossRef]

47. Huth, U.S.; Schubert, R.; Peschka-Suss, R. Investigating the uptake and intracellular fate of pH-sensitive liposomes by flow cytometry and spectral bio-imaging. *J. Control. Release* **2006**, *110*, 490–504. [CrossRef] [PubMed]

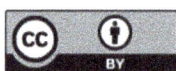

pharmaceutics

MDPI

Article

Development of Parvifloron D-Loaded Smart Nanoparticles to Target Pancreatic Cancer

Ana Santos-Rebelo [1,2], Catarina Garcia [1,2], Carla Eleutério [3], Ana Bastos [3,4],
Sílvia Castro Coelho [5], Manuel A. N. Coelho [5], Jesús Molpeceres [2], Ana S. Viana [6],
Lia Ascensão [7], João F. Pinto [3,4], Maria M. Gaspar [3,4], Patrícia Rijo [1,4] and
Catarina P. Reis [3,4,8,*]

[1] Centro de Investigação em Biociências e Tecnologias da Saúde (CBIOS),
   Universidade Lusófona de Humanidades e Tecnologias, Campo Grande 376, 1749-024 Lisboa, Portugal;
   ana.rebelo1490@gmail.com (A.S.-R.); catarina.g.garcia@gmail.com (C.G.); p1609@ulusofona.pt (P.R.)
[2] Department of Biomedical Sciences, Faculty of Pharmacy, University of Alcalá,
   Ctra. A2 km33,600 Campus Universitario, 28871 Alcalá de Henares, Spain; jesus.molpeceres@uah.es
[3] Faculdade de Farmácia, Universidade de Lisboa (FFUL), Av. Prof. Gama Pinto, 1649-003 Lisboa, Portugal;
   carlavania@ff.ul.pt (C.E.); anacarrerabastos@gmail.com (A.B.); jfpinto@ff.ulisboa.pt (J.F.P.);
   mgaspar@ff.ulisboa.pt (M.M.G.)
[4] iMed.ULisboa-Faculdade de Farmácia, Universidade de Lisboa, Av. Prof. Gama Pinto,
   1649-003 Lisboa, Portugal
[5] Laboratory for Process Engineering, Environment (LEPABE), Department of Chemical Engineering,
   Faculty of Engineering, University of Porto, 4200-135 Porto, Portugal; silviac@fe.up.pt (S.C.C.);
   mcoelho@fe.up.pt (M.A.N.C.)
[6] Centro de Química e Bioquímica (CQB), Centro de Química Estrutural (CQE), Faculdade de Ciências,
   Universidade de Lisboa, Campo Grande 1749-016 Lisboa, Portugal; apsemedo@fc.ul.pt
[7] Centre for Environmental and Marine Studies (CESAM), Faculdade de Ciências, Universidade de Lisboa,
   Campo Grande 1749-016 Lisboa, Portugal; lmpsousa@fc.ul.pt
[8] Institute of Biophysics and Biomedical Engineering (IBEB), Faculdade de Ciências, Universidade de Lisboa,
   1749-016 Lisboa, Portugal
* Correspondence: catarinareis@ff.ulisboa.pt; Tel.: +351-217-946-400, Fax: +351-217-946-470

Received: 21 September 2018; Accepted: 1 November 2018; Published: 4 November 2018

Abstract: Pancreatic cancer is the eighth leading cause of cancer death worldwide. For this reason, the development of more effective therapies is a major concern for the scientific community. Accordingly, plants belonging to *Plectranthus* genus and their isolated compounds, such as Parvifloron D, were found to have cytotoxic and antiproliferative activities. However, Parvifloron D is a very low water-soluble compound. Thus, nanotechnology can be a promising delivery system to enhance drug solubility and targeted delivery. The extraction of Parvifloron D from *P. ecklonii* was optimized through an acetone ultrasound-assisted method and isolated by Flash-Dry Column Chromatography. Then, its antiproliferative effect was selectivity evaluated against different cell lines (IC$_{50}$ of 0.15 ± 0.05 µM, 11.9 ± 0.7 µM, 21.6 ± 0.5, 34.3 ± 4.1 µM, 35.1 ± 2.2 µM and 32.1 ± 4.3 µM for BxPC3, PANC-1, Ins1-E, MCF-7, HaCat and Caco-2, respectively). To obtain an optimized stable Parvifloron D pharmaceutical dosage form, albumin nanoparticles were produced through a desolvation method (yield of encapsulation of 91.2%) and characterized in terms of size (165 nm; PI 0.11), zeta potential (−7.88 mV) and morphology. In conclusion, Parvifloron D can be efficiently obtained from *P. ecklonii* and it has shown selective cytotoxicity to pancreatic cell lines. Parvifloron D nanoencapsulation can be considered as a possible efficient alternative approach in the treatment of pancreatic cancer.

Keywords: *Plectranthus ecklonii*; Parvifloron D; cytotoxicity; pancreatic cancer; nanoparticles

1. Introduction

Pancreatic cancer is one of the most deadly oncologic disease and it is estimated that it will be the second most common cause of death due to cancer in the United States (USA) in 2030 [1].

This type of cancer is difficult to diagnose early, and currently, the treatment options available are very limited, being surgical resection the only potentially curative treatment. Nevertheless, surgery may be not possible in 80–90% of the cases, and long-term survival after surgical resection is very low [2–4].

Chemotherapy has demonstrated a positive impact on overall survival when prescribed after surgery with curative intent, and may reduce the risk of recurrence [5]. Gemcitabine and erlotinib are some examples of approved drugs in use and nab-paclitaxel has been approved in the USA and in Europe for metastasis [6]. However, chemotherapy with classical therapeutic agents has many side effects, such as nausea and vomiting, loss of appetite, hair loss, ulcers nozzles and higher chance of infection, as it promotes a shortage of white blood cells. In order to improve the long-term survival and improve the quality of life of patients with pancreatic cancer, it is imperative to find new therapeutic agents.

The use of medicinal plants and their constituents has proved their potential as clinical alternatives to synthetized drugs, leading to the discovery of new bioactive compounds [7]. These compounds have generated a strong interest in pharmacological research, towards the development of new anticancer agents. In fact, more than 50% of the compounds with different mechanisms of action used in chemotherapy are extracted from plant materials [4,6].

Many *Plectranthus* species are used as plants with medicinal interest against a variety of diseases, such as cancer. Abietane diterpenoids have been reported as the main constituents of some species in this *genus* and are responsible for its potential therapeutic value [8]. These naturally occurring compounds display a vast array of biological activities including cytotoxic and antiproliferative activities against human tumor cells [8,9]. Diterpenoids containing an abietane skeleton have proven to be strongly cytotoxic against human leukemia cells [10].

Burmistrova et al. confirmed that Parvifloron D (Figure 1) has strong cytotoxic properties against several human tumor cell lines [8]. Parvifloron D was isolated from *P. ecklonii* and thus, this plant can be associated as a good source of this abietane diterpenoid. In addition, it was also found that Parvifloron D anti-proliferative effect is generally associated with an increase in the intracellular level of Reactive Oxygen Species (ROS) that seems to play a crucial role in the apoptotic process of cells [11].

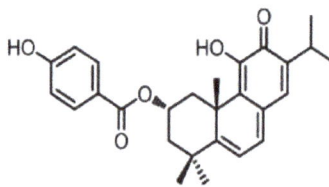

Figure 1. Molecular structure form Parvifloron D.

Nanotechnology has the potentiality of controlling and manipulating matter at the nanoscale by designing and engineering new systems [4]. Advances in nanoscience and nanotechnology can transform what has been done until today since new strategies will enhance and upgrade solutions to the formulation problems raised [12]. Besides improving solubility and stability of active compounds, nanoparticles may extend a formulation's action and successfully combine active substances with different degrees of hydrophilicity [12–14]. Its targeting abilities to deliver drugs directly to the affected organs and tissues are another advantage of these systems that can be used in medicine [12,15].

Nanocarriers can improve the efficiency of drugs by changing their body distribution, decreasing acute toxicity, increasing their dissolution rate and in vivo stability concerning the risk of earlier metabolism and degradation [12,14,16,17].

The present study focuses on the optimization of the extraction and isolation of Parvifloron D, given its cytotoxic potential. Therefore, new approaches to target pancreatic cancer cells will be performed to improve its selectivity. Moreover, the development of a novel diterpene-encapsulated nanosystem will be done in order to optimize the Parvifloron D stability.

2. Materials and Methods

2.1. Materials

Plant material *P. ecklonii* Benth was given by the Faculty of Pharmacy of the University of Lisbon and it was collected from seeds provided by the herbarium of the National Botanical Garden of Kirstenbosch, South Africa. Voucher specimens (S/No. LISC) have been deposited in the herbarium of the Tropical Research Institute in Lisbon [8]. Acetone, hexane and ethyl acetate were supplied by VWR Chemicals (VWR international S.A.S., Briare, France); Silica was obtained from Merck (grade 60, 230–400 mesh, Merck KGaA, Darmstadt, Germany); Bovine serum albumin was purchased to Sigma-Aldrich (Steinheim, Germany). Culture media and antibiotics were obtained from Invitrogen (Life Technologies Corporation, Carlsbad, CA, USA). All cell lines were obtained from the American Type Culture Collection (LGC Standards S.L.U. Barcelona, Spain). Reagents for cell proliferation assays were purchased from Promega (Madison, WI, USA). All reagents used for the nanoparticles preparation were of analytical grade and purified water obtained by a Millipore system (Millipore, Burlington, MA, USA).

2.2. Extraction and Isolation

2.2.1. Extraction

The whole plant-dried powdered *P. ecklonii* (197.55 g) was used to perform the Parvifloron D exhaustive extraction followed by thin-layer chromatography (TLC) (hexane: ethyl acetate, 7:3 (*v*/*v*)). The ultrasound-assisted extraction was performed using the acetone (10 × 600 mL) as the extraction solvent. The extract was obtained (28.54 g) by filtration and evaporation of acetone under vacuum (<40 °C) [9].

2.2.2. Isolation

Repeated Flash-Dry Column Chromatography of *P. ecklonii* extract (25 g), over silica gel (Merck 9385, 75 g), using n-hexane: ethyl acetate mixtures of increasing polarity, allowed the isolation of pure Parvifloron D (0.882 g) [18]. The chemical structure of Parvifloron D was elucidated comparing the ^{1}H-NMR spectroscopic data (Table S1: NMR data of PvD, (CDCl3, [1]H 400 MHz, [13]C 100 MHz; δ in ppm, J in Hz) and Table S2: Significant assignments observed on Heteronuclear Multiple Bond Correlation (HMBC) experiment for Parvifloron D) which was almost identical to those in the literature [9,19].

2.3. Parvifloron D Quantification by HPLC-DAD Analysis

The High-Performance Liquid Chromatography (HPLC) quantification of Parvifloron D from *P. ecklonii* extract was carried out as previously described [20]. It was used as a Liquid Chromatograph Agilent Technologies 1200 Infinity Series Liquid Chromatography (LC) System equipped with diode array detector (DAD), using a ChemStation Software (Agilent Technologies, Waldbronn, Germany) and a LiChrospher, 100 RP-18 (5 mm) column from Merck (Darmstadt, Germany). Parvifloron D was determined and quantified by injecting 20 μL of the sample at 1 mg/mL, using a gradient composed of Solution A (methanol), Solution B (acetonitrile) and Solution D (0.3% trichloroacetic acid in water) as follows: 0 min, 15% A, 5% B and 80% D; 20 min, 80% A, 10% B and 10% D; 25 min, 80% A, 10% B and 10% D. The flow rate was set at 1 mL/min. The authentic sample of Parvifloron D was run under the same conditions in methanol, and the detection was carried out between 200 and 600 nm with a diode array detector (DAD). All analyses were performed in triplicate.

2.4. Cell Culture and Cytotoxicity Assays

In order to evaluate Parvifloron D selectivity and antiproliferative effects against human tumor cells, different cell lines were tested: three pancreatic (BxPC3, PANC-1 and Ins1-E) and three non-pancreatic (MCF-7, HaCat and Caco-2) cell lines.

All cell lines tested, BxPC3 (human pancreas adenocarcinoma), PANC-1 (human pancreas adenocarcinoma), Ins1-E (rat pancreas insulinoma), MCF-7 (human breast cancer), HaCat (human keratinocyte) and Caco-2 (colon adenocarcinoma), are typically adherent cell cultures. Evaluations were made in different conditions regarding the different types of cells. Thus, BxPC3 cells were maintained in Roswell Park Memorial Institute (RPMI)-1640 medium with 10% heat-inactivated FBS; Ins1-E cells were maintained in RPMI medium supplemented with 10% fetal bovine serum, 100 IU/mL of penicillin, 100 µg/mL streptomycin and β-mercaptoethanol (50 µM) 1:1000; MCF-7, PANC-1 and HaCat cells were maintained in Dulbecco's Modified Eagle's medium (DMEM) with high-glucose (4500 mg/L), supplemented with 10% fetal bovine serum and 100 IU/mL of penicillin and 100 µg/mL streptomycin; and Caco-2 cells were maintained in RPMI medium supplemented with 10% fetal bovine serum and 100 IU/mL of penicillin and 100 µg/mL streptomycin all at 37 °C in a humidified atmosphere of 5% CO_2 incubator.

The effects of Parvifloron D on cell growth were evaluated by different assays, namely, for BxPC3 cells, the sulforhodamine B (SRB) assay (colorimetric) was used [21] and for Ins1-E, MCF-7, PANC-1, HaCat and Caco-2 cells the MTT test was used [10]. Briefly, cells were seeded in 96-well plates (using a cell concentration of 800 cells per well for BxPC3, 1×10^4 cell/mL per well for Ins1-E, MCF-7, PANC-1, HaCat and Caco-2) under normal conditions (5% CO_2 humidified atmosphere at 37 °C) and allowed to adhere for 24 h. The cells were then incubated with Parvifloron D at different concentrations: between 0.5 and 25.0 µM for BxPC3 and to Ins1-E, MCF-7, PANC-1, HaCat and Caco-2 between 10.0 and 60.0 µM. Following this incubation period, and once the cells were analyzed through different assays, they were processed under different conditions. BxPC3 cells were fixed with 10% trichloroacetic acid for 1 h on ice, and washed and stained with 50 µL 0.4% SRB dye for 30 min. The cells were then washed repeatedly with 1% acetic acid to remove unbound dye. After, the cells were dried, and the protein-bound stain was solubilized with 10 mM Tris solution.

The SRB absorbance was measured at 560 nm using the microplate reader Model 680 (Bio-Rad, Hercules, CA, USA). The concentration that inhibits cell survival in 50% (IC_{50}) was determined using the SRB assay. The absorbance of the wells containing the drug and the absorbance of the wells containing untreated cells, following a 24 h incubation period, were subsequently compared with that of the wells containing the cells that had been fixed at time zero (when Parvifloron D was added). Similarly, Ins1-E, MCF-7, PANC-1, HaCat and Caco-2 cells medium was removed, and the wells were washed with Phosphate-Buffered Saline (PBS). Then, 50 µL of a 10% MTT solution was added to the cells and the plates were incubated for 4 h. After the incubation time, 100 µL of DMSO were added to each well to solubilize the formazan crystals formed during the incubation period.

The absorbance of all samples was again measured at 570 nm using the microplate reader and IC_{50} was determined.

The cytotoxic effect was evaluated by determining the percentage of viable/death cells for each Parvifloron D studied concentration. Based on these values, the IC_{50} (Parvifloron D concentration that induces a 50% inhibition of cell growth) was calculated, according to an equation proposed by Hills and co-workers [22]. For IC_{50} determination, two concentrations, X_1 and X_2, and the respective cell densities, Y_1 and Y_2, that correspond to higher or lesser than half cell density in negative control (Y_0), were established, according to the following equation:

$$\text{Log } IC_{50} = \text{Log } X_1 + \{[(Y_1 - (Y_0)/2)]/(Y_1 - Y_2)\} \times (\text{Log } X_2 - \text{Log } X_1) \tag{1}$$

where, $Y_0/2$ is the half-cell density of the negative control; Y_1 is the cell density above $Y_0/2$; X_1 is the concentration corresponding to Y_1; Y_2 is the cell density below $Y_0/2$; X_2 is the concentration corresponding to Y_2; The IC_{50} was determined by linear interpolation between X_1 and X_2.

2.5. Parvifloron D Solubility Assays

Parvifloron D solubility in PBS (pH 7.4, European Pharmacopoeia 7.0) was determined at two different temperatures, 25 °C and 37 °C, by measuring the amount of compound dissolved in a saturated solution (~30 µg/mL) after 24 h, with constant stirring (200 rpm). Three independent measurements at each condition were conducted (n = 3) [23].

2.6. Parvifloron D Encapsulation into a Biocompatible and Hydrophilic Nanomaterial

In previous studies, Parvifloron D has showed low water-solubility, probably due to its long carbon chains and the presence of aromatic rings, giving Parvifloron D lipophilic characteristics [24,25], along with an apparent lack of selectivity to cancer cells [23]. Therefore, the encapsulation of Parvifloron D into a biocompatible and hydrophilic nanomaterial as a drug delivery system had the main objective of the achievement of optimized bioavailability and stability of the drug and thus, optimal drug loading and release properties, a long shelf life and higher therapeutic efficacy, with lower side effects [26].

Albumin was chosen as the encapsulating material to Parvifloron D due to its biocompatibility and affinity to the liver. The technology used to produce nanoparticles was the desolvation method, suitable to a wide range of polymers, especially heat-sensitives ones such as albumin, being the main advantage that it does not require an increase in temperature [27,28]. Briefly, bovine serum albumin was dissolved in purified distilled water with the pH adjusted to 8.2 with NaOH 0.1 M. Subsequently, Parvifloron D was dissolved in acetone and added to the albumin solution, which was added dropwise into a solution of absolute ethanol under magnetic stirring (500 rpm). After stirring, an opalescent suspension was spontaneously formed at room temperature. After this desolvation process, glucose in water (1.8%, v/v) was added to cross-link the desolvated albumin nanoparticles. The cross-linking process was performed under stirring of the colloidal suspension over a time period of 30 min. Measurement of pH was conducted with a pH electrode meter (827 pH lab Metrohm) calibrated daily with buffer solutions pH 4.00 ± 0.02 and 7.00 ± 0.02 (25 °C).

2.7. Determination of the Parvifloron D Encapsulation Efficiency by HPLC Analysis

Parvifloron D encapsulation efficiency (EE%) was determined using a reverse-phase HPLC chromatographic method (stationary phase—LiChrospher RP 18 (5 µm), Lichrocart 250–4.6) for the drug quantification at a detection wavelength of 254 nm. Briefly, a HPLC (Hitachi system LaCrom Elite, Column oven, Diode Array Detector (UV-Vis) (Hitachi High Technologies America, San Jose, CA, USA)) was used with a mobile phase comprising methanol and trichloroacetic acid 0.1% (80:20, v/v) (flow rate of 1.0 mL/min). Column conditions were maintained at 30 °C, with an injection volume of 20 µL and a run-time of 15 min. Measurements were carried out in duplicate and according to the described formula:

$$EE\ (\%) = (\text{Amount of encapsulated drug/Initial drug amount}) \times 100\% \tag{2}$$

2.8. In Vitro Release Studies

After determining Parvifloron D solubility, to maintain sink conditions during the in vitro release studies, empty nanoparticles and Parvifloron D-loaded nanoparticles were freeze-dried (24 h at −50 ± 2 °C, Freezone 2.5 L Benchtop Freeze Dry System, Labconco, MO, USA) and weighted according to the drug solubility. As an approximation to the blood pH, each sample of weighted nanoparticles was placed in a glass recipient, containing 250 mL of PBS (pH 7.4, European Pharmacopoeia 7.0), under constant stirring (200 rpm), in order to simulate the in vivo conditions [23]. At appropriate time intervals, aliquots of the release medium were collected from three different points of the dissolution medium, in order to obtain a homogenous collection of the sample. Nanoparticles were isolated from the supernatant by centrifugation (20,000 rpm for 15 min). The Parvifloron D amount collected from the in vitro release medium, at each time point, was determined by HPLC (see Section 2.7). The assay was conducted for 72 h, to assure that all Parvifloron D was released. ($n = 3$, mean $\pm$ SD).

2.9. Physical and Morphological Characterization of the Nanoparticles: Dynamic Light Scattering (DLS), Scanning Electron Microscopy (SEM) and Atomic Force Microscopy (AFM)

Freshly prepared empty nanoparticles and Parvifloron D-loaded nanoparticles were studied in terms of their structure, surface morphology, shape and size by DLS, SEM and AFM.

Physical characterization of the nanoparticles was carried out by evaluation of mean particle size, polydispersity index (PI) and zeta potential by DLS and electrophoretic mobility (Coulter nano-sizer Delsa Nano™ (Beckman Coulter, Brea, CA, USA)) of the nanoparticles' concentrated suspension ($n = 3$).

For SEM, the aqueous suspensions containing empty and loaded nanoparticles were fixed with 2.5% glutaraldehyde in 0.1 M sodium phosphate buffer at pH 7.2 (European Pharmacopoeia 7.0) during 1 h. After centrifugation, the pellets were washed three times in the fixative buffer. Then, aliquots (10 µL) of the two samples suspensions were scattered over a round glass coverslip previously coated with poly-L-lysine and left to dry in a desiccator. Subsequently, the material was coated with a thin layer of gold and observed on a JEOL 5200LV scanning electron microscope (JEOL Ltd., Tokyo, Japan) at an accelerating voltage of 20 kV. Images were recorded digitally.

AFM images were acquired on an atomic force microscope, Multimode 8 coupled to Nanoscope V Controller, from Bruker, UK, by using peak force tapping and ScanAssist mode. In order to offer a clean and flat surface for AFM analysis, an aliquot of each sample (~30 µL) was mounted on a freshly cleaved mica sheet and left to dry before being analyzed. The images were obtained in ambient conditions, at a sweep rate close to 1 Hz, using scanasyst-air 0.4 N/m tips, from Bruker.

2.10. Physicochemical Characterization of Nanoparticles Interaction Analysis by Fourier Transform Infrared (FT-IR)

To study the possible interactions between Parvifloron D and bovine serum albumin polymer of the developed nanoparticles, FT-IR spectroscopy was conducted on freeze-dried nanoparticles samples and on each isolated compound, using potassium bromide (KBr). The FT-IR spectra was recorded by using a Nicolet FT-IR Spectrometer (Thermo Electron Corporation, Beverly, MA, USA) from 4000 to 400 cm^{-1}, at a scanning speed of cm^{-1} for 256 scans by placing the KBr pellet on the attenuated total reflection objective. The final data is reported as a data average of 256 scans. The pellet was prepared in a ratio of 1:10 (w/w) of KBr to sample (nanoparticles or other component) and left to dry in a desiccator for 24 h before the analysis. The following samples were compared: empty nanoparticles (i.e., without Parvifloron D), Parvifloron D-loaded nanoparticles, physical mixture of Parvifloron D and bovine serum albumin (1:1, w/w), the polymer (bovine serum albumin), the cross-linking agent (glucose) and the drug (Parvifloron D).

2.11. Differential Scanning Calorimetry

In an attempt to check the purity of the drug and to confirm possible physicochemical interactions between nanoparticles and their raw components, thermal transformations and phase transitions of the nanoparticles were studied by calorimetry (Diferential Scanning Calorimetry, Q200, TA Instruments, New Castle, DE, USA) under a nitrogen gas flow of 50 mL/min (AirLiquide, Algés, Portugal). Samples (1–5 mg) were analyzed in hermetic aluminum pans at a heating rate of 10 °C /min from 40 to 400 °C. The endothermic and exothermic events were analyzed using TA-Universal Analysis software (Universal Analysis 2000 version 4.7A, TA Instruments, New Castle, DE, USA).

3. Results and Discussion

3.1. Extraction and Isolation

The diterpenoid Parvifloron D was isolated from a *P. ecklonii* extract in a total amount of 166.1 µg/mg, quantified by HPLC. This extraction yield of Parvifloron D with acetone was optimized when compared with Burmistrova et al. extraction (136.75 µg/mg) [8]. Here, the ultrasound-assisted extraction showed a higher extraction yield when compared with the previous described maceration method. The optimized isolation of Parvifloron D (882 mg, 0.45% on the dry plant) showed to be a successful isolation process which presented a higher yield of Parvifloron D in comparison with M Simões et al. results (0.27% on the dry plant) [9].

The isolated compound peak was verified by HPLC, as Figure 2 shows.

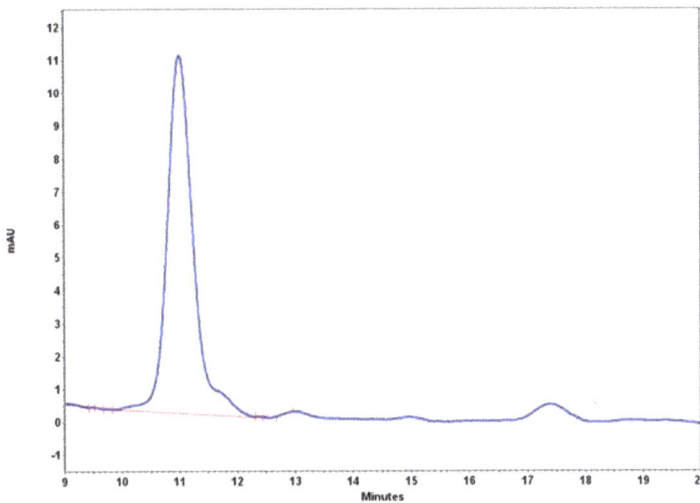

Figure 2. Isolated Parvifloron D spectra by High-Performance Liquid Chromatography (HPLC) analysis.

3.2. Parvifloron D Quantification by HPLC-DAD

The phytochemical analysis of *P. ecklonii* extract was performed by HPLC-DAD as represented in Figure 3. The presence of Parvifloron D was revealed (Retention Time (RT) = 27.63 min) as the principal constituent was obtained and its absorption spectra was performed, as previously described [29].

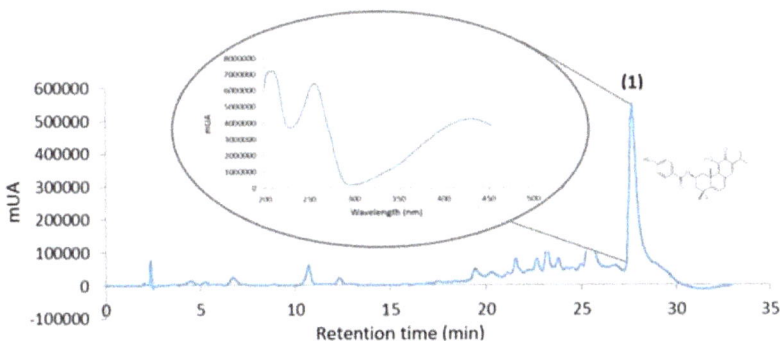

Figure 3. HPLC profile of *P. ecklonii* extract (254 nm): (1) Parvifloron D peak and absorption spectra.

3.3. Cell culture and Cytotoxicity Assays

To study the cytotoxicity of free Parvifloron D, SRB and MTT assays were conducted. The results have shown that free Parvifloron D was more cytotoxic to pancreatic cell lines (BxPC3, PANC-1 and Ins1-E) than to non-pancreatic cell lines (MCF-7, Caco-2 and HaCat), displaying more selectivity to our target tumor cells than to others. Parvifloron D presented the lowest value of IC_{50} of 0.15 ± 0.05 µM for BxPC3 (human pancreatic tumor cells), and a high value of 32.1 ± 4.3 µM for Caco-2 cells (colon adenocarcinoma) according Table 1. Even in tumor cells, Parvifloron D had a higher selectivity to human tumor pancreatic cells. Cell viability in different time points, 24 h and 48 h, for Ins1-E, MCF7 and Caco-2 cells were measured and the results were added to supplementary material (Table S3—IC_{50} (µM) values in different time points, 24 h and 48 h, of different cell lines–cytotoxicity assays).

Table 1. IC_{50} ($\pm$ Standard deviation (SD)) values of different cell lines—cytotoxicity assays.

Cell line	IC_{50} (µM) $\pm$ SD
MCF-7 (breast cancer)	35.1 ± 2.2
HaCat (human keratinocyte)	34.3 ± 4.1
Caco-2 (Colon adenocarcinoma)	32.1 ± 4.3
INS-1E (rat pancreatic insulinoma)	21.6 ± 0.5
BxPC3 (human pancreatic adenocarcinoma)	0.15 ± 0.1
PANC-1 (human pancreatic adenocarcinoma)	11.9 ± 0.7

Considering some previously published results such as X. Yu et al. (IC_{50} = 0.2 µM to gemcitabine in BxPC3 cell line) [30], A. Singh et al. (IC_{50} = 123.9 µM to gemcitabine in PANC-1 cell line) [31], A. Acuna et al. (IC_{50} = 46.5 µM to PH-427 in BxPC3 cell line) [32], S. Mukai et al. (IC_{50} = 19.5 µM and 20.4 µM to gefitinib in BxPC3 and PANC-1 cell lines, respectively) [33], L. Wang et al. (IC_{50} = 39.86 µM and 83.76 µM to Pemetrexed in BxPC3 and PANC-1 cell lines, respectively) [34] or even A. Wright et al. (IC_{50} = 70.9 µM and 22.8 µM to Aphrocallistin in BxPC3 and PANC-1 cell lines, respectively) [35], we can suggest that Parvifloron D has a higher cytotoxic potential (IC_{50} = 0.15 ± 0.05) to these pancreatic tumor cells.

Despite these results and concerning the Parvifloron D mechanism of action, our group work is studding Parvifloron D-induced cell death and they have observed that Parvifloron D induces an increase in Sub-G1 and a reduction of G2/M populations in MDA-MB-231 (human breast tumor cells), as Burmistrova et al. already described in leukemia HL-60 and U-937 cells [8]. These results lead us to believe that Parvifloron D-induced cell death can be through this mechanism independently of the cell line tested. Although, this data is still in progress, and thus it has not been published yet. Nevertheless, our group has tested the internalization of polymeric nanoparticles with Parvifloron D, observing that it had occurred by endocytosis within 2 h [23]. Moreover, according to the literature, seven membrane-associated albumin-binding proteins have been discovered, namely: albondin/glycoprotein60 (gp60), glycoprotein18 (gp18), glycoprotein30 (gp30), the neonatal Fcreceptor (FcRn), heterogeneous nuclear ribonucleoproteins (hnRNPs), calreticulin, cubilin, and megalin [36]. This leads us to believe that our nanoparticles may internalize via endocytosis [37]. This assumption must be confirmed with future experiments of nanoparticles co-localization and nanoparticles cellular quantification.

3.4. Nanoparticles Encapsulation Efficiency by HPLC Analysis

In order to determine Parvifloron D encapsulation efficiency, a calibration curve was made using previously isolated Parvifloron D as a calibration standard. Parvifloron D standards ranging from 3 to 75 µg/mL were evaluated and a calibration curve (y = 7589.9x − 12798) was obtained with $R^2 = 0.999$. Limit of Detection (LOD) and Limit of Quantification (LOQ) were calculated to be 2.6 µg/mL and 7.9 µg/mL, respectively.

Encapsulation efficiency (%) was determined by measuring the non-encapsulated drug. Non-encapsulated drug was measured (8.79 µg/mL) (i.e., indirect quantification) and the value obtained was subtracted from the amount of drug initially added, being the encapsulation efficiency value for Parvifloron D 91.2 ± 5.51% (mean value ± SD, $n = 3$).

3.5. Parvifloron D Solubility Assays and In Vitro Release Studies

HPLC studies were carried out to determine the solubility of Parvifloron D in PBS (pH 7.4) before performing in vitro release studies of Parvifloron D after entrapment into the albumin nanoparticles.

After 24h incubation in PBS pH 7.4, at two different temperatures, 25 °C and 37 °C, Parvifloron D solubility was 3.7 ± 0.8 µg/mL and 4.9 ± 0.3 µg/mL, respectively ($n = 3$).

Concerning the in vitro release studies, all entrapped Parvifloron D was released from albumin nanoparticles in 72 h in PBS at pH 7.4. As illustrated in Figure 4, after 24 h, approximately 40% of Parvifloron D was released from the nanoparticles and no burst release was observed. Besides, Parvifloron D degradation was evaluated as the in vitro release studies went by. The release profile was continually sustained over the assay and all of the drug was been released in less than 72 h.

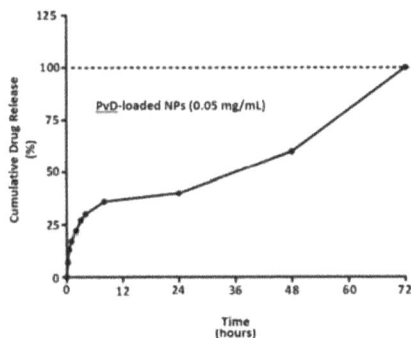

Figure 4. In vitro drug release of Parvifloron D-loaded nanoparticles at 0.05 mg/mL, for 72 h, in phosphate buffered saline (PBS) pH 7.4 solution. Results are expressed as mean of measurements of three independent nanoparticles lots ± Standard Deviation (SD) ($n = 3$).

3.6. Physical and Morphological Characterization of the Nanoparticles: DLS, AFM, SEM

In terms of mean size value, Parvifloron D-loaded nanoparticles were smaller than empty nanoparticles (165 nm (PI 0.11) and 250 nm (PI 0.37), respectively). This fact is probably due to electrostatic interactions, which may reduce and compact the particle structure. It should also be noted that there was a color change of nanoparticles from white to orange, when Parvifloron D was entrapped inside the particles. The pH value was around 8.5 in both formulations. Zeta potential was negative in both cases (−19.65 and −7.88 mV to empty nanoparticles and Parvifloron D-loaded nanoparticles, respectively) and the difference might be attributed to the presence of Parvifloron D, suggesting some interaction between the albumin and the drug, which can be related to the intrinsic charge of Parvifloron D (pKa values of 8.9, 9.9, calculated values by ChemDraw Professional).

AFM analysis has confirmed particles size. Figure 5 shows that the particle size of the prepared nanoparticles was approximately 210 nm and 190 nm for empty and Parvifloron D-loaded nanoparticles, respectively, as measured by DLS. AFM can offer a significant contribution to understand surface and interface properties, thus allowing for the optimization of biomaterials performance, processes, and physical and chemical properties even at the nanoscale [38]. In addition, we can notice that particles, especially the empty nanoparticles, were monodispersed. Figure 6 shows the 3D images highlighting the shape and morphology of the prepared nanoparticles.

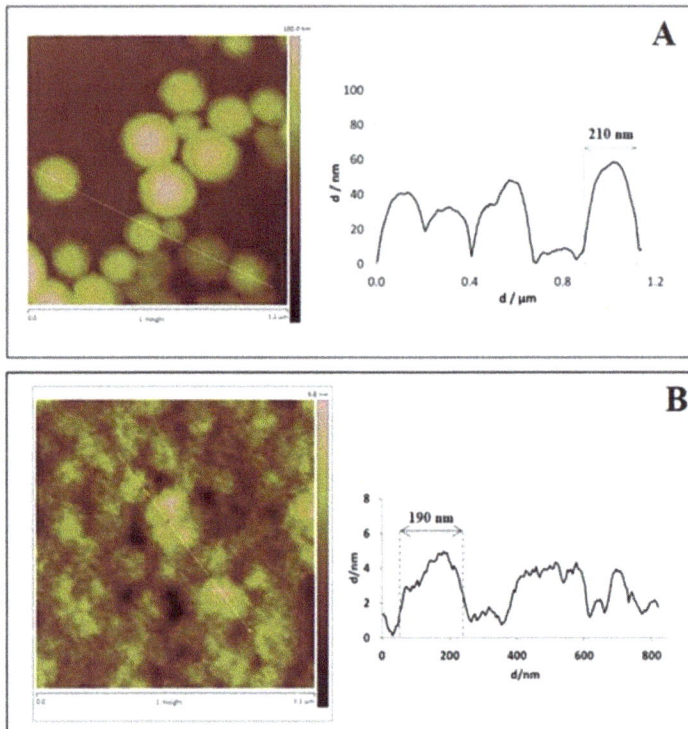

Figure 5. Atomic Force Microscopy (AFM) sectorial analysis of: (**A**) Albumin empty nanoparticles and (**B**) Parvifloron D-loaded nanoparticles. Particle sizes of 210 nm and 190 nm are also represented, for A and B, respectively.

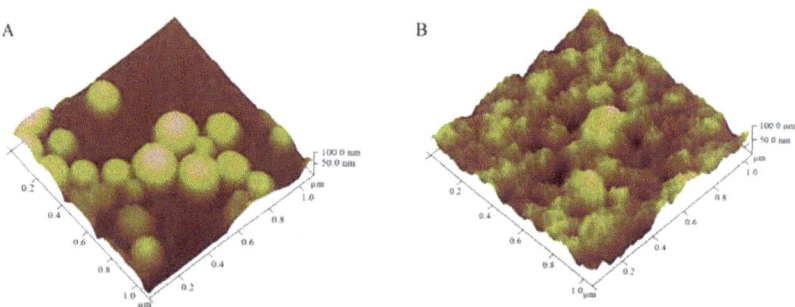

Figure 6. Atomic Force Microscopy (AFM) analysis 3D images of: (**A**) Albumin empty nanoparticles and (**B**) Parvifloron D-loaded nanoparticles.

In the current study, SEM observations showed that nanoparticles in both formulations had a uniform distribution and exhibited a spherical shape with a smooth surface. It is also clearly seen that the particles size is different, the empty nanoparticles being slightly larger than the Parvifloron D-loaded nanoparticles (Figure 7). Here, SEM provides information on surface topography, size, and size distribution of nanoparticles [39].

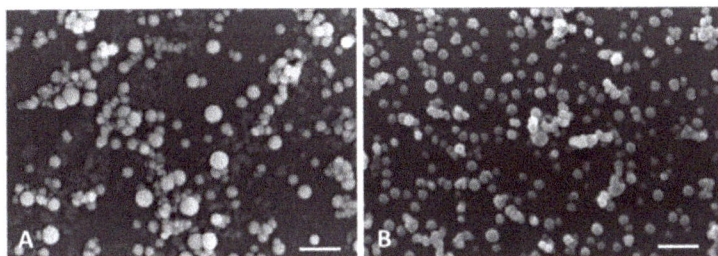

Figure 7. Scanning Electron Microscopy (SEM) micrographs of: (**A**) Albumin empty nanoparticles (scale bar: 1 μm) and (**B**) Parvifloron D-loaded nanoparticles (scale bar: 1 μm).

3.7. Physicochemical Characterization of Nanoparticles Interaction Analysis by FT-IR

FT-IR spectra main peaks and the corresponding functional groups were identified for all tested samples. For physical mixtures and nanoparticles, the peaks were identified based on the functional groups of the raw components (wavenumbers: 4000–400 cm^{-1}), as it is shown in Table 2. This analysis has demonstrated to be a useful method to interpret intra- and inter-material interactions in raw materials and their combination to obtain nanoparticles.

After the analysis of the spectra, it was confirmed the bovine serum albumin structure by the presence of specific bands for amides (I and II). Also, Parvifloron D analysis showed its specific bands, confirming its structure previously done by NMR (supplementary material). When albumin empty nanoparticles were analyzed, the same specific bands were identified in the raw bovine serum albumin spectra, although the N–H amide II band has shifted, suggesting some structure modification of bovine serum albumin chains when aggregated to provide nanoparticles. In addition, a new band at 3000 cm^{-1} appears in empty nanoparticles, probably due to the cross-linking with glucose. As for the interactions between drug and nanoparticles, it was possible to differentiate the spectra of albumin nanoparticles loaded with Parvifloron D and the physical mixture of bovine serum albumin and free Parvifloron D (at 1:1, w/w). This fact can indicate that the drug was successfully entrapped inside the nanoparticles, and observing the distinct peaks in the nanostructures analysis, some kind of drug–albumin interaction during nanoparticles formation might have occurred.

3.8. Differential Scanning Calorimetry

Differential scanning calorimetry was used to characterize the different properties of the developed nanosystems, such as Parvifloron D polymorphism, interactions between drug and nanoparticles and the effect on their thermal events, compared to raw materials. Figure 8 shows an exothermic peak near to 170 °C, indicating a crystallization and an endothermic peak close to 300 °C, which can represent a crystal melting, suggesting that Parvifloron D is a polymorphic drug. Anyway, to better understand the thermal behavior of Parvifloron D, more crystallographic studies have to be conducted in the future. Bovine serum albumin endothermic peaks were observed around 215 °C while exothermic peaks appeared around 310 °C. Analyzing albumin at nanoparticles form, its spectra changed, showing a lower melting point, once the endothermic peak appeared near to 190 °C, suggesting some structure modification of albumin chains to organize nanoparticles arrangement. For albumin nanoparticles loaded with Parvifloron D, the spectra show two endothermic peaks which probably represents both bovine serum albumin and Parvifloron D melting points, but due to some rearrangement between these raw materials into nanoparticles, these endothermic events had occurred at lower temperatures (136 °C and 219 °C).

Table 2. FT-IR analysis of spectra of all tested samples (cm^{-1}).

Functional Groups Compound	O-H Carboxylic Acid (Stretching)	C-H Alkane (Stretching)	C=O Carbonyl (Stretching)	C=O Amide I (Stretching)	N-H Amide II (Bending)	C=C Aromatic (Stretching)	C-H Alkane (Bending)	C-O Alcohol (Stretching)	=C-H Alkene (Bending)
BSA [1]	—	—	—	1654	1590	—	—	—	—
PvD [2]	—	2871	1693	—	—	1510	—	—	850
Glucose	3350	—	—	—	—	—	1456	1032	—
Physical mixture BSA + PvD	—	2871	1690	1658	1590	1515	—	—	—
Empty BSA-NPs [3]	3000	—	—	1654	1540	—	—	—	—
BSA-NPs loaded With PvD	3000	2873	—	1654	1540	1540	—	—	910

[1] BSA: Bovine serum albumin; [2] PvD: Parvifloron D; [3] NPs: nanoparticles.

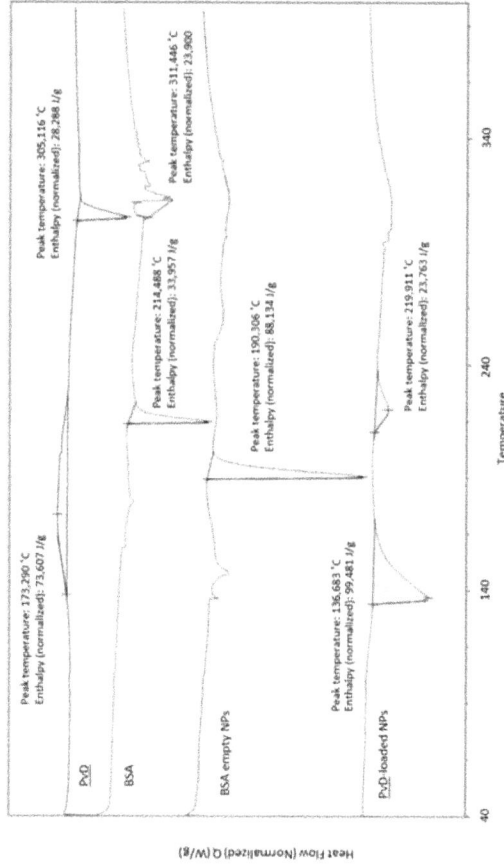

Figure 8. Differential Scanning Calorimetry (DSC) thermal transformations in free Parvifloron D, bovine serum albumin polymer, albumin empty nanoparticles and Parvifloron D-loaded nanoparticles, respectively. The major peak temperatures (°C) and the difference in Gibbs energy (J/g), for each sample, are also represented.

4. Conclusions

Parvifloron D has been efficiently extracted and isolated from *P. ecklonii*. Cell cultures have shown that Parvifloron D may have more selectivity to human pancreatic tumor cells than healthy cells or breast cancer cells. Parvifloron D-loaded small and spherical nanoparticles (water soluble particles) have been formulated with high encapsulation efficiency. Those nanoparticles led to a controlled release of the drug encapsulation over 72 h. Parvifloron D nanoparticles were stable, and therefore, they can be considered a suitable and promising carrier to deliver the drug to the tumor site, improving the treatment of pancreatic cancer.

Supplementary Materials: The following are available online at http://www.mdpi.com/1999-4923/10/4/216/s1, Table S1: NMR data of PvD, (CDCl$_3$, ^{1}H 400 MHz, ^{13}C 100 MHz; δ in ppm, J in Hz); Table S2: Significant assignments observed on HMBC experiment for PvD and Table S3: IC$_{50}$ (μM) values in different time points, 24 h and 48 h, of different cell lines—cytotoxicity assays.

Author Contributions: Conceptualization: A.S.-R. and C.P.R.; methodology and formal analysis: A.S.-R., C.G., C.E., A.B., S.C.C., M.A.N.C., J.M., A.S.V., L.A., J.F.P., M.M.G., P.R. and C.P.R.; investigation: A.S.-R.; writing—original draft preparation, A.S.-R.; writing, review and editing: C.P.R., J.M., J.F.P., A.S.V., M.M.G. and L.A.; supervision, C.P.R., P.R. and J.M.; project administration: A.S.-R. and C.P.R.; funding acquisition: ULHT/CBIOS and UAH.

Funding: In this research, phytochemical section was funded by Fundação para a Ciência e Tecnologia (FCT) under the reference UID/DTP/04567/2016 and SEM analysis was funded by Fundação para a Ciência e Tecnologia (FCT) with financial support to CESAM (UID/AMB/50017), through FCT/MEC National funds, and the co-funding by the FEDER, within the PT2020 Partnership Agreement and Compete 2020.

Acknowledgments: The authors would like to thank to P. Fonte for kindly donating the Ins1-E cell line used in this paper, and to A. S. Fernandes and N. Saraiva (CBIOS/ULHT) for sharing their unpublished results, allowing us to better discuss the mechanism of action of Parvifloron D. The authors would also like to thank to M. Minas da Piedade and C. Bernardes for their help in FT-IR analysis.

Conflicts of Interest: The authors declare no conflict of interest.

References

1. Rahib, L.; Smith, B.D.; Aizenberg, R.; Rosenzweig, A.B.; Fleshman, J.M.; Matrisian, L.M. Projecting cancer incidence and deaths to 2030: The unexpected burden of thyroid, liver, and pancreas cancers in the united states. *Cancer Res.* **2014**, *74*, 2913–2921. [CrossRef] [PubMed]

2. Niess, H.; Kleespies, A.; Andrassy, J.; Pratschke, S.; Angele, M.K.; Guba, M.; Jauch, K.-W.; Bruns, C.J. Pancreatic cancer in the elderly: Guidelines and individualized therapy. *Der Chir.* **2013**, *84*, 291–295. [CrossRef]

3. Oberstein, P.E.; Olive, K.P. Pancreatic cancer: Why is it so hard to treat? *Ther. Adv. Gastroenterol.* **2013**, *6*, 321–337. [CrossRef] [PubMed]

4. Rebelo, A.; Molpeceres, J.; Rijo, P.; Reis, C.P. Pancreatic Cancer Therapy Review: From Classic Therapeutic Agents to Modern Nanotechnologies. *Curr. Drug Metab.* **2017**, *18*, 346–359. [CrossRef] [PubMed]

5. Neoptolemos, J.P.; Stocken, D.D.; Friess, H.; Bassi, C.; Dunn, J.A.; Hickey, H.; Beger, H.; Fernandez-Cruz, L.; Dervenis, C.; Lacaine, F.; et al. A Randomized Trial of Chemoradiotherapy and Chemotherapy after Resection of Pancreatic Cancer. *N. Engl. J. Med.* **2004**, *350*, 1200–1210. [CrossRef] [PubMed]

6. Gourav, L.; Deepak-K., S.; Pawan-K., S.; Chand, M.P. Anticancer, antimicrobial and antifertility activities of some medicinal plants: A review. *Med. Drug Res.* **2015**, *3*, 7–11.

7. Nicolai, M.; Pereira, P.; Vitor, R.F.; Pinto, C.; Roberto, A.; Rijo, P. Antioxidant activity and rosmarinic acid content of ultrasound-assisted ethanolic extracts of medicinal plants. *Measurement* **2016**, *89*, 328–332. [CrossRef]

8. Burmistrova, O.; Perdomo, J.; Simões, M.F.; Rijo, P.; Quintana, J.; Estévez, F. The abietane diterpenoid parvifloron D from *Plectranthus ecklonii* is a potent apoptotic inducer in human leukemia cells. *Phytomedicine* **2015**, *22*, 1009–1016. [CrossRef] [PubMed]

9. Simões, M.F.; Rijo, P.; Duarte, A.; Matias, D.; Rodríguez, B. An easy and stereoselective rearrangement of an abietane diterpenoid into a bioactive microstegiol derivative. *Phytochem. Lett.* **2010**, *3*, 234–237. [CrossRef]

10. Burmistrova, O.; Simões, M.F.; Rijo, P.; Quintana, J.; Bermejo, J.; Estévez, F. Antiproliferative activity of abietane diterpenoids against human tumor cells. *J. Nat. Prod.* **2013**, *76*, 1413–1423. [CrossRef] [PubMed]

11. Rosa, S.; Correia, V.; Ribeiro, I.; Rijo, P.; Saraiva, N.; Fernandes, A. In vitro antioxidant properties of the diterpenes Parvifloron D and 7α-acetoxy-6β-hydroxyroyleanone. *Biomed. Biopharm. Res.* **2015**, *12*, 59–67. [CrossRef]

12. Bonifácio, B.V.; Silva, P.B.; Aparecido dos Santos Ramos, M.; Maria Silveira Negri, K.; Maria Bauab, T.; Chorilli, M. Nanotechnology-based drug delivery systems and herbal medicines: A review. *Int. J. Nanomed.* **2014**, *9*, 1–15. [CrossRef]

13. Reis, C.P.; Figueiredo, I.V.; Carvalho, R.A.; Jones, J.; Nunes, P.; Soares, A.F.; Silva, C.F.; Ribeiro, A.J.; Veiga, F.J.; Damgé, C.; et al. Toxicological assessment of orally delivered nanoparticulate insulin. *Nanotoxicology* **2008**, *2*, 205–217. [CrossRef]

14. Kouchakzadeh, H.; Shojaosadati, S.A.; Maghsoudi, A.; Farahani, E.V. Optimization of PEGylation Conditions for BSA Nanoparticles Using Response Surface Methodology. *AAPS PharmSciTech* **2010**, *11*, 1206–1211. [CrossRef] [PubMed]

15. Abrantes, G.; Duarte, D.; Reis, C.P. An Overview of Pharmaceutical Excipients: Safe or Not Safe? *J. Pharm. Sci.* **2016**, *105*, 2019–2026. [CrossRef] [PubMed]

16. Reis, C.P.; Damgé, C. Nanotechnology as a promising strategy for alternative routes of insulin delivery. *Methods Enzymol.* **2012**, *508*, 271–294. [CrossRef] [PubMed]

17. Pinto Reis, C.; Silva, C.; Martinho, N.; Rosado, C. Drug carriers for oral delivery of peptides and proteins: Accomplishments and future perspectives. *Ther. Deliv.* **2013**, *4*, 251–265. [CrossRef] [PubMed]

18. Harwood, L. "Dry-Column" Flash Chromatography. *Aldrichim. Acta* **1985**, *18*, 25.

19. Gaspar-Marques, C.; Simões, M.F.; Valdeira, M.L.; Rodríguez, B. Terpenoids and phenolics from *Plectranthus strigosus*, bioactivity screening. *Nat. Prod. Res.* **2008**, *22*, 167–177. [CrossRef] [PubMed]

20. Rijo, P.; Falé, P.L.; Serralheiro, M.L.; Simões, M.F.; Gomes, A.; Reis, C. Optimization of medicinal plant extraction methods and their encapsulation through extrusion technology. *Measurement* **2014**, *58*, 249–255. [CrossRef]

21. Coelho, S.C.; Almeida, G.M.; Santos-Silva, F.; Pereira, M.C.; Coelho, M.A.N. Enhancing the efficiency of bortezomib conjugated to pegylated gold nanoparticles: An in vitro study on human pancreatic cancer cells and adenocarcinoma human lung alveolar basal epithelial cells. *Expert Opin. Drug Deliv.* **2016**, *13*, 1075–1081. [CrossRef] [PubMed]

22. Hills, M.; Hudson, C.; Smith, P.G. Global monitoring of the resistance of malarial parasites to drugs: Statistical treatment of micro-test data. In *Working Paper No. 2.8. 5 for the Informal Consultation on the Epidemiology of Drug Resistance of Malaria Parasites*; World Health Organisation: Geneva, Switzerland, 1986.

23. Silva, C.O.; Molpeceres, J.; Batanero, B.; Fernandes, A.S.; Saraiva, N.; Costa, J.G.; Rijo, P.; Figueiredo, I.V.; Faísca, P.; Reis, C.P. Functionalized diterpene parvifloron D-loaded hybrid nanoparticles for targeted delivery in melanoma therapy. *Ther. Deliv.* **2016**, *7*, 521–544. [CrossRef] [PubMed]

24. Smith, R.; Tanford, C. Hydrophobicity of Long Chain n-Alkyl Carboxylic Acids, as Measured by Their Distribution Between Heptane and Aqueous Solutions. *Proc. Natl. Acad. Sci. USA* **1973**, *70*, 289–293. [CrossRef] [PubMed]

25. Silva, P.J. Inductive and resonance effects on the acidities of phenol, enols, and carbonyl α-hydrogens. *J. Org. Chem.* **2009**, *74*, 914–916. [CrossRef] [PubMed]

26. Bilia, A.R.; Piazzini, V.; Guccione, C.; Risaliti, L.; Asprea, M.; Capecchi, G.; Bergonzi, M.C. Improving on Nature: The Role of Nanomedicine in the Development of Clinical Natural Drugs. *Planta Med.* **2017**, *83*, 366–381. [CrossRef] [PubMed]

27. Pinto Reis, C.; Neufeld, R.J.; Ribeiro, A.J.; Veiga, F. Nanoencapsulation I. Methods for preparation of drug-loaded polymeric nanoparticles. *Nanomed. Nanotechnol. Biol. Med.* **2006**, *2*, 8–21. [CrossRef] [PubMed]

28. Weber, C.; Coester, C.; Kreuter, J.; Langer, K. Desolvation process and surface characterisation of protein nanoparticles. *Int. J. Pharm.* **2000**, *194*, 91–102. [CrossRef]

29. Figueiredo, N.L.; Falé, P.L.; Madeira, P.J.A.; Florêncio, M.H.; Ascensão, L.; Serralheiro, M.L.M.; Lino, A.R.L. Phytochemical Analysis of Plectranthus sp. Extracts and Application in Inhibition of Dental Bacteria, Streptococcus sobrinus and Streptococcus mutans. *Eur. J. Med. Plants* **2014**, *4*, 794–809. [CrossRef]

30. Yu, X.; Di, Y.; Xie, C.; Song, Y.; He, H.; Li, H.; Pu, X.; Lu, W.; Fu, D.; Jin, C. An in vitro and in vivo study of gemcitabine-loaded albumin nanoparticles in a pancreatic cancer cell line. *Int. J. Nanomed.* **2015**, *10*, 6825–6834. [CrossRef] [PubMed]

31. Singh, A.; Xu, J.; Mattheolabakis, G.; Amiji, M. EGFR-targeted gelatin nanoparticles for systemic administration of gemcitabine in an orthotopic pancreatic cancer model. *Nanomed. NBM* **2015**, *12*, 589–600. [CrossRef] [PubMed]

32. Acuna, A.; Jeffery, J.J.; Abril, E.R.; Nagle, R.B.; Guzman, R.; Pagel, M.D.; Meuillet, E.J. Nanoparticle delivery of an AKT/PDK1 inhibitor improves the therapeutic effect in pancreatic cancer. *Int. J. Nanomed.* **2014**, *9*, 5653–5665. [CrossRef]

33. Mukai, S.; Moriya, S.; Hiramoto, M.; Kazama, H.; Kokuba, H.; Che, X.F.; Yokoyama, T.; Sakamoto, S.; Sugawara, A.; Sunazuka, T.; et al. Macrolides sensitize EGFR-TKI-induced non-apoptotic cell death via blocking autophagy flux in pancreatic cancer cell lines. *Int. J. Oncol.* **2016**, *48*, 45–54. [CrossRef] [PubMed]

34. Wang, L.I.N.; Zhu, Z.; Zhang, W.; Zhang, W. Schedule-dependent cytotoxic synergism of pemetrexed and erlotinib in BXPC-3 and PANC-1 human pancreatic cancer cells. *Exp. Ther. Med.* **2011**, *2*, 969–975. [CrossRef] [PubMed]

35. Wright, A.E.; Roth, G.P.; Hoffman, J.K.; Divlianska, D.B.; Pechter, D.; Sennett, S.H.; Guzmán, E.A.; Linley, P.; McCarthy, P.J.; Pitts, T.P.; et al. Isolation, synthesis, and biological activity of aphrocallistin, an adenine-substituted bromotyramine metabolite from the hexactinellida sponge *Aphrocallistes beatrix*. *J. Nat. Prod.* **2009**, *72*, 1178–1183. [CrossRef] [PubMed]

36. Merlot, A.M.; Kalinowski, D.S.; Richardson, D.R. Unraveling the mysteries of serum albumin—More than just a serum protein. *Front. Physiol.* **2014**, *5*, 1–7. [CrossRef] [PubMed]

37. Yameen, B.; Choi, W.I.; Vilos, C.; Swami, A.; Shi, J.; Farokhzad, O.C. Insight into nanoparticle cellular uptake and intracellular targeting. *J. Control. Release* **2015**, *28*, 485–499. [CrossRef] [PubMed]

38. Marrese, M.; Guarino, V.; Ambrosio, L. Atomic Force Microscopy: A Powerful Tool to Address Scaffold Design in Tissue Engineering. *J. Funct. Biomater.* **2017**, *8*, 7. [CrossRef] [PubMed]

39. Kowoll, T.; Müller, E.; Fritsch-Decker, S.; Hettler, S.; Störmer, H.; Weiss, C.; Gerthsen, D. Contrast of backscattered electron SEM images of nanoparticles on substrates with complex structure. *Scanning* **2017**, *2017*. [CrossRef] [PubMed]

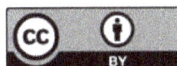

pharmaceutics

MDPI

Article

SPC Liposomes as Possible Delivery Systems for Improving Bioavailability of the Natural Sesquiterpene β-Caryophyllene: Lamellarity and Drug-Loading as Key Features for a Rational Drug Delivery Design

Antonella Di Sotto [1,*], Patrizia Paolicelli [2,*], Martina Nardoni [2], Lorena Abete [1], Stefania Garzoli [2], Silvia Di Giacomo [1], Gabriela Mazzanti [1], Maria Antonietta Casadei [2] and Stefania Petralito [2,*]

1   Department of Physiology and Pharmacology "V. Erspamer", Sapienza University of Rome, P.le Aldo Moro 5, 00185 Rome, Italy; lorena.abete@uniroma1.it (L.A.); silvia.digiacomo@uniroma1.it (S.D.G.); gabriela.mazzanti@uniroma1.it (G.M.)
2   Department of Chemistry and Technology of Drugs, Sapienza University of Rome, P.le Aldo Moro 5, 00185 Rome, Italy; martina.nardoni@uniroma1.it (M.N.); stefania.garzoli@uniroma1.it (S.G.); mariaantonietta.casadei@uniroma1.it (M.A.C.)
*   Correspondence: antonella.disotto@uniroma1.it (A.D.S.); patrizia.paolicelli@uniroma1.it (P.P.); stefania.petralito@uniroma1.it (S.P.)

Received: 27 November 2018; Accepted: 11 December 2018; Published: 13 December 2018

Abstract: The natural sesquiterpene β-caryophyllene (CRY) has been highlighted to possess interesting pharmacological potentials, particularly due to its chemopreventive and analgesic properties. However, the poor solubility of this sesquiterpene in aqueous fluids can hinder its uptake into cells, resulting in inconstant responses of biological systems, thus limiting its application. Therefore, identifying a suitable pharmaceutical form for increasing CRY bioavailability represents an important requirement for exploiting its pharmacological potential. In the present study, the ability of soybean phosphatidylcholine (SPC) liposomes to improve bioavailability and absorption of CRY in cancer cells has been evaluated. Liposomal formulations of CRY, differing for lamellarity (i.e., unilamellar and multilamellar vesicles or ULV and MLV) and for the drug loading (i.e., 1:0.1, 1:0.3 and 1:0.5 mol/mol between SPC and CRY) were designed with the aim of maximizing CRY amount in the liposome bilayer, while avoiding its leakage during storage. The low-loaded formulations significantly potentiated the antiproliferative activity of CRY in both HepG2 and MDA-MB-468 cells, reaching a maximum IC_{50} lowering (from two to five folds) with 1:0.3 and 1:0.1 SPC/CRY MLV. Conversely, increasing liposome drug-loading reduced the ability for CRY release, likely due to a possible interaction between SPC and CRY that affects the membrane properties, as confirmed by physical measures.

Keywords: lipophilic compound; caryophyllene sesquiterpene; antiproliferative activity; liposomes; lamellarity; drug loading

1. Introduction

β-caryophyllene or *trans*-caryophyllene (CRY), a bicyclic sesquiterpene with a rare cyclobutane ring (Figure 1), is a volatile compound found in large amounts in the essential oil of many different spice and food plants, particularly *Eugenia caryophyllata* L., *Copaifera multijuga* (copaiba) and *Cannabis sativa* L [1].

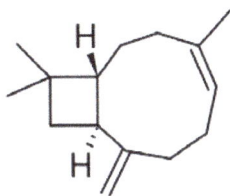

Figure 1. Chemical structure of β-caryophyllene (CRY).

In nature, β-caryophyllene is usually found together with small amount of its isomers α-caryophyllene and γ-caryophyllene or in a mixture with its oxidation product, β-caryophyllene oxide. Several biological activities have been reported for β-caryophyllene, including antimicrobial, antileishmanial, antimalarial, local anesthetic, spasmolytic and anticonvulsivant activities [2]. It has been reported to partly act as an agonist of the CB2 receptor, which represents a therapeutic target for the treatment of inflammation, pain, atherosclerosis, and inflammatory-based diseases, including colitis, cerebral ischemia and brain inflammation [3–7]. Also, it has been recently shown to possess chemopreventive properties [1,8–11] and displayed a chemosensitizing power when administered in combination with anticancer drugs, thus resensitizing chemoresistant cancer cells [12]. It was found to be able to interfere with targeted signalling pathways involved in inflammation and cancer, including HMGB1/TLR4 signalling and STAT3 [10,13,14].

Despite these promising biological activities, β-caryophyllene is characterized by high lipophilicity and poor stability in hydrophilic media (such as biological fluids), which limit its bioavailability and absorption into cells. Bioavailability depends on the nature and chemical-physical properties of a molecule and is mainly due to water solubility (or dissolution rate) and membrane permeability [15]. Low bioavailability is a common feature of different natural substances, defined as "poorly water-soluble drugs", and can hinder their administration, clinical application and market entry. In this context, improving bioavailability represents an important requirement for exploiting the pharmacological potential of such natural substances and meeting the need for suitable pharmaceutical formulations.

To this end, various strategies, including formulation in complex forms as micelles, liposomes, polymeric nanoparticles and lipid nanoparticles, have been approached. Among them, liposomes have been extensively applied in the years as biomembrane models and as drug carriers in the pharmaceutical and medical fields, owing to their excellent biocompatibility and biodegradability, low toxicity and lack of immunogenicity [16,17]. They have also been adopted as efficient systems for incorporating natural compounds, such as essential oil components, and improving their solubility and chemical stability [18].

Liposome structure allows the incorporation of different types of drugs: hydrophilic substances are encapsulated in the inner aqueous compartments, while lipophilic drugs are mainly entrapped within the lipid bilayer [19]. According to lamellarity and size, they are usually classified as multilamellar vesicles (MLV; greater than 0.5 µm), small unilamellar vesicles (SUV; between 20 and 100 nm) and large unilamellar vesicles (LUV; greater than 100 nm) [20].

Taking into account the strong lipophilicity of CRY and its low dissolution rate in biological fluids, in the present study we propose a rational design of soy phosphatidylcholine (SPC) liposomal formulations for improving cellular uptake of CRY and then its antiproliferative activity in cancer cells, focusing on lamellarity and drug-loading as major key features to develop optimized delivery systems. SPC is commonly used in different types of drug delivery formulations, due to its structural similarity with biomembrane phospholipids, and seems to represent an interesting molecule to be used for designing liposomal chemotherapy formulations, since it could enhance the antiproliferative activity of anticancer drugs by affecting the cholesterol-induced stiffening of cancer cell biomembrane, thus favoring drug permeability. It is well accepted that cancer cells, respect to normal cells, are characterized by changes in biomembrane phospholipid composition and a constitutive activation of the fatty acid biosynthesis seems to support the increased cell proliferation [21]. Particularly, higher accumulation of cholesterol leads to a more rigid and low-permeable membrane, with increased resistance to cancer chemotherapy.

In order to characterize the best features of SPC liposomes in improving the dissolution of CRY in biological fluids and its cellular uptake, both unilamellar (ULV) and multilamellar (MLV) formulations were studied. In fact, due to the physico-chemical properties of CRY, it is expected that the drug is incorporated within the phospholipid bilayer of liposomes. Therefore, liposomal formulations of CRY have been rationally designed taking into account that the loading of CRY in the bilayer of liposomes, while avoiding its leakage during storage, requires special consideration in product development and represents a key feature for optimizing the formulation. The lipid composition, lamellarity, the manufacturing process and drug incorporation can all influence the physicochemical properties of a liposomal formulation, including the drug release performance. Therefore, when liposomes are investigated as drug delivery vehicles of hydrophobic drugs, the influence of the drug–lipid ratio on the arrangement of the nonpolar region of the vesicles membrane should be considered to design a delivery vehicle that is at the same time able to catch and release the encapsulated payload in order to achieve the therapeutic purpose [22].

In line with this evidence, in the present study different formulations at three loading degrees, characterized by SPC phospholipid and CRY molar ratio of 1:0.1, 1:0.3 and 1:0.5 as well as different lamellarity were prepared. A physicochemical characterization by dynamic light scattering, fluorescence anisotropy and entrapment efficiency of CRY were performed. The increased bioavailability was evaluated on the basis of the cytotoxicity potency of the formulations encapsulating CRY with respect to the substance alone. In specific, the antiproliferative activity of CRY-loaded SPC ULV and MLV with respect to that of CRY alone was studied in liver cancer HepG2cells. Also, triple negative MDA-MB-468 breast cancer cells were used being high-responsive to CRY cytotoxicity respect to HepG2 cells.

2. Materials and Methods

2.1. Chemicals

β-Caryophyllene (CRY; >98.5% purity), soybean phosphatidylcholine (Phospholipon90; SPC), HEPES [4-(2-hydroxyethyl) piperazine-1-ethane-sulfonic acid], thiocyanatoiron (III), 1,6-diphenyl-1,3,5-hexatriene (DPH) and (4,5-dimethyl-2-thiazolyl)-2,5-diphenyl-2H-tetrazolium bromide (MTT; ≥97.5% purity) and cholesterol (Chol) were purchased from Sigma-Aldrich Co (St. Louis, MO, USA). Dulbecco's Modified Eagle's medium (DMEM) was from Aurogene (Rome, Italy). Chloroform, dimethyl sulfoxide, ethanol, 1,2-dicloroethane and hydrochloric acid were supplied by Carlo Erba Reagents (Arese, Italy) and were of analytical grade. All solutions were prepared in the better solvent, sterilized by filtration and stored for a just conservation time at recommended temperature, i.e., room temperature (RT) or refrigerated conditions (from 4 °C to −20 °C).

For the cytotoxicity assay, the sesquiterpene was dissolved in absolute EtOH (100% v/v): at the tested concentrations, and the percentage of ethanol was less than 1% v/v in the final mixture, in order to exclude a potential toxicity due to the solvent. Conversely, both the CRY-loaded and plain SPC liposomes were directly dispersed in the culture medium at different concentrations.

2.2. Liposome Preparation

Liposomes were prepared by the thin-film hydration method followed by extrusion [23]. Specifically, 250 mg of SPC and different amount of CRY (7, 20 or 33 mg) were dissolved in a 50 mL round-bottom flask in the minimum volume of chloroform to give lipid-to-drug molar ratio of 1:0.1, 1:0.3 and 1:0.5.

The solvent was removed by rotary evaporation under reduced pressure to form a thin layer on the flask wall. The resultant thin film was further dried with a high vacuum oil pump for at least 2 h.

Dried film was hydrated in 5 mL of a 10 mM HEPES buffer solution (pH 7.4) at 25 °C and the dispersion was shaken vigorously with a vortex mixer to form multi-lamellar vesicles (MLV).

The generated multilamellar vesicles were repeatedly extruded at 25 °C through polycarbonate membranes of decreasing pore size using a thermobarrel Extruder, (Lipex Biomembrane, Vancouver, BC, Canada) until a defined size distribution was achieved (2 times through 400 nm membranes and finally 6 times through 200 nm membranes). All liposome formulations were flushed with nitrogen gas, stored at 4 °C and used within two weeks.

2.3. Gas Chromatographic/Mass Spectrometric (GC/MS)

Purity of CRY and its concentration obtained in the liposomal dispersion was determined by the gas chromatographic/mass spectrometric (GC/MS) technique. The GC/MS analyses were performed on a Clarus 500 series from Perkin Elmer instruments (Waltham, MA, USA) operating in the electron impact mode (70 eV) and equipped with NIST (National Institute of Standards and Technology) libraries. A Stabilwax fused-silica capillary column (Restek, Bellefonte, PA, USA) (60 m × 0.25 mm, 0.25 mm film thickness) was used with helium as carrier gas (1.0 mL/min). 1 μL of sample was injected into the GC injector at the temperature of 280 °C and in splitless mode. The oven of GC was programmed to rise from 90 °C to 200 °C at 3 °C/min and then held at 200 °C for 2 min. All analyses were performed at constant flow. A calibration curve was generated by running various solutions containing graded amounts of the CRY and injecting a constant volume of each standard solution exactly measured. The calibration curve was obtained by plotting the peaks area (automatically calculated by the computer) on the ordinate and the amounts on the abscissa.

2.4. Physicochemical Characterization of Liposomes

2.4.1. Dynamic Light Scattering (DLS) and Zeta-Potential Measurements

Particle size distribution and zeta-potential were measured with a Zetasizer Nano ZS90 (Malvern Panalytical, Malvern, UK). Hydrodynamic diameter and polydispersity index were evaluated by dynamic light scattering (DLS) experiments, whereas zeta-potential was measured by electrophoretic light scattering (ELS) experiments. The DLS and ELS techniques used a photon correlator spectrometer equipped with a 4 mW He/Ne laser source operating at 633 nm. All measurements were performed at a scattering angle of 90° and were thermostatically controlled at 25 °C. The samples were opportunely diluted with 10 mM HEPES (pH 7.4) before analysis. Size, polydispersity index and zeta-potential values of the liposome formulations are the mean of three different preparation batches ± standard deviation.

2.4.2. Assay of Phospholipids

Phospholipid content in liposomes was quantified as reported in literature [24]. Briefly, 0.4 mL of sample (20–200 nmol) was mixed with 0.2 mL of ethanol, 1 mL of thiocyanatoiron (III) and 0.6 mL of 0.17 N hydrochloric acid. 3 mL of 1,2-dichloroethane were added to extract the thiocyanatoiron–phospholipid complex formed after shaking for 2 min. The sample was then centrifuged for 5 min at 12,000 rpm. The absorbance of the organic phase was read at a wavelength of 470 nm in a Lambda 25 spectrophotometer (Perkin Elmer, Waltham, USA). The calibration curve was obtained with several solutions of known SPC concentration.

2.4.3. Evaluation of Total Amount of β-Caryophyllene (CRY) in Liposomal Suspensions

Phospholipids and drug molecules dissolved in the organic phase may be get lost during solvent removal under vacuum and high-pressure extrusion steps. Considering that CRY is a liquid with an initial boiling point of 129 °C, to evaluate the amount of the sequiterpene actually present in the different liposomal formulations, it was first extracted from vesicles and then its concentration was determined by the GC/MS technique reported in Section 2.3. In particular, 5 mL of CRY-loaded SPC

ULV were diluted with 10 mL of 10 mM HEPES (pH 7.4) and extracted with $CHCl_3$ (5 mL). To promote the separation of the two phases, $CaCl_2$ (460 mg) was added to the biphasic system and the organic phase then collected. The extraction procedure was repeated three times, all the organic phases were mixed and made up to known volume before GC/MS analysis.

2.4.4. Steady-State and Time-Resolved Fluorescence Measurements

Steady state anisotropy of DPH in liposomes was measured to assess the effect of CRY and its concentration on the fluidity of SPC liposome membranes. To this end, DPH-loaded SPC liposomes were prepared by the thin-film hydration method reported in Section 2.2, dissolving SPC (250 mg) and DPH (0.15 mg; 6.46×10^{-4} mmol) in a 50 mL round-bottom flask in the minimum volume of chloroform to give a lipid-to-DPH molar ratio of 1:0.002.

The solvent was removed as previously described and the resultant thin film was hydrated in 5 mL of a 10 mM HEPES buffer solution (pH 7.4) at 25 °C. The generated multilamellar vesicles were repeatedly extruded at 25 °C through polycarbonate membranes of decreasing pore size.

DPH normally is located within the hydrophobic region of the bilayer membrane. DPH responds to changes in physical properties of the acyl chain region of the membrane that affect its ability to rotate. Probe movement is quantified by measuring the degree to which DPH fluorescence emission is depolarized following excitation by polarized light. These fluorescence anisotropy measurements respond to changes in the order degree of the DPH surrounding environment: changes in the liquid–crystalline state organization of the liposome membrane alter the rate of probe movement; in particular, the more disordered the membrane environment, the greater is the motional freedom of the fluorophore and hence the lower the observed anisotropy. An increase in steady state anisotropy of DPH in membranes may imply a reduction in mobility of lipids.

Steady-state fluorescence anisotropy measurements, for DPH-loaded liposomes, were carried out at room temperature with a Perkin-Elmer LS50B spectrofluorometer. The excitation and emission wavelengths were 350 and 450 nm, respectively, and all slits were set to a width of 2.5/2.5 nm.

Samples, opportunely diluted with 10 mM HEPES buffer pH 7.4, were illuminated by vertically (V) or horizontally (H) polarized monochromatic light at $\lambda = 350$ nm and the emitted fluorescence intensities (I) parallel or perpendicular to the direction of the excitation beam were recorded at $\lambda = 450$ nm. Total fluorescence intensity $\left[I_f = (I_{//})V + 2G(I_{\perp})H\right]$ is obtained by addition of the respectively horizontally $[I_{\perp}]$ and vertically $[I_{//}]$ intensities polarised light emission. The stationary fluorescence anisotropy (r) was determined using the typical calculation:

$$r = \frac{(I_{//})V - G(I_{\perp})H}{I_f}$$

Total fluorescence intensity and anisotropy measurements required correction for the gain of photomultipler detector $[G = (I_{//})H/(I_{\perp})H]$.

The effect of CRY incorporation on the phospholipid bilayer of SPC liposomes was evaluated by comparison with the well-known effect produced by cholesterol (Chol) on the membrane behavior.

Anisotropy data are represented as the mean $\pm$ standard deviation (SD).

2.5. Cytotoxicity Studies

2.5.1. Human Cancer Cell Lines

Liver cancer HepG2 cells were a kind gift of Prof. Eufemi (Sapienza University of Rome, Italy), while triple negative MDA-MB-468 breast cancer cells were purchased from IRCCS AOU San Martino -IST (Genoa, Italy). The cells were grown under standard conditions (37 °C and 5% CO_2) in DMEM-F12 medium containing L-glutamine (1% v/v) and HEPES (15 mM) and supplemented with 10% heat-inactivated FBS, 100 U/mL penicillin and 100 µg/mL streptomycin in 75 cm² flasks.

Subcultures were prepared every 4 days, renewing growth medium every 2–3 days. All experiments were performed when cells reached the logarithmic growth phase.

2.5.2. Cytotoxicity Assay

The cultured cells were seeded into 96-well microplates (20,000 cells/well), allowed to grow for 24 h, then treated with CRY (1–75 µg/mL in EtOH 1% *v*/*v*) or CRY loaded SPC liposomes. The concentrations of pure CRY were prepared by progressive dilution in EtOH 100% *v*/*v*, then added to cells at 1% *v*/*v* in the final mixture, at which ethanol was nontoxic. A vehicle control (EtOH 1% *v*/*v* in the final mixture for CRY and 10 mM HEPES for SPC ULV and MLV), corresponding to 100% cell viability and a standard cytotoxic agent (i.e., doxorubicin, 10 µg/mL in the final mixture) were also included in the experiments.

After 24 h incubation, the cytotoxicity of the treatment was measured by the 3-[4,5-dimethylthiazol-2-yl]-2,5-diphenyl tetrazolium bromide (MTT) assay according to previous published methods [25]. The assay was carried out at least in three biological replicates, and in each experiment each concentration was tested in six technical triplicates. The treatment was considered cytotoxic when the cell viability was lower than 70% with respect to vehicle treated cells [26].

The results were expressed as percentage of cell viability (about three experiments including 8-10 replicates for each treatment) with respect to the vehicle.

Results of cytotoxicity studies are expressed as mean ± standard error (SE). The concentration–response curves were constructed using the Hill equation:

$$E = \frac{E_{max}}{[1 + (10 log IC_{50} - A) Hill\ Slope]}$$

where E is the effect at a given concentration of the substance, E_{max} is the maximum activity, IC_{50} is the concentration that produces a 50% of the inhibitory response, A is the substance molar concentration, $HillSlope$ is the curve slope.

2.6. Statistical Analysis

Statistical analysis was performed by GraphPad Prism™ (Version 4.00) software (GraphPad Software, Inc., San Diego, CA, USA). The one-way analysis of variance (one-way ANOVA), followed by Dunnett's multiple comparison post-test, was used to analyze the difference among different treatments, while the Student's *t*-test was applied to determine the statistical significance between two different experimental conditions. The values of $p < 0.05$ were considered significant.

3. Results

3.1. Physicochemical Characterization of Soybean Phosphatidylcholine (SPC) Unilamellar and Multilamellar Vesicles (ULV and MLV)

Results obtained by DLS measurements highlighted that high pure CRY did not alter the vesicles formation, since no significant changes in physicochemical features (i.e., mean diameter, zeta-potential and size distribution) of CRY-loaded SPC ULV and MLV, compared to conventional liposomes, were found even at the highest molar ratio tested (1:0.5 mol/mol) (Tables 1 and 2). Moreover, no loss of CRY was observed during the preparation process. In fact, GC/MS analysis performed after the extraction of CRY from liposomes evidenced a perfect overlap of the actual recovered amount with the theoretical one, thus indicating that no losses of sesquiterpene occurred. When the physicochemical features of liposomes were evaluated in the presence of cell medium, no interference with the dimensional analysis was highlighted, thus suggesting a suitable stability of the formulation in cell culture environment (data not shown). The amount of structured phospholipids in the liposomal suspensions, with and without CRY, resulted in not being affected by the presence of the sesquiterpene, thus suggesting their compatibility.

Table 1. Physicochemical features of soybean phosphatidylcholine (SPC) unilamellar vesicles (ULV) liposomes.

Sample	Hydrodynamic Diameter (nm)	PdI	ζ-Potential (mV)	SPC Recovery (%)
Unloaded SPC vesicles	180.6 ± 4.7	0.079 ± 0.015	−15.3 ± 0.4	92.2 ± 1.7
SPC/CRY vesicles (mol/mol)				
1:0.1	185.5 ± 4.2	0.076 ± 0.006	−14.1 ± 0.2	89.5 ± 1.2
1:0.3	176.7 ± 7.5	0.075 ± 0.005	−14.3 ± 0.5	88.5 ± 0.5
1:0.5	181.4 ± 2.1	0.085 ± 0.012	−13.5 ± 0.6	85.2 ± 2.2

Hydrodynamic diameter (Z-Average, nm); polydispersity index (PdI); ζ-potential (mV) and % of SPC recovery.

Table 2. Physicochemical features of SPC multilamellar vesicles (MLV) liposomes.

Sample	Hydrodynamic Diameter (nm)	PdI
Unloaded SPC vesicles	699.7 ± 6.6	0.359 ± 0.069
SPC/CRY vesicles (mol/mol)		
1:0.1	643.9 ± 13.6	0.339 ± 0.045
1:0.3	631.5 ± 21.1	0.371 ± 0.005
1:0.5	497.1 ± 7.9	0.387 ± 0.025

Hydrodynamic diameter (Z-Average, nm); polydispersity index (PdI).

3.2. Cytotoxicity of CRY and Plain SPC-Based Liposomes

Under our experimental conditions, CRY did not affect the cell viability of HepG2 cells up to 10 µg/mL, although a slight cell viability reduction (about 10%) was found starting from 5 µg/mL. A significant decrease of cell viability (about 45% reduction respect to control) was found at 25 µg/mL, reaching a greatest inhibition of about 90% at 75 µg/mL (Figure 2). In MDA-MB-468 cells, CRY produced early toxicity signs (inhibition of 10%) at 2.5 µg/mL, with a biologically significant effect at 15, 25 and 50 µg/mL (inhibition of 38%, 84% and 98% respectively) (Figure 2). The IC$_{50}$ values were 44.7 (C.L. 19.5–96.8) and 19.2 (C. L. 15.4–23.8) µg/mL in HepG2 and MDA-MB-468 cells, respectively.

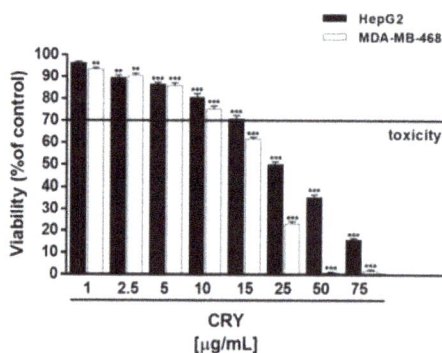

Figure 2. Effect of CRY on the viability of HepG2 and MDA-MB-468 cells. ** $p < 0.01$ and *** $p < 0.001$ (analysis of variance (ANOVA) + multiple Dunnett's comparison post-test); denotes a statistically significant reduction of cell viability compared to control (i.e., vehicle-treated cells). A cell viability lower than 70% respect to control was considered as cytotoxic [26].

The cytotoxicity of plain SPC ULV and MLV (1–1000 µg/mL) in HepG2 and MDA-MB-468 cells was preliminarily evaluated, in order to define the maximum concentration at which liposomal formulations did not affect cell viability. Plain SPC ULV were nontoxic up to the concentration of 100 µg/mL in both HepG2 and MDA-MB-468 cells, with biologically significant cytotoxic effects (from 40% to 56% inhibition of cell viability) starting from 200 µg/mL (Figure 3). Conversely, plain SPC MLV produced biologically significant cytotoxic effects (from 40% to 50% inhibition of cell viability) at

1000 μg/mL in both HepG2 and MDA-MB-468 cells, with early toxicity signs (about 25% inhibition of cell viability) at 500 μg/mL (Figure 3).

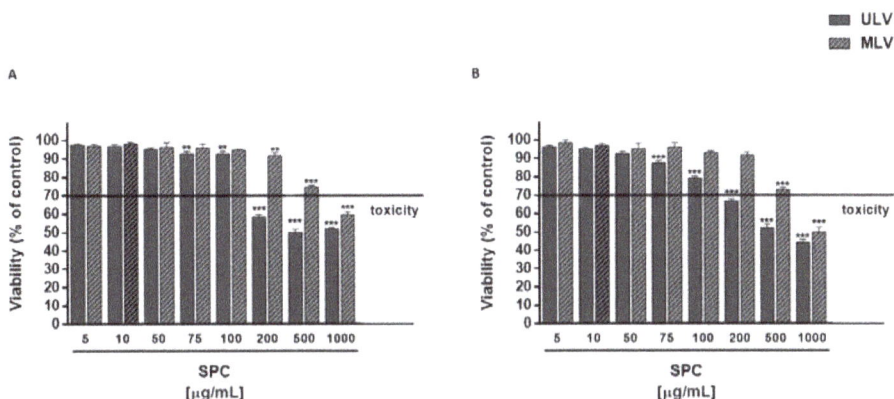

Figure 3. Effect of SPC ULV and MLV on the viability of HepG2 (**A**) and MDA-MB-468 (**B**) cells. ** $p < 0.01$ and *** $p < 0.001$ vs. control (i.e., vehicle-treated cells), denotes a statistically significant reduction of cell viability compared to control (ANOVA + multiple Dunnett's comparison post-test). A cell viability lower than 70% respect to control was considered as cytotoxic [26].

3.3. Cytotoxicity of CRY-Loaded SPC ULV at Different Molar Ratio

When assessed in HepG2 cells, different behaviour was found for CRY-loaded SPC ULV respect to pure CRY, as a function of their molar ratio (Figure 4). In particular, the 1:0.1 molar ratio between SPC and CRY produced about a 40% cytotoxicity increase of CRY at low concentrations of 0.1, 1, 5 and 10 μg/mL, which were non-effective when CRY was administered as pure compound. Conversely, a progressive loss of the cytotoxic effect of CRY was found at highest concentrations of 25, 50 and 75 μg/mL of 1:0.1 SPC/CRY ULV, reaching a maximum 40% inhibition (Figure 4). In spite of a biologically significant cytotoxicity of low-dose 1:0.1 SPC/CRY ULV, the 1:0.3 and 1:0.5 unilamellar formulations produced non-biologically relevant cytotoxic effects and progressively reduced the antiproliferative activity of pure CRY at all the tested concentrations, reaching a maximum of 63% inhibition (Figure 4)

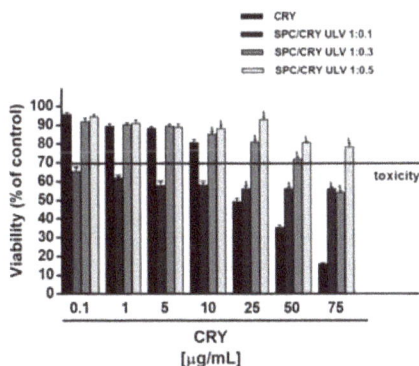

Figure 4. Cytotoxicity of SPC ULV differently loaded with CRY (1:0.1, 1:0.3 and 1:0.5 mol/mol) in HepG2 cells after 24 h incubation. *** $p < 0.001$ vs CRY; denotes a statistically significant increase of cytotoxicity respect to pure CRY (ANOVA + multiple Dunnett's comparison post-test). § $p < 0.001$ vs. CRY, denotes a statistically significant reduction respect to CRY cytotoxicity (ANOVA + multiple Dunnett's comparison post-test). A cell viability lower than 70% respect to control (i.e., vehicle-treated cells) was considered as cytotoxic [26].

Furthermore, the highest doses of loaded liposomes (starting from 25 μg/mL of 1:0.1 and 1:0.3 SPC/CRY ULV) significantly reduced the cytotoxicity of plain SPC ULV, at the corresponding concentrations (Figure 4). This evidence suggested that increasing molar ratio between SPC and CRY in ULV formulations can hinder CRY release and retain the molecule into liposomes; also, some interactions between SPC and CRY could be expected, so explaining the reduced toxicity of plain SPC ULV. A similar behaviour was observed in MDA-MB-468 cells for 1:0.5 SPC/CRY ULV, which did not potentiate CRY cytotoxicity in all the experimental conditions, while inhibiting the antiproliferative activity of pure CRY by about 20%, at concentrations of 25 and 50 μg/mL (Figure 5). Conversely, the 1:0.1 loaded formulation induced a significant potentiation of CRY cytotoxicity (from about 20 to 30%) at concentrations of 2.5 and 5 μg/mL, which disappeared at the highest tested concentrations.

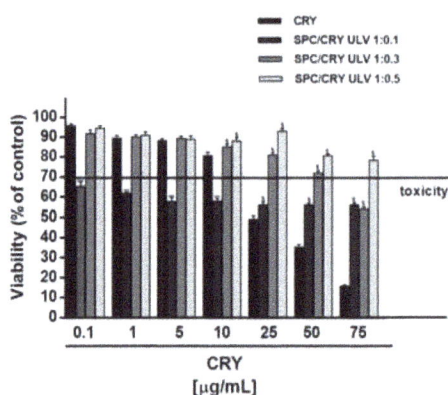

Figure 5. Cytotoxicity of SPC ULV differently loaded with CRY (1:0.1, 1:0.3 and 1:0.5 mol/mol) in MDA-MB-468 cells after 24 h incubation. *** $p < 0.001$ vs. CRY, denotes a statistically significant increase of cytotoxicity respect to pure CRY (ANOVA + multiple Dunnett's comparison post-test). § $p < 0.001$ vs. CRY, denotes a statistically significant reduction respect to CRY cytotoxicity (ANOVA + multiple Dunnett's comparison post-test). A cell viability lower than 70% respect to control (i.e., vehicle-treated cells) was considered as cytotoxic [26].

Similarly, the 1:0.3 SPC/CRY ULV produced a slight (about 10%) but significant increase of CRY toxicity at concentrations of 2.5 and 5 μg/mL. It is noteworthy that potentiation occurred at non-effective concentrations of CRY administered as a pure compound. For all loaded formulations, the highest concentrations of 25 and 50 μg/mL induced a significant inhibition (from about 10 to 28%) of CRY antiproliferative activity, thus suggesting a possible loss of activity of the drug or the loss of the carrier's ability to deliver the incorporated substance (Figure 5). When CRY was administered as 1:0.1 SPC ULV, the IC_{50} values were not evaluable in HepG2 cells, while a slight reduction (about 1.5 folds) was obtained in MDA-MB-468 cells (Table 3).

Table 3. IC$_{50}$ values of CRY administered as pure compound or as ULV and MLV formulations in HepG2 and MDA-MB-468 cells.

	HepG2	MDA-MB-468
	IC$_{50}$ (CL) µg/mL	
	RR	
CRY	44.7 (19.5–96.8)	19.2 (15.4–23.8)
	SPC/CRY ULV (mol/mol)	
1:0.1	ne	12.4 (6.4–109.9)
		1.5
1:0.3	ne	ne
1:0.5	ne	ne
	SPC/CRY MLV (mol/mol)	
1:0.1	ne	4.9 (2.4–9.9)
		3.9
1:0.3	9.1 (2.6–32.0)	8.3 (6.1–11.2)
	4.9	2.3
1:0.5	ne	ne

CL, confidential limits; RR, reversal ratio (ratio between the IC$_{50}$ values of CRY alone and CRY-loaded SPC liposomes); ne, not evaluable as a lower than 80% inhibition of cell viability was reached.

3.4. Cytotoxicity of CRY-Loaded SPC MLV at Different Molar Ratio

Under our experimental conditions, multilamellar liposomes produced different cytotoxic effects as a function of drug loading. In HepG2 cells, 1:0.1 SPC/CRY MLV did not affect the cell viability up to 1 µg/mL, while it produced a marked potentiation of CRY cytotoxicity, at concentrations from 5 to 25 µg/mL, reaching the greatest effect of about 45% at 5 µg/mL (Figure 6). A significant and progressive increase of CRY antiproliferative activity, with a maximum potentiation of about 40%, was also produced by 1:0.3 loaded multilamellar formulation (Figure 6) within the concentrations of 1 and 50 µg/mL: the IC$_{50}$ value of CRY was reduced about five-fold (Table 3). Conversely, the 1:0.5 molar ratio between SPC and CRY increased the biological activity of CRY at concentrations of 5 and 10 µg/mL, with a maximum potentiation of 30% at 5 µg/mL (Figure 6). At the highest concentration of 75 µg/mL, all the CRY-loaded multilamellar formulations markedly reduced the antiproliferative activity of pure CRY, reaching a maximum 26% inhibition (Figure 6).

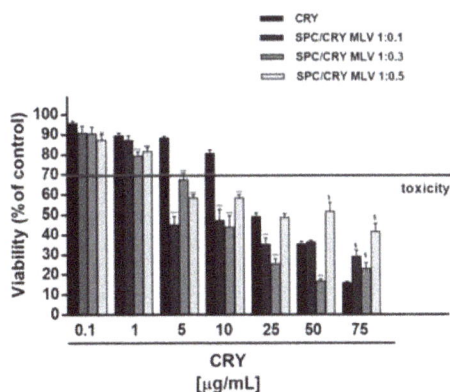

Figure 6. Cytotoxicity of SPC MLV differently loaded with CRY (1:0.1, 1:0.3 and 1:0.5 mol/mol) in HepG2 cells after 24 h incubation. ** $p < 0.01$ and *** $p < 0.001$ vs CRY; denotes a statistically significant increase of cytotoxicity respect to pure CRY (ANOVA + multiple Dunnett's comparison post-test). § $p < 0.001$ vs. CRY, denotes a statistically significant reduction respect to CRY cytotoxicity (ANOVA + multiple Dunnett's comparison post-test). A cell viability lower than 70% respect to control (i.e., vehicle-treated cells) was considered as cytotoxic [26].

Analogously, in MDA-MB-468 cells, the 1:0.1 SPC/CRY MLV induced a significant potentiation of CRY cytotoxicity from 0.1 to 10 µg/mL, with a maximum increase of about 30% at 5 and 10 µg/mL (Figure 7). The 1:0.3 and 1:0.5 loaded formulations produced lower potentiation of CRY activity (about 10–25%) from 0.1 to 10 µg/mL. Conversely, the highest concentrations of 25 and 50 µg/mL reduced the antiproliferative activity of pure CRY, reaching a maximum 30% inhibition (Figure 7).

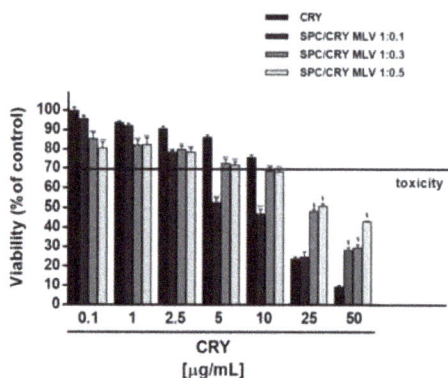

Figure 7. Cytotoxicity of SPC MLV differently loaded with CRY (1:0.1, 1:0.3 and 1:0.5 mol/mol) in MDA-MB-468 cells after 24 h incubation. ** $p < 0.01$ and *** $p < 0.001$ vs. CRY, denotes a statistically significant increase of cytotoxicity respect to pure CRY (ANOVA + multiple Dunnett's comparison post-test). § $p < 0.001$ vs. CRY, denotes a statistically significant reduction respect to CRY cytotoxicity (ANOVA + multiple Dunnett's comparison post-test). A cell viability lower than 70% respect to control (i.e., vehicle-treated cells) was considered as cytotoxic [26].

Within the concentrations from 0.1 to 25 µg/mL, the IC_{50} value of CRY was reduced about four-fold when CRY was administered as 1:0.1 MLV, while about two-fold when CRY was administered as 1:0.3 MLV (Table 3).

Furthermore, the highest dose (75 µg/mL) of 1:0.5 SPC/CRY MLV significantly reduced the cytotoxicity of plain SPC MLV at the corresponding concentration, thus displaying a behaviour similar to that found for CRY-loaded ULV (Figure 7). Accordingly, a possible segregation of CRY into liposome due to its interaction with SPC could be expected.

3.5. Evaluation of the Potential Interaction between CRY and SPC ULV

In order to better characterize the possible interaction between CRY and SPC ULV, additional experiments in which the two separate components were co-administered to cells, at the same concentrations found in liposome formulations, were performed in HepG2 cells.

When administered in the presence of SPC ULV, CRY exhibited a lower cytotoxic behaviour with respect to the pure compound. Despite a biologically relevant toxicity of the pure compound alone, the presence of SPC ULV induced a significant loss of CRY bioactivity. About a 30% reduction of its antiproliferative effect is observed (Figure 8) probably due to the high hydrophobic nature of CRY, which is therefore carried off by liposomes.

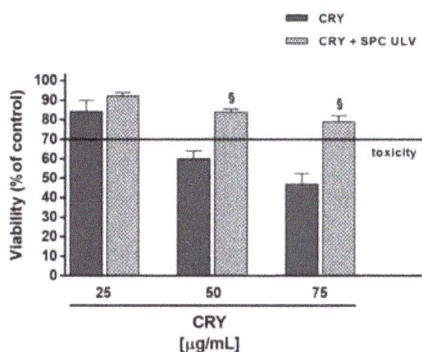

Figure 8. Cytotoxicity of CRY and the combination of SPC/CRY ULV (1:0.5 mol/mol) in HepG2 cells after 24 h incubation. § $p < 0.001$ vs. CRY, denotes a statistically significant reduction respect to CRY cytotoxicity (ANOVA + multiple Dunnett's comparison post-test). A cell viability lower than 70% respect to control (i.e., vehicle-treated cells) was considered as cytotoxic [26].

Similar results were reported by Botré et al. [27], who observed that the addition of empty liposomes to urine samples containing free steroids interfere with the recovery of the drugs, with consequent important implication on doping analysis. These results support our hypothesis that the reduced bioactivity of CRY, when administered as SPC ULV with low molar ratio or at high concentration of the drug, could be due to a close interaction of the substance with phospholipid components as a consequence of its high-grade lipophilicity.

To test this hypothesis, fluorescence anisotropy studies were carried out in order to evaluate the effect of CRY and its concentration on the fluidity of the SPC bilayer membrane of liposomes. The results obtained were compared with that produced by cholesterol (Chol) on the membrane behavior (Figure 9). Fluorescence anisotropy studies have found that lipophilic molecules, such as cholesterol and caryophyllene sesquiterpene, can affect the typical fluidity of SPC-based vesicles and reduce the mobility of the hydrocarbon chains of membrane fatty acids. In order to determine how CRY affects membrane structure, we analyze the extent to which this molecule mimics the behavior of cholesterol in L_d liposomes. Liposomes made of SPC, SPC/Chol and SPC/CRY respectively were tested.

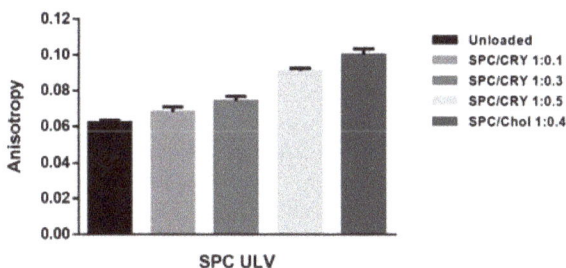

Figure 9. Anisotropy measures obtained by DPH-probe fluorescence for 1:0.1, 1:0.3 and 1:0.5 SPC/CRY ULV and 1:0.4 SPC/cholesterol (Chol) ULV.

As shown in Figure 9, conventional SPC ULV liposomes produced an average anisotropy value of 0.062. SPC bilayer was expected to be in a homogenous liquid disordered (L_d) state; the low anisotropy value obtained reflects the freedom of movement of the DPH fluorophore in the fluid disordered state of plain SPC liposome.

The thickening effect obtained as a result of cholesterol addition to a fluid bilayer is well documented [27] and the results reported in Figure 9 are in good agreement with previous published data. When cholesterol 40% mol/mol was incorporated in L_d SPC/Chol bilayer, in fact, the DPH fluorescence anisotropy increases, thus indicating that at this cholesterol amount, a greater order level exists for the phospholipid acyl chain packing. According to Marsh [28], cholesterol in the liposomal fluid bilayer promotes the formation of a phase that coexists with the L_d phase. In SPC/Chol liposomes the close contact between the sterol and adjacent phospholipids results in the formation of the so called liquid-ordered (L_o) phase. This new intermediate fluid phase exhibits translational degrees of freedom of the lipid molecules that are similar to those in a conventional fluid bilayer state, while the conformational degrees of freedom of the lipid hydrocarbon chains resemble those of the gel state. In contrast, a progressive increase of the anisotropy value appeared for CRY-loaded liposomes that is proportional to the amount of drug incorporated into the vesicles bilayer.

Increasing the mixing ratios between SPC and CRY, the fluorescence anisotropies of DPH were increased almost linearly, suggesting that rotational motion of DPH in SPC liposomes was restricted by CRY entrapment. Comparing the behaviour of SPC/CRY ULV with a 1:0.5 molar ratio and that of SPC/Chol ULV, very similar anisotropy values were found (Figure 9).

In line with these results, our hypothesis is that liposome formulations with a higher than 1:0.1 molar ratio between SPC and CRY can modify the phospholipid bilayer organization, thus hindering drug release.

4. Discussion

Low solubility of the natural sesquiterpene β-caryophyllene (CRY) in aqueous fluids and the subsequent poor bioavailability represent key aspects limiting its use in therapy. CRY also exhibited sensitivity to light, oxygen, humidity, and high temperatures [29]: these conditions decrease its stability and limit its biological effectiveness. A possible strategy to overcome these problems is the use of drug delivery systems, which may provide much higher bioavailability of this compound and ensure obtaining desired biological effects. Previous studies proposed cyclodextrin complexation to improve the bioavailability of CRY [30–32]. Recently, oil/water microemulsions have been also reported to possess suitable properties for effective topical delivery of β-caryophyllene [33].

Many synthetic and herbal drugs possess the problem of poor oral bioavailability, due to their very low water solubility or poor permeation through the biological membranes, thus leading to a limited dissolution profile in biological fluids and inefficacy in therapy. Increased reports highlighted the promising role of phospholipid-based formulations as effective drug delivery systems for natural bioactive constituents [34]. Being the main components of cellular membrane, phospholipids are characterized by an excellent biocompatibility; also, they possess amphiphilic structures and surface-active wetting characteristics, which allow enhancing the hydrophilicity of hydrophobic compounds. In water, phospholipids self-assemble into supramolecular aggregates, among which liposomes displayed high cell affinity and tissue compatibility, improving drug stability and ability to deliver both hydrophilic and lipophilic substances [34].

In line with this evidence, in the present study the internalization of CRY into the cells was increased using soybean phosphatidylcholine (SPC) liposomes Our hypothesis was that CRY, when administered as liposomal formulations, rationally designed in term of drug to lipid ratio, can be easily uptaken from cells, thus leading to an improved antiproliferative activity. SPC has been used as phospholipid molecule forming the lipid bilayer not only for its structural similarity with cell biomembrane constituents, but also for its ability to affect the cholesterol-induced stiffening of cancer cell biomembrane, which has been found responsible for reduced drug permeability and chemoresistance development in cancer cells [21].

In our cancer cell models, high concentrations of SPC exhibited early cytotoxicity signs, likely due to its ability to increase the permeability of cancer cell biomembrane, through the interference with cholesterol accumulation. In line with this evidence and considering that previous studies highlighted the ability of phosphatidylcholine to induce cholesterol depletion and to be inversely related to cholesterol amount [35,36], we hypothesize that the cytotoxicity found at higher concentrations of plain SPC liposomes can be, at least in part, due to a cholesterol transfer between liposomes and cells. Liposomes could reduce the cholesterol/phospholipid ratio and increase lipid disorder in cell membrane. Depletion of cholesterol in cell thus, could make cell more vulnerable, also to physical stress [37]; similarly, methyl-beta-cyclodextrin has been used for cholesterol removal, although the effect was incomplete [38].

Under our experimental conditions, the encapsulation of CRY within SPC liposomes highlighted that the cellular uptake of CRY can be improved or reduced as a function of the molar ratio between SPC and CRY.

Characterizing the optimal concentration of CRY in liposomal formulations represents a key point for the increase of its antiproliferative effectiveness. Both ULV and MLV liposomes loaded with the highest molar ratio between SPC and CRY (i.e., 1:0.5) induced a progressive loss of the antiproliferative potential of the sesquiterpene. The results obtained highlighted that, despite a possible improvement of low-dose CRY cytotoxicity, increased molar ratio between SPC and CRY markedly interfere with the biological activity of pure compound. This phenomenon suggests that the substance can be greatly retained and become stuck into liposomes, likely due to a stable interaction between CRY and phosphatidylcholine and a stiffening of the membrane structure, which hinders the sesquiterpene release by vesicles and its uptake into cells. Accordingly, Sarpietro et al. [39] showed that CRY possessed a great capacity to interact with membrane phospholipids and to spread through the lipophilic matrix, determining an alteration of the cooperativity. This hypothesis is also in agreement with the more accepted ordering effect induced by cholesterol in biomembrane bilayer and SPC ULV [28]. Therefore, we hypothesize that incorporating high concentrations of CRY in the ULV bilayer can alter membrane packing of SPC liposomes by inducing conformational phospholipid ordering, thus leading to a decreased fluidity and permeability of the bilayer of the phospholipid carrier.

The enhanced rigidity of the membrane, that could be generated by the inclusion of hydrophobic CRY, might seal the system and reduce the drug release. Moreover, the release of high CRY concentrations embedded within the lipid bilayers could be compromised due to strong hydrophobic interactions that might develop between the drug and the phospholipid acyl chains.

The trend displayed by SPC multilamellar vesicles support the hypothesis of the reduced bioactivity of CRY due to a condensing effect of this molecule on the bilayer. In fact, the results observed with the MLV system were partly similar to SPC ULV only at the highest CRY concentrations. We reasonable speculate that CRY reduces the fluidity of the SPC MLV bilayer to a lesser extent with respect to SPC ULV. In fact, for a fixed SPC/CRY ratio, the number of CRY molecules included in each of the lamella of the multilamellar carrier was smaller with respect to ULV, thus leading to a reduced extent of the stiffness effect.

5. Conclusions

In the present study, SPC liposomes have been developed as potential effective delivery systems to increase the in vitro bioavailability and stability of the natural sesquiterpene CRY. According to widely accepted evidence that release is governed by molecule lipophilicity and liposome features, our results allow us to hypothesize that CRY release by SPC liposomes is strictly dependent on lamellarity and drug-to-lipid ratio. Lipid-to-drug ratio is a critical parameter as it may influence the therapeutic efficacy of the drug, in particular with lipophilic drugs. The increase of drug encapsulation could be not a valid strategy in liposomal formulation, as the drug release properties of the liposomal product could be negatively affected by the molar concentration of drug in liposomes. In fact, as SPC liposome loading increases, a condensing effect of the loaded molecule on the fluid bilayer occurs. As a consequence, the substance can be greatly retained, and its release restrained. In the case of CRY, this feature can negatively affect and hinder its anticancer effectiveness. Therefore, the SPC to CRY ratio seems to represent a key tool for the development of optimized liposomal formulation to control membrane fluidity and permeability of SPC liposomes, and thus predict the release abilities. In fact, low-loaded MLV appears to induce the maximum increase of CRY antiproliferative activity in both HepG2 and

MDA-MB-468 cells, thus suggesting the ability of these formulations to better carry the lipophilic cargo inside cells. However, further in vitro studies are necessary to measure the CRY release by SPC vesicles and the achieved intracellular levels effectively.

In conclusion, our results highlight the importance of rationally designing formulations to develop the optimal liposomal composition, taking into account not only the chemical nature of the payload but also that the high drug loading in liposomes could be critical for the maximum usefulness of its therapeutic potential.

Author Contributions: Conceptualization, A.D.S., P.P. and S.P.; Formal analysis, A.D.S., P.P. and M.N.; Funding acquisition, A.D.S.; Investigation, A.D.S., P.P., M.N., L.A., S.G., S.D.G. and S.P.; Methodology, A.D.S., P.P., S.D.G., M.A.C. and S.P.; Project administration, A.D.S., P.P. and S.P.; Supervision, G.M. and M.A.C.; Visualization, A.D.S. and M.N.; Writing–original draft, A.D.S., P.P., G.M., M.A.C. and S.P.

Funding: This research was partly funded by Sapienza University grant number C26A14MWNR (A. Di Sotto). Fellowships of A.D.S. and S.D.G. were funded by the Enrico and Enrica Sovena Foundation (Italy).

Conflicts of Interest: The authors declare no conflict of interest.

References

1. Di Sotto, A.; Evandri, M.G.; Mazzanti, G. Antimutagenic and mutagenic activities of some terpenes in the bacterial reverse mutation assay. *Mutat. Res.* **2008**, *653*, 130–133. [CrossRef]
2. Fidyt, K.; Fiedorowicz, A.; Strządała, L.; Szumny, A. β-caryophyllene and β-caryophyllene oxide-natural compounds of anticancer and analgesic properties. *Cancer Med.* **2016**, *5*, 3007–3017. [CrossRef] [PubMed]
3. Gertsch, J. Antiinflammatory cannabinoids in diet—Towards a better understanding of CB2 receptor action? *Commun. Integr. Biol.* **2008**, *1*, 26–28. [CrossRef] [PubMed]
4. Bento, A.F.; Marcon, R.; Dutra, R.C.; Claudino, R.F.; Cola, M.; Leite, D.F.; Calixto, J.B. β-Caryophyllene inhibits dextran sulfate sodium-induced colitis in mice through CB2 receptor activation and PPARγ pathway. *Am. J. Pathol.* **2011**, *178*, 1153–1166. [CrossRef] [PubMed]
5. Chang, H.J.; Kim, J.M.; Lee, J.C.; Kim, W.K.; Chun, H.S. Protective effect of betacaryophyllene; a natural bicyclic sesquiterpene; against cerebral ischemic injury. *J. Med. Food* **2013**, *16*, 471–480. [CrossRef] [PubMed]
6. Liu, H.; Song, Z.; Liao, D.; Zhang, T.; Liu, F.; Zhuang, K.; Luo, K.; Yang, L. Neuroprotective effects of trans-caryophyllene against kainic acid induced seizure activity and oxidative stress in mice. *Neurochem. Res.* **2015**, *40*, 118–123. [CrossRef]
7. Viveros-Paredes, J.M.; González-Castañeda, R.E.; Gertsch, J.; Chaparro-Huerta, V.; López-Roa, R.I.; Vázquez-Valls, E.; Beas-Zarate, C.; Camins-Espuny, A.; Flores-Soto, M.E. Neuroprotective Effects of β-Caryophyllene against Dopaminergic Neuron Injury in a Murine Model of Parkinson's Disease Induced by MPTP. *Pharmaceuticals* **2017**, *10*, 60. [CrossRef]
8. Di Sotto, A.; Mazzanti, G.; Carbone, F.; Hrelia, P.; Maffei, F.; Mazzanti, G. Inhibition by beta-caryophyllene of ethyl methanesulfonate-induced clastogenicity in cultured human lymphocytes. *Mutat. Res.* **2010**, *699*, 23–28. [CrossRef]
9. Di Giacomo, S.; Mazzanti, G.; Di Sotto, A. Mutagenicity of cigarette butt waste in the bacterial reverse mutation assay: The protective effects of β-caryophyllene and β-caryophyllene oxide. *Environ. Toxicol.* **2016**, *31*, 1319–1328. [CrossRef]
10. Di Giacomo, S.; Abete, L.; Cocchiola, R.; Mazzanti, G.; Eufemi, M.; Di Sotto, A. Caryophyllane sesquiterpenes inhibit DNA-damage by tobacco smoke in bacterial and mammalian cells. *Food Chem. Toxicol.* **2018**, *111*, 393–404. [CrossRef]
11. Hanušová, V.; Caltová, K.; Svobodová, H.; Ambrož, M.; Skarka, A.; Murínová, N.; Králová, V.; Tomšík, P.; Skálová, L. The effects of β-caryophyllene oxide and trans-nerolidol on the efficacy of doxorubicin in breast cancer cells and breast tumor-bearing mice. *Biomed. Pharmacother.* **2017**, *95*, 828–836. [CrossRef]
12. Di Giacomo, S.; Di Sotto, A.; El-Readi, M.Z.; Mazzanti, G.; Wink, M. Chemosensitizing Properties of β-Caryophyllene and β-Caryophyllene Oxide in Combination with Doxorubicin in Human Cancer Cells. *Anticancer Res.* **2017**, *37*, 1191–1196. [PubMed]

13. Fontes, L.B.A.; Dias, D.D.S.; Aarestrup, B.J.V.; Aarestrup, F.M.; Da Silva Filho, A.A.; Corrêa, J.O.D.A. β-Caryophyllene ameliorates the development of experimental autoimmune encephalomyelitis in C57BL/6 mice. *Biomed. Pharmacother.* **2017**, *91*, 257–264. [CrossRef] [PubMed]

14. Zhou, L.; Zhan, M.L.; Tang, Y.; Xiao, M.; Li, M.; Li, Q.S.; Yang, L.; Li, X.; Chen, W.W.; Wang, Y.L. Effects of β-caryophyllene on arginine ADP-ribosyltransferase 1-mediated regulation of glycolysis in colorectal cancer under high-glucose conditions. *Int. J. Oncol.* **2018**, *53*, 1613–1624. [CrossRef]

15. Kawabata, Y.; Wada, K.; Nakatani, M.; Yamada, S.; Onoue, S. Formulation design for poorly water-soluble drugs based on biopharmaceutics classification system: Basic approaches and practical applications. *Int. J. Pharm.* **2011**, *420*, 1–10. [CrossRef] [PubMed]

16. Sarfraz, M.; Afzal, A.; Raza, S.M.; Bashir, S.; Madni, A.; Khan, M.W.; Ma, X.; Xiang, G. Liposomal co-delivered oleanolic acid attenuates doxorubicin-induced multi-organ toxicity in hepatocellular carcinoma. *Oncotarget* **2017**, *8*, 47136–47153. [CrossRef]

17. Yang, G.; Yang, T.; Zhang, W.; Lu, M.; Ma, X.; Xiang, G. In vitro and in vivo antitumor effects of folatetargeted ursolic acid stealth liposome. *J. Agric. Food Chem.* **2014**, *62*, 2207–2215. [CrossRef]

18. Coimbra, M.; Isacchi, B.; van Bloois, L.; Torano, J.S.; Ket, A.; Wu, X.; Broere, F.; Metselaar, J.M.; Rijcken, C.J.; Storm, G.; et al. Improving solubility and chemical stability of natural compounds for medicinal use by incorporation into liposomes. *Int. J. Pharm.* **2011**, *416*, 433–442. [CrossRef]

19. Rodríguez, J.; Martín, M.J.; Ruiz, M.A.; Clares, B. Current encapsulation strategies for bioactive oils: From alimentary to pharmaceuical perspectives. *Food Res. Int.* **2016**, *83*, 41–59. [CrossRef]

20. Mishra, G.P.; Bagui, M.; Tamboli, V.; Mitra, A.K. Recent applications of liposomes in ophthalmic drug delivery. *J. Drug Deliv.* **2011**, *2011*, 863734. [CrossRef] [PubMed]

21. Lladó, V.; López, D.J.; Ibarguren, M.; Alonso, M.; Soriano, J.B.; Escribá, P.V.; Busquets, X. Regulation of the cancer cell membrane lipid composition by NaCHOleate: Effects on cell signaling and therapeutical relevance in glioma. *Biochim. Biophys. Acta* **2014**, *1838*, 1619–1627. [CrossRef] [PubMed]

22. Kannan, V.; Balabathula, P.; Divi, M.K.; Thoma, L.A.; Wood, G.C. Optimization of drug loading to improve physical stability of paclitaxel-loaded long-circulating liposomes. *J. Liposome Res.* **2015**, *25*, 308–315. [CrossRef] [PubMed]

23. Bangham, A.D. Properties and uses of lipid vesicles: An overview. *Ann. N. Y. Acad. Sci.* **1978**, *308*, 2–7. [CrossRef] [PubMed]

24. Yoshida, Y.; Furuya, E.; Tagawa, K. A direct colorimetric method for the determination of phospholipids with dithiocyanatoiron reagent. *J. Biochem.* **1980**, *88*, 463–468. [CrossRef] [PubMed]

25. Di Sotto, A.; Mazzanti, G.; Savickiene, N.; Staršelskyte, R.; Baksenskaite, V.; Di Giacomo, S.; Vitalone, A. Antimutagenic and antioxidant activity of a protein fraction from aerial parts of Urtica dioica. *Pharm. Biol.* **2014**, *53*, 935–938. [CrossRef] [PubMed]

26. International Organization for Standardization. *Biological Evaluation of Medical Devices—Part 5: Tests for In Vitro Cytotoxicity (ISO 10993-5)*; International Organization for Standardization: Geneva, Switzerland, 2009.

27. Botrè, F.; Esposito, S.; de la Torre, X. How we risk: Liposomes and steroids. In *Recent Advances in Doping Analysis*; Schanzer, W., Geyer, H., Gotzmann, A., Mareck, U., Eds.; Sport und Buch Strauß: Koln, Germany, 2011; Volume 19, pp. 24–33.

28. Marsh, D. Liquid-ordered phases induced by cholesterol: A compendium of binary phase diagrams. *Biochim. Biophys. Acta* **2010**, *1798*, 688–699. [CrossRef] [PubMed]

29. Sköld, M.; Karlberg, A.T.; Matura, M.; Börje, A. The fragrance chemical β-caryophyllene-air oxidation and skin sensitization. *Food Chem. Toxicol.* **2006**, *44*, 538–545. [CrossRef] [PubMed]

30. Liu, H.; Yang, G.; Tang, Y.; Cao, D.; Qi, T.; Qi, Y.; Fan, G. Physicochemical characterization and pharmacokinetics evaluation of β-caryophyllene/β-cyclodextrin inclusion complex. *Int. J. Pharm.* **2013**, *450*, 304–310. [CrossRef]

31. Lou, J.; Teng, Z.; Zhang, L.; Yang, J.; Ma, L.; Wang, F.; Tian, X.; An, R.; Yang, M.; Zhang, Q.; et al. β-Caryophyllene/Hydroxypropyl-β-Cyclodextrin Inclusion Complex Improves Cognitive Deficits in Rats with Vascular Dementia through the Cannabinoid Receptor Type 2—Mediated Pathway. *Front. Pharmacol.* **2017**, *8*, 2. [CrossRef]

32. Quintans-Júnior, L.J.; Araújo, A.A.; Brito, R.G.; Santos, P.L.; Quintans, J.S.; Menezes, P.P.; Serafini, M.R.; Silva, G.F.; Carvalho, F.M.; Brogden, N.K.; et al. β-caryophyllene; a dietary cannabinoid; complexed with β-cyclodextrin produced anti-hyperalgesic effect involving the inhibition of Fos expression in superficial dorsal horn. *Life Sci.* **2016**, *149*, 34–41. [CrossRef]

33. De Oliveira Neves, J.K.; Apolinário, A.C.; Alcantara Saraiva, K.L.; da Silva, D.T.C.; de Freitas Araújo Reis, M.Y.; de Lima Damasceno, B.P.G.; Pessoa, A.; Moraes Galvão, M.A.; Soares, L.A.L.; Veiga Júnior, V.F.; et al. Microemulsions containing Copaifera multijuga Hayne oil-resin: Challenges to achieve an efficient system for β-caryophyllene delivery. *Ind. Crops Prod.* **2018**, *111*, 185–192. [CrossRef]

34. Li, C.; Zhang, J.; Zu, Y.J.; Nie, S.F.; Cao, J.; Wang, Q.; Nie, S.P.; Deng, Z.Y.; Xie, M.Y.; Wang, S. Biocompatible and biodegradable nanoparticles for enhancement of anti-cancer activities of phytochemicals. *Chin. J. Nat. Med.* **2015**, *13*, 641–652. [CrossRef]

35. Akopian, D.; Kawashima, R.L.; Medh, J.D. Phosphatidylcholine-Mediated Aqueous Diffusion of Cellular Cholesterol Down-Regulatesthe ABCA1 Transporter in Human Skin Fibroblasts. *Int. J. Biochem. Res. Rev.* **2015**, *5*, 214–224. [CrossRef] [PubMed]

36. Nuñez-Garcia, M.; Gomez-Santos, B.; Buqué, X.; García-Rodriguez, J.L.; Romero, M.R.; Marin, J.J.G.; Arteta, B.; García-Monzón, C.; Castaño, L.; Syn, W.K.; et al. Osteopontin regulates the cross-talk between phosphatidylcholine and cholesterol metabolism in mouse liver. *J. Lipid Res.* **2017**, *58*, 1903–1915. [CrossRef]

37. Simons, K.; Ehehalt, R. Cholesterol lipid rafts and disease. *J. Clin. Investig.* **2002**, *110*, 597–603. [CrossRef]

38. Litz, J.P.; Thakkar, N.; Portet, T.; Keller, S.L. Depletion with Cyclodextrin Reveals Two Populations of Cholesterol in Model Lipid Membranes. *Biophys. J.* **2016**, *110*, 635–645. [CrossRef]

39. Sarpietro, M.G.; Di Sotto, A.; Accolla, M.L.; Castelli, F. Differential Scanning Calorimetry Study on the Interaction of β-Caryophyllene and β-Caryophyllene Oxide with Phospholipid Bilayers. *Thermochim. Acta* **2015**, *600*, 28–34. [CrossRef]

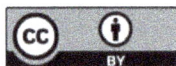

pharmaceutics

MDPI

Article

In Vitro Anticancer Activity of Extracellular Vesicles (EVs) Secreted by Gingival Mesenchymal Stromal Cells Primed with Paclitaxel

Valentina Coccè [1,†], Silvia Franzè [2,†], Anna Teresa Brini [1,3], Aldo Bruno Giannì [1,4], Luisa Pascucci [5], Emilio Ciusani [6], Giulio Alessandri [7], Giampietro Farronato [1,8], Loredana Cavicchini [1], Valeria Sordi [9], Rita Paroni [10], Michele Dei Cas [10], Francesco Cilurzo [2,*] and Augusto Pessina [1,*]

[1] CRC StaMeTec, Department of Biomedical, Surgical and Dental Sciences, University of Milan, 20133 Milan, Italy; valentina.cocce@guest.unimi.it (V.C.); anna.brini@unimi.it (A.T.B.); aldo.gianni@unimi.it (A.B.G.); giampietro.farronato@unimi.it (G.F.); loredana.cavicchini@unimi.it (L.C.)
[2] Department of Pharmaceutical Science, University of Milan, 20133 Milan, Italy; silvia.franze@unimi.it
[3] IRCCS Orthopedic Institute Galeazzi, 20161 Milan, Italy
[4] Maxillo-Facial and Dental Unit, Fondazione Ca' Granda IRCCS Ospedale Maggiore Policlinico, 20122 Milan, Italy
[5] Department of Veterinary Medicine, University of Perugia, 06123 Perugia, Italy; luisa.pascucci@unipg.it
[6] Laboratory of Clinical Pathology and Medical Genetics, Fondazione IRCCS Istituto Neurologico "C. Besta", 20133 Milan, Italy; emilio.ciusani@istituto-besta.it
[7] Cellular Neurobiology Laboratory, Department of Cerebrovascular Diseases, IRCCS Neurological Institute C. Besta, 20133 Milan, Italy; giulio.alessandri@istituto-besta.it
[8] Unit of Orthodontics and Paediatric Dentistry, Fondazione Ca' Granda IRCCS Ospedale Maggiore Policlinico, 20122 Milan, Italy
[9] Diabetes Research Institute, IRCCS San Raffaele Scientific Institute, 20132 Milan, Italy; sordi.valeria@hsr.it
[10] Department of Health Sciences of the University of Milan, 20142 Milan, Italy; rita.paroni@unimi.it (R.P.); michele.deicas@unimi.it (M.D.C.)
[*] Correspondence: francesco.cilurzo@unimi.it (F.C.); augusto.pessina@unimi.it (A.P.); Tel.: +39-0250315072 (A.P.)
[†] These authors contributed equally to this work.

Received: 6 December 2018; Accepted: 26 January 2019; Published: 1 February 2019

Abstract: Interdental papilla are an interesting source of mesenchymal stromal cells (GinPaMSCs), which are easy to isolate and expand in vitro. In our laboratory, GinPaMSCs were isolated, expanded, and characterized by studying their secretome before and after priming with paclitaxel (PTX). The secretome of GinPaMSCs did not affect the growth of cancer cell lines tested in vitro, whereas the secretome of GinPaMSCs primed with paclitaxel (GinPaMSCs/PTX) exerted a significant anticancer effect. GinPaMSCs were able to uptake and then release paclitaxel in amounts pharmacologically effective against cancer cells, as demonstrated in vitro by the direct activity of GinPaMSCs/PTX and their secretome against both human pancreatic carcinoma and squamous carcinoma cells. PTX was associated with extracellular vesicles (EVs) secreted by cells (EVs/PTX), suggesting that PTX is incorporated into exosomes during their biogenesis. The isolation of mesenchymal stromal cells (MSCs) from gingiva is less invasive than that from other tissues (such as bone marrow and fat), and GinPaMSCs provide an optimal substrate for drug-priming to obtain EVs/PTX having anticancer activity. This research may contribute to develop new strategies of cell-mediated drug delivery by EVs that are easy to store without losing function, and could have a superior safety profile in therapy.

Keywords: gingiva mesenchymal stromal cells; paclitaxel; squamous cell carcinoma; drug delivery; exosomes

1. Introduction

A large number of sources have been considered to isolate and expand mesenchymal stromal cells (MSCs), by taking into account the accessibility and availability of stem cells as well as their biological characteristics [1,2]. Most of these studies were conducted on MSCs derived from bone marrow, adipose tissue, umbilical cord blood, and, more recently, also from oral material [3–5]. Among MSCs from the oral compartment, gingival MSCs can be easily isolated, since this tissue can be removed during dental crown lengthening and periodontal surgical procedures [4,6]. As reported, MSCs from gingival papilla (GinPaMSCs) have an interesting phenotype previously described in detail [7], a relatively low osteogenic differentiation ability [8], and have significant wound healing properties that allow tissue repair without producing significant scarring [9]. Of course, most studies on MSCs have been addressed to clinical applications for regenerative medicine. The ability of MSCs to incorporate molecules and use them as a tool for drug delivery has also been proposed and intensively studied in the last years. In fact, the drug delivery mediated by MSCs can have significant advantages in comparison to the systemic administration of free chemotherapy drugs, because MSCs may migrate towards inflammatory microenvironments and accumulate in the tumor sites [10], opening up the possibility of new therapeutic anticancer strategies based on MSCs, including engineered MSCs [11,12]. Furthermore, when used in loco-regional treatments, these systems can improve the effective drug concentration in the cancer tissue and, therefore, reduce the adverse toxic effects. Moreover, vesicles might be involved in the clearance of drugs. In fact, harmful substances such as cytotoxic drugs may be associated to the vesicles, and vesicle shedding acts as a mechanism of drug expulsion. In particular, lipophilic drugs are shuttled to the plasma membrane via vesicle-mediated traffic for the final elimination [13,14]. MSCs from different sources can uptake and release drugs without any genetic manipulation, and can incorporate a significant amount of a chemotherapeutic drug (e.g., paclitaxel) that is subsequently released in quantities sufficient to affect cancer cell proliferation both in vitro and in vivo [15,16]. This capacity has also been demonstrated for mesodermal cells isolated from gingival interdental papilla [17] and dental pulp [18], suggesting that GinPaMSCs could be an interesting potential tool for cytotherapy based on cell-mediated drug delivery. Furthermore, MSC secretomes (including extracellular vesicles (EVs)) have been recently reported to be a possible alternative to MSCs for therapeutic purposes [19], being able to release accumulated drugs not only as free molecules, but also associated to exosomes and/or microvesicles [20]. Based on these observations, the present study aimed to assess the anticancer activity of secretomes from both untreated and paclitaxel (PTX)-primed GinPaMSCs, by demonstrating that both PTX-loaded GinPaMSCs and the corresponding extracellular vesicles (EVs/PTX) were active against cancer cells. This study, performed on tongue squamous cell carcinoma cell line SCC154, provides a strong proof of concept, suggesting a possible application of the procedure to collect PTX-associated EVs from drug-primed GinPaMSC working as "natural anticancer liposomes". Among the possible different MSC sources, gingiva could be the source of choice, since MSCs obtained with minimal invasive procedures are easy to expand, with high anatomical homology to treat oral neoplasia.

2. Materials and Methods

2.1. Mesenchymal Stromal Cells

Human MSCs were isolated from gingival papilla, and after expansion were characterized as previously described [7,17]. Briefly, samples of gingival tissue obtained from reductive gingivoplasty were minced with surgical scissors, treated for 3 h with type I Collagenase (50 U/mL, Life Technologies, Monza, Italy) at 37 °C under stirring conditions, and the cells were centrifuged at $300\times g$ for 10 min. The cells present in the pellets were cultured in a 25 cm² flask in Dulbecco's modified Eagle's medium with high glucose (DMEM HG) + 10% foetal bovine serum (FBS) and 1% L-glutamine (Euroclone, UK), at 37 °C in atmosphere of air + 5% CO_2. Primary cultures were then studied to evaluate the population doubling time (PDT), clonogenicity (CFU-F), and expression of the mesenchymal stem cell markers (CD73, CD90, and CD105). GinPaMSCs showed a mild expression of CD14, but they were CD45-negative and able to differentiate into osteogenic, adipogenic, and chondrogenic lineages.

2.2. PTX Loading in GinPaMSCs

To load GinPaMSCs with PTX, the cells were primed with a high amount of drug according to a standardized procedure previously described [7,15,17]. Briefly, cultures were obtained by seeding 2×10^4 cells/cm^2, and after 72 h, cells were exposed to 2 µg/mL PTX for 24 h. Then, after washing twice with phosphate buffered saline (PBS), the cell monolayer was trypsinized, washed in Hank's solution (HBSS)(Euroclone, Pero, Italy), and the PTX-primed cells (GinPaMSCs/PTX) were seeded in a 25 cm^2 flask in DMEM HG with 10% FBS and 2 mM L-glutamine (Euroclone, Pero, Italy) to release the drug. After 48 h of incubation into conditioned media (CM), PTX-loaded GinPaMSCs (GinPaMSCs/PTX/CM) were collected and tested in vitro for their anti-proliferative activity on different tumor cell lines (see Section 2.7). In particular, human pancreatic adenocarcinoma cell line CFPAC-1 was used as a standard laboratory assay according to the method reported below. CM from untreated MSCs were used as control.

2.3. Cell Cycle Analysis

A cell cycle study was performed by starting from GinPaMSCs after synchronization, obtained by serum starvation (48 h of culture in medium containing 0.5% FBS). Then, the cells were treated with PTX in 25 cm^2 flasks according to the above described standard conditions. DNA content for cell cycle phase detection was estimated by comparing untreated cells, 24 h PTX-primed cells, and cells trypsinized (i.e., drug uptake-phase), washed, and subcultured in the absence of PTX for 24 h (i.e., drug releasing phase). Briefly, cells were suspended in phosphate buffered saline (PBS) and fixed with 96% (v/v) ethanol for 1 h at 4 °C. After a PBS wash, cells were suspended in propidium iodide (50 µg/mL) in PBS. Cells were incubated overnight at 4 °C and analyzed by FC (FacsVantageSE, Becton-Dikinson, Franklin Lakes, NJ, USA).

2.4. Secretome Analysis and Extracellular Vesicles (EVs) Collection

To collect EVs, the medium of 72 h cultures of GinPaMSCs (6×10^4 cells/cm^2; both not primed and primed with PTX, as above described) was replaced with basal medium, namely DMEM HG + 1% L-glutamine without foetal bovine serum. Then, CM of cell cultures, the secretome, were collected at 24 and 48 h of incubation at 37 °C, 5% CO$_2$. To separate the PTX-loaded EVs from free PTX, aliquots of secretome were centrifuged on a 100 kDa filter device (Microsep Advance Centrifugal Devices, Life Sciences, Port Washington, NY, USA) at 5000× g for 15 min. The two fractions (i.e., EV: F > 100 kDa; free PTX: F < 100 kDa) were collected and characterized by the physico-chemical and biological assays reported below, using the whole secretome as control.

2.5. Extracellular Vesicles (EVs) Characterization

2.5.1. Phospholipids

The phospholipid concentrations present in the EVs were estimated as phosphate content, using the Rouser method and sodium dihydrogen phosphate as standard [21]. Test and standard samples were inserted in separate Pyrex glass tubes and heated at 100 °C until complete evaporation. An empty tube was used as control. To liberate phosphates, samples and standards were cleaved by addition of 300 µL of 70% perchloric acid and heated at 200 °C for 20 min. Then, 1 mL of purified water and 400 µL 1.25% w/v ammonium molybdate were added to each tube and mixed vigorously. Finally, 400 µL of 5% w/v ascorbic acid (Sigma-Aldrich, Darmstadt, Germany) was added and mixed before heating at 100 °C for 5 min. In the presence of phosphate, samples turned blue and the absorbance at 820 nm was measured. The phospholipid concentration in EVs were estimated to be proportional to the absorbance of a 40 nmol/µL standard. All analyses were performed at least in triplicate.

2.5.2. Particle Size and ζ-Potential

Particle size distribution and ζ-potentials of samples were determined using a Zetasizer (Nano-ZS, Malvern Instrument, Malvern, Worcestershire, UK). To perform dynamic light scattering (DLS) analyses, samples were opportunely diluted with ultrapure MilliQ® water to avoid the interference due to the culture medium coloration. Particle size measurements were carried out using a disposable cuvette and a detection angle of 173°. ζ-potentials were measured in the same sample. The results are expressed as the mean and standard deviation of three measurements.

2.5.3. EVs Concentration

The concentration of EVs was determined by a nanoparticle tracking assay (NTA, Nanosight NS300, Malvern Instrument, Malvern, Worcestershire, UK). A 25 µL sample was diluted with PBS to 1 mL and analyzed at 25 °C. The capture of the images was performed according to the following setting: Camera shutter 31.48 ms; 24.98 fps; detection threshold 7 multi. The results are expressed as the mean of five determinations.

2.5.4. Transmission Electron Microscopy (TEM)

The CM were analysed by a previously described TEM procedure [22]. Briefly, 20 µL of EV suspension was placed on Parafilm. A formvar-coated copper grid (Electron Microscopy Sciences, Hatfield, PA, USA) was gently placed on the top of the drop for about 60 min in a humidified chamber. Grids were then washed in 0.1 M cacodylate buffer (CB) at pH 7.3 and finally fixed for 10 min with 2.5% glutaraldehyde (Fluka, St. Louis, MO, USA) in CB. After washing in CB, EVs were contrasted with 2% uranyl acetate. The grids were then air dried and observed under a Philips EM208 transmission electron microscope (TEM) equipped with a digital camera (University Centre for Electron Microscopy (CUME), Perugia, Italy).

2.6. Mass Spectrometry Analysis

PTX extraction and purification from secretomes was performed by liquid–liquid extraction (LLE). Aliquots of 500 µL of secretome, or fractions, were added with 100 µL of internal standard (0.1 µg/mL PTX-d5, Cayman Chemicals, Ann Arbor, MI, USA) and with toluene in a ratio of 1:2 (v/v). After sonication for 30 min at 40 °C, samples were vigorously shaken at 50 oscillations/s for 15 min, then centrifuged at 10,000 rpm for 2 min. The organic phase was evaporated and re-dissolved with 100 µL methanol, and 10 µL was injected for LC–MS/MS analysis. The multiple reaction monitoring (MRM) analysis was run on a HPLC Dionex 3000 UltiMate (Thermo Fisher Scientific, Waltham, MA, USA) coupled to a tandem mass spectrometer AB Sciex 3200 QTRAP (AB Sciex S.r.l., Milan, Italy). Separation was attained on a reversed-phase analytical column (Luna®, 3 µm, C18(2) 50 × 2 mm, Phenomenex, CA, USA), with a linear gradient between eluent A (water + 5 mM ammonium formate + 0.1% formic acid) and eluent B (acetonitrile + 0.1% formic acid). After 2 min at 20%, eluent B was increased to 95% in 4 min, held for 0.5 min, taken back to the initial conditions in 0.5 min, and kept for 2 min at 20%. The flow rate was 0.4 mL/min, and the autosampler and the column oven were kept at 15 °C and 30 °C, respectively. The representative MRM transitions were 854.5 > 286.1 (PTX) and 859.4 > 291.5 (IS, PTX-d5).

2.7. Tumor Cell Lines

Human pancreatic adenocarcinoma cell line CFPAC-1 [23,24], glioblastoma multiforme cell line T98G [25], human meshotelioma cell line M20 [26], and human squamous cell carcinoma line SCC154 [27] were provided by Centro Substrati Cellulari (ISZLER, Brescia, Italy). Cells were maintained in the complete medium (Iscove modified Dulbecco's medium (IMDM) for CFPAC-1, T98G, and M20; DMEM HG for SCC154) supplemented with 10% FBS, by 1:5 weekly dilution. All reagents were provided by Euroclone, Pero, Italy.

2.8. In Vitro Anticancer Assays

The inhibitory effects of secretomes from drug-loaded GinPaMSCs, as well as the F > 100 kDa and F < 100 kDa fractions, were evaluated on the proliferation of different cancer cell lines by the MTT assay as previously described [15], taking the optical density (OD) of the cancer cell treated with EVs-unloaded GinPaMSCs as a control. The inhibitory concentration (IC_{50}) was determined according to the Reed & Muench formula [28]. To study the interaction between CFPAC-1 and GinPaMSCs, a rosette adherence assay was performed [29,30]. Briefly, 5×10^5 CFPAC-1 were mixed with GinPaMSCs or GinPaMSCs/PTX in a conical tube with 0.5 ml of IMDM + 5% foetal bovine serum (FBS; Lonza, I). The cell suspension was incubated at 37 °C in air + 5% CO_2 without stirring. After 24 h, 20 µL suspensions were collected by a micropipette from the pellet lying on the tube bottom, and then transferred on a slide in order to evaluate the rosette formation under inverted microscope (Leitz, Germany) at 100× and 200× magnifications.

2.9. Statistical Analysis

Data are expressed as average ± standard deviation (SD). Differences between mean values were evaluated according to Student's *t*-test performed by the GRAPHPADINSTAT program (GraphPad Software Inc., San Diego, CA, USA) or ANOVA, followed by the Tukey post-hoc analysis (OriginPro 2017, Origin US, Nothampton, MA, USA). *p* values ≤ 0.05 were considered statistically significant. The linearity of response and the correlation were studied using regression analysis, by Excel 2013 software.

3. Results

3.1. Sensitivity of GinPaMSCs to the Cytotoxic Activity of PTX

The sensitivity of GinPaMSCs to PTX, tested by a 24 h cytotoxic MTT assay at three logarithmic dosages of 0.1–1 and 10 µg/mL (Figure 1A), confirmed the significant resistance of MSCs to the toxic effect of PTX that did not affect significantly the cell viability. The cell cycle analysis, studied on GinPaMSCs treated with a standard dosage of 2 µg/mL for 24 h (Figure 1B), indicated a decreased number of cells in phase G0, accompanied by a significant ($p < 0.05$) increase of cells in the G2/M phase. This is compatible with the known mechanism of action of PTX, which inhibits the cell proliferation in G2/M.

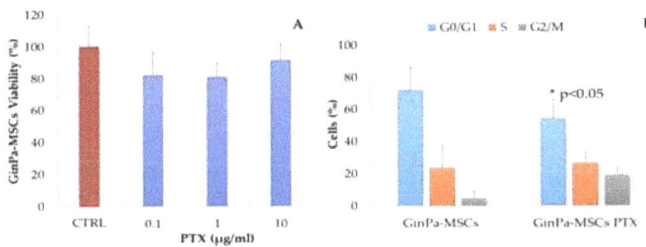

Figure 1. (**A**) Sensitivity of gingival papilla mesenchymal stem cells (GinPaMSCs) to cytotoxic activity of paclitaxel (PTX) was evaluated as cell viability at 24 h of treatment in the presence of three increasing logarithmic concentrations of the drug. The effect is expressed as percentage of the optical density measured in cultures that did not receive PTX (considered as 100%). The histogram shows the mean ± standard deviation (SD) of three independent experiments. (**B**) The histograms show the cell cycle-phase distributions of GinPaMSCs before and after treatment with 2000 ng/ml of PTX for 24 h (GinPaMSCs/PTX). Each value represents the mean ± standard deviation (*n* = 3).

3.2. Effects Exerted on Tumor Cell Growth by Cytokines Detected in the GinPaMSCs Secretome

The treatment of GinPaMSCs with PTX did not significantly modify the pattern of cytokine production, except for an increase of IL8 and MIF and a decrease of SCGFb. The secretome of

GinPaMSCs did not modulate the in vitro cancer cell proliferation independently of the cell line (Figure 2A). On the contrary, the secretome of cells primed with PTX (GinPaMSCs/PTX) exerted a dramatic dose–response inhibition of CFPAC-1 (pancreatic carcinoma) and SCC-154 (squamous carcinoma). Indeed, for both the cell lines, the regression analysis showed high coefficients of correlation (R^2), comparable to that of PTX (Figure 2B,C).

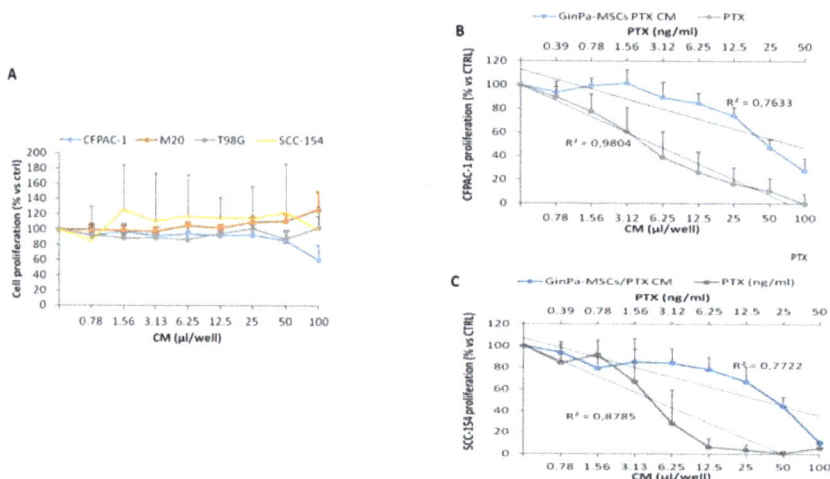

Figure 2. The activity of the GinPaMSc secretome was tested on the proliferation of four cancer cell lines (**A**). The GinPaMSCs/PTX secretome anticancer activity (blue line) and PTX solution (black line) against (**B**) pancreatic cancer cells CFPAC-1 and (**C**) squamous cell carcinoma SCC-154. The data represents the mean ± standard deviation of three independent experiments.

3.3. Direct Anticancer Activity by GinPaMSCs/PTX

The anticancer activity against CFPAC-1 and SCC-154 was confirmed by a 24 h co-culture of MSCs and cancer cells (Figure 3). Cancer cells co-cultured with GinPaMSCs did not show any sign of toxicity (Figure 3A,C), whereas many dead cancer cells were detected in the presence of GinPaMSCs/PTX, as confirmed by intracellular trypan blue uptake (Figure 3B,D).

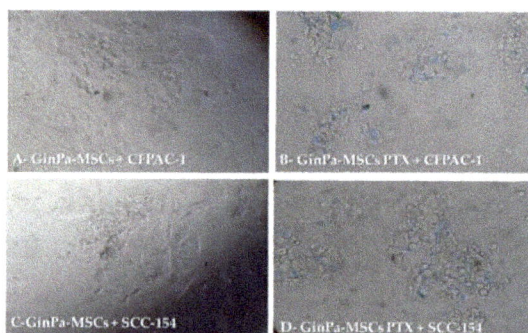

Figure 3. Direct anticancer activities of GinPaMSCs and GinPaMSCs/PTX secretomes against pancreatic cancer cells CFPAC-1 and squamous cell carcinoma SCC-154, evaluated by trypan blue in a MSCs–tumor cells co-culture system. (Panels A and C = 100× magnification, panels B and D = 200× magnification).

3.4. Characterization of EVs from GinPaMSCs and GinPaMSCs/PTX Secretome

TEM analysis of the GinPaMSCs secretome suggested the presence of EVs and exosomes with different sizes ranging from 50 to 500 nm. The treatment of GinPaMSCs with PTX did not modify the morphology of the EVs/exosome presence in either of the conditioned media (Figure 4).

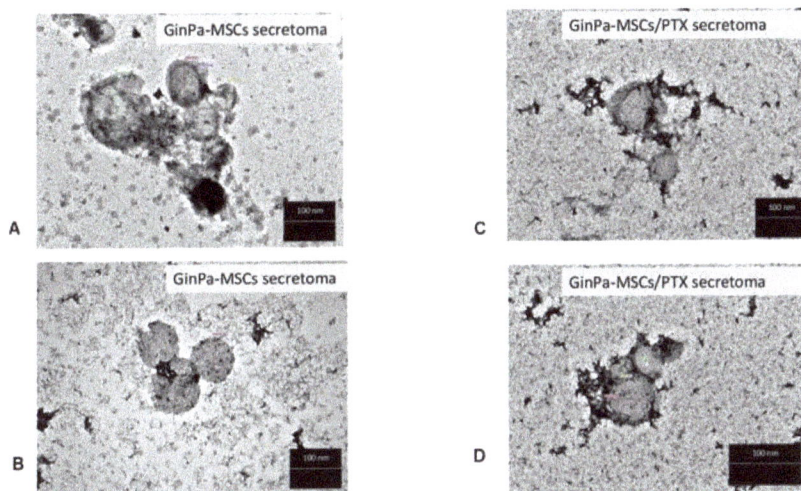

Figure 4. TEM analysis of extracellular vesicles (EVs) isolated from the secretome of cell cultures. No differences are evidenced in round-shaped morphologies of EVs from GinPaMSCs (**A,B**) and GinPaMSCs/PTX (**C,D**) with regard to size, shape, or electron density. Scale bar 100 nm.

The size distribution analysis of the isolated secretomes of GinPaMSCs was deepened both by DLS and NTA. The results of DLS analysis showed the presence of a population of microvesicles, with a particle size ranging between 200 and 300 nm, in the samples obtained from both the control and PTX-treated MSCs (Table 1). Purification by ultrafiltration led to the formation of large particles, but this increment of particle size was significant only in the case of GinPaMSCs samples (Tukey test $p = 0.0003$). This variation was not considered as a sign of particle aggregation, since the ζ-potentials showed only slight changes after purification values, maintaining the same trend (Table 1). The ζ-potential of the isolated EVs was quite negative (Table 1), and this is in line with the abundance of phosphatidylserine [31].

Table 1. Main physico-chemical features of the secretome.

	Samples	D_H (nm)	ζ-potential (mV)	Phospholipids (mM)
GinPaMSCs	unfractionated	242 ± 34	-16.6 ± 0.2	0.32 ± 0.06
	Ultra-filtrated (F > 100 kDa)	430 ± 33	-20.9 ± 0.3	0.49 ± 0.07
GinPaMSCs/PTX	unfractionated	303 ± 23	-18.1 ± 2.3	0.33 ± 0.09
	Ultra-filtrated (F > 100 kDa)	385 ± 19	-22.7 ± 0.3	0.62 ± 0.15

The presence of phospholipids, which do not represent the totality of the lipid composition of extracellular vesicles, was confirmed by the Rouser assay (Table 1). No trace of vesicles was instead found in the filtrate, confirming that the purification process did not lead to the loss of some secretomes, but only allowed the removal of free PTX.

NTA analysis of the secretome evidenced the presence of different populations of vesicles and allowed us to clarify their number distribution in the samples. In particular, the whole secretome showed three different populations at about 135 nm, 200–300 nm, and 435 nm (Figure 5). The latter was not detected in the samples obtained by GinPaMSCs/PTX, which in general showed a narrowed particle size distribution, as exemplified in Figure 5. GinPaMSCs/PTX released a higher number of extracellular vesicles than untreated GinPaMSCs ($3.01 \times 10^9 \pm 1.19 \times 10^8$ versus $2.37 \times 10^9 \pm 6.80 \times 10^7$ particles/mL, respectively) but the difference was not statistically relevant.

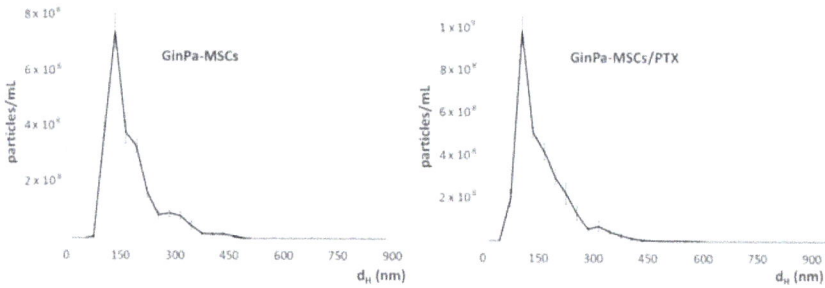

Figure 5. Size distribution analysis of the secretomes of GinPaMSCs and GinPaMSCs/PTX, analyzed by nanoparticle tracking assay (NTA). In both samples, several populations of vesicles were present at 200–300 nm.

3.5. Paclitaxel Dosage in EV Fractions of GinPaMSCs and GinPaMSCs/PTX Secretomes

The validated LC–MS/MS method was successfully applied to quantify PTX in the different samples of conditioned media from GinPaMSCs and GinPaMSCs/PTX: Unfractionated secretomes and ultra-filtered fractions (F > 100 kDa and F < 100kDa). PTX was present in both the whole secretome and the F > 100kDa fraction of PTX-treated GinPaMSCs, suggesting the incorporation or the unspecific bind of PTX to EVs (Figure 6A). No signal related to PTX was detected in the secretome of untreated GinPaMSCs used as negative controls (data not shown) or in ultra-filtered <100 GinPaMSCs/PTX samples (Figure 6C).

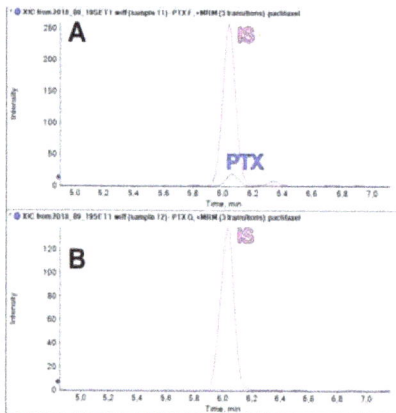

Sample	PTX (ng/ml)
Culture CM	< LOQ
GinPa MSCs CM	< LOQ
GinPa MSCs/PTX CM	54.2 ± 0.3
GinPa MSCs CM (F>100Kd)	< LOQ
GinPa MSCs CM (F<100Kd)	< LOQ
GinPa MSCs/PTX CM (F>100Kd)	36.8 ± 3.6
GinPa MSCs/PTX CM (F<100Kd)	< LOQ

LOQ (Limit of Quantification)= 1 ng/ml

Figure 6. PTX dosage by mass spectrometry in EV fractions. The chromatogram identification of PTX peaks by LC–MS/MS retention time: (**A**) F > 100 kDa fraction and (**B**) F < 100 kDa fraction, in which no PTX peaks were appreciable. PTX was quantified successfully in both the unfractioned secretome and the F > 100 kDa fraction of PTX-treated GinPaMSCs (**C**).

3.6. Anticancer Activity of EVs from GinPaMSCs and GinPaMSCs/PTX Secretomes

The anticancer activity of EVs secreted by GinPaMSCs/PTX was tested against squamous cancer cells (SCC154) (Figure 7). The activity is expressed as percentage of cell growth, normalized on the effect of EVs secreted by untreated GinPaMSCs used as controls. The fraction F < 100 kDa did not exert any activity against the cancer cell proliferation, with a non-significant coefficient of correlation ($R^2 = 0.13$). The fraction F > 100 KDa produced a significant dose-dependent inhibition of cancer cell growth, also confirmed by regression analysis ($R^2 = 0.99$), that is similar to the inhibition produced by the unfractioned secretome (CM) ($R^2 = 0.95$). These results agree with the mass spectrometry analysis that demonstrated the presence of PTX in both CM and in the F > 100 kDa (Figure 6).

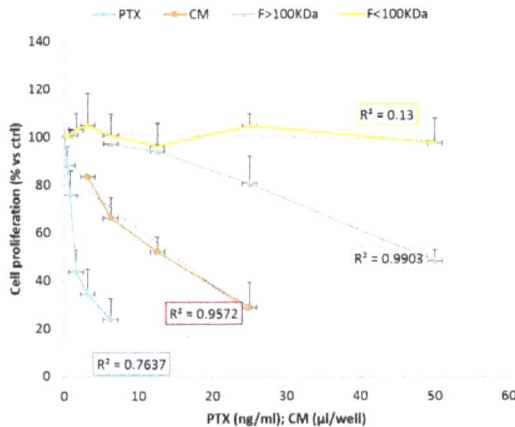

Figure 7. The anticancer activity of EVs from GinPaMSCs and GinPaMSCs/PTX tested against squamous cancer cells (SCC154). The activity is expressed as percentage of cell growth, normalized on the effect of EVs secreted by untreated GinPaMSCs used as controls (OD: 1.28 ± 0.09 was considered 100% proliferation). Data is reported as the mean ± standard deviation of three independent experiments.

4. Discussion

Our data confirm that MSCs from gingival papilla (GinPaMSCs) have a significant resistance to PTX that tested until 10,000 ng/ml, reducing the cell viability by about 20% and blocking cells in the G2/M cycle phase (Figure 1). This evidence agrees with literature data which demonstrated that the treatment of MSCs with PTX reduces their proliferation activity, migration ability, and some differentiation potentials, without significantly affecting their viability [32,33]. Of course, the analyses of secretomes of GinPaMSCs identified the presence of cytokines that did not modulate, stimulate, or inhibit the growth of four different tumor cell lines (Figure 2A). On the contrary, the secretome from the cells primed with PTX exerted a dramatic dose–response inhibition on both CFPAC-1 (pancreatic carcinoma cells) and SCC-154 (squamous carcinoma cells) (Figure 2B,C). After priming of GinPaMSCs by PTX, a little modulation of cytokine production was observed that may be considered ineffective on cancer cell growth, suggesting that the dramatic anticancer activity exerted by GinPaMSC/PTX secretomes can be mainly due to the presence of the drug secreted by PTX-primed GinPaMSCs. This result is also confirmed by the significant toxicity of GinPaMSCs/PTX only against CFPAC-1 and SCC-154, whereas cancer cells co-cultured in the presence of unprimed GinPaMSCs showed no sign of toxicity (Figure 3). Based on our previous experience with an established murine MSC line (SR4987) [20], we here investigated if primary human MSCs, particularly the gingival-derived MSCs, were able to process and then deliver PTX associated to exosomes or microvesicles. TEM analysis of GinPaMSCs secretomes demonstrated the presence of microvesicles at different sizes (Figure 4). This result was further confirmed both by dynamic light scattering (DLS) and nanoparticle tracking assay (NTA). In particular, DLS indicated the presence of a population of microvesicles ranging between 200 and 300 nm both in the secretome of GinPaMSCs and that of GinPaMSCs/PTX. Moreover, it can be assumed that isolated microvesicles shared the same origin, since the same amount of phospholipids was detected in both types of cells (Table 1). The study on size distribution by NTA evidenced three different populations in the GinPaMSCs secretome, whereas the population at about 435 nm was not detected in the Gin-PaMSCs/PTX secretome (Figure 5). This small discrepancy between NTA and DLS data depends only on the scattering intensity, because the larger the particle, the higher the contribution to the total signal. Instead, NTA allows us to provide a more reliable distribution in number. In any case, besides the slight differences in particle size distributions, it is important to highlight that the GinPaMSCs treated with PTX released a slightly higher number of EVs with respect to untreated GinPaMSCs. This difference in not statistically relevant, but this trend confirmed that PTX treatment did not affect the microvesicle biogenesis of GinPaMSCs.

The anti-proliferation activity of EVs was studied in both the unfractioned secretome (i.e., CM) and its fractions. The results confirmed that the anticancer activity was due only to the fraction containing MVs (F > 100KDa). As expected, no activity was found in the unfractioned secretomes of untreated MSCs (Figure 7), while it was a little surprising that the F < 100KDa fraction from GinPaMSCs/PTX did not contain PTX and did not present activity. This apparent discrepancy can be explained considering that a lipophilic drug, such as PTX, can be easily adsorbed and retained by filters. However, the present research was designed as a qualitative study with the main purpose to demonstrate the ability of GinPaMSCs to secrete PTX associated with EVs. A deep investigation is currently in progress to optimize the incorporation and/or release of PTX in the attempt to produce large batches of EVs by using bioreactors.

The microvesicles secreted by GinPaMSCs/PTX were active against two tumor cell lines, namely pancreatic carcinoma (CFPAC1) and tongue squamous cell carcinoma (SCC154) cell lines. As found in the preliminary screening (Figure 1), CM from GinPaMSCs/PTX was active on different tumor cell lines, and we focused the study on a human SCC model that could express an important anatomical/histological homology with the origin of MSCs generated by gingival tissue. In general, MSCs are considered as an important source of EVs and/or exosomes, and are under investigation for their role both in tumor progression and in drug delivery for tumor therapy and regenerative medicine [34–37]. As reported [20,38], upon in vitro exposure to high concentrations of PTX, MSCs can "load" the drug and deliver it by means of EVs so that the PTX-loaded EVs acquire strong anti-tumor effects on human cancers both in vitro and in vivo. Even if cancer cell-derived exosomes were proposed as effective carriers of PTX to their parental cells [39], our results demonstrated for the first time that human gingival MSCs produce a significant amount of EVs and can be considered an ideal candidate for the large production of EVs and/or exosomes. If primed with PTX, these cells can also release the drug associated to EVs and/or exosomes acting as "natural anticancer liposomes". Among the different MSC sources, our study suggests that gingival MSCs, which present an important homology with tumors originated from oral tissues (such as SCC), could be obtained with a minimally invasive procedure and easily expanded.

Currently, of paramount importance are preclinical studies, which can further corroborate the advantages of EVs. As a matter of fact, EVs could be easily manufactured in large batches by reducing the cost due to the need to personalize the cellular products, and have a superior safety profile in therapy (e.g., reduced risk related to ectopic tissue formation, microvasculature infusion toxicity, rejection) with respect to MSCs. Furthermore, the use of EVs in therapy gives the possibility to manage high drug concentrations in a minimal volume, improving the storage, the transport, and the infusion procedures [40,41].

Author Contributions: Conceptualization, A.P., G.A. and F.C.; Methodology, S.F., V.C., L.P., E.C. and V.S.; Formal Analysis, V.C., S.F.; Investigation, S.F., V.C., L.P., M.C.D. and L.C.; Data Curation, A.P., F.C. and V.C.; Vriting—Original Draft Preparation, A.P., F.C.; Writing—Review & Editing, A.P., F.C.; Supervision, R.P., A.T.B., A.B.G. and G.F.; Funding Acquisition, A.T.B., A.B.G. and G.F.

Funding: This research received no external funding.

Conflicts of Interest: The authors declare no conflict of interest.

References

1. Bortolotti, F.; Ukovich, L.; Razban, V.; Martinelli, V.; Ruozi, G.; Pelos, B.; Dore, F.; Giacca, M.; Zacchigna, S. In vivo therapeutic potential of mesenchymal stromal cells depends on the source and the isolation procedure. *Stem Cell Rep.* **2015**, *4*, 332–339. [CrossRef]

2. Liu, Q.; Zhang, X.; Jiao, Y.; Liu, X.; Wang, Y.; Li, S.L.; Zhang, W.; Chen, F.M.; Ding, Y.; Jiang, C.; et al. In vitro cell behaviors of bone mesenchymal stem cells derived from normal and postmenopausal osteoporotic rats. *Int. J. Mol. Med.* **2018**, *41*, 669–678. [CrossRef]

3. Xiao, L.; Nasu, M. From regenerative dentistry to regenerative medicine: Progress, challenges, and potential applications of oral stem cells. *Stem Cells Cloning* **2014**, *7*, 89–99. [CrossRef] [PubMed]

4. Egusa, H.; Sonoyama, W.; Nishimura, M.; Atsuta, I.; Akiyama, K. Stem cells in dentistry–part I: Stem cell sources. *J. Prosthodont. Res.* **2012**, *56*, 151–165. [CrossRef]

5. Bakopoulou, A.; Apatzidou, D.; Aggelidou, E.; Gousopoulou, E.; Leyhausen, G.; Volk, J.; Kritis, A.; Koidis, P.; Geurtsen, W. Isolation and prolonged expansion of oral mesenchymal stem cells under clinical-grade, GMP-compliant conditions differentially affects stemness properties. *Stem Cell Res. Ther.* **2017**, *8*, 247. [CrossRef]

6. Fawzy El-Sayed, K.M.; Mekhemar, M.K.; Beck-Broichsitter, B.E.; Bähr, T.; Hegab, M.; Receveur, J.; Heneweer, C.; Becker, S.T.; Wiltfang, J.; Dörfer, C.E. Periodontal regeneration employing gingival margin-derived stem/progenitor cells in conjunction with IL-1ra-hydrogel synthetic extracellular matrix. *J. Clin. Periodontol.* **2015**, *42*, 448–457. [CrossRef] [PubMed]

7. Brini, A.T.; Coccè, V.; Ferreira, L.M.; Giannasi, C.; Cossellu, G.; Giannì, A.B.; Angiero, F.; Bonomi, A.; Pascucci, L.; Falchetti, M.L.; et al. Cell-mediated drug delivery by gingival interdental papilla mesenchymal stromal cells (GinPaMSCs) loaded with paclitaxel. *Expert Opin. Drug Deliv.* **2016**, *13*, 789–798.

8. Moshaverinia, A.; Chen, C.; Xu, X.; Akiyama, K.; Ansari, S.; Zadeh, H.H.; Shi, S. Bone regeneration potential of stem cells derived from periodontal ligament or gingival tissue sources encapsulated in RGD-modified alginate scaffold. *Tissue Eng. Part A* **2014**, *20*, 611–621. [CrossRef] [PubMed]

9. Larjava, H.; Wiebe, C.; Gallant-Behm, C.; Hart, D.A.; Heino, J.; Häkkinen, L. Exploring scarless healing of oral soft tissues. *J. Can. Dent. Assoc.* **2011**, *77*, b18. [PubMed]

10. Reagan, M.R.; Kaplan, D.L. Concise review: Mesenchymal stem cell tumor-homing: Detection methods in disease model systems. *Stem Cells* **2011**, *29*, 920–927. [CrossRef] [PubMed]

11. Sasportas, L.S.; Kasmieh, R.; Wakimoto, H.; Hingtgen, S.; van de Water, J.A.; Mohapatra, G.; Figueiredo, J.L.; Martuza, R.L.; Weissleder, R.; Shah, K. Assessment of therapeutic efficacy and fate of engineered human mesenchymal stem cells for cancer therapy. *Proc. Natl. Acad. Sci. USA* **2009**, *106*, 4822–48277. [CrossRef] [PubMed]

12. Stuckey, D.W.; Shah, K. TRAIL on trial: Preclinical advances in cancer therapy. *Trends Mol. Med.* **2013**, *19*, 685–694. [CrossRef] [PubMed]

13. Shedden, K.; Xie, X.T.; Chandaroy, P.; Chang, Y.T.; Rosalia, G.R. Expulsion of small molecules in vesicles shed by cancer cells: Association with gene expression and chemosensitivity profiles. *Cancer Res.* **2003**, *63*, 4331–4337. [PubMed]

14. Chen, V.Y.; Posada, M.M.; Blazer, L.L.; Zhao, T.; Rosania, G.R. The role of the VPS4A-exosome pathway in the intrinsic egress route of a DNA-binding anticancer drug. *Pharm. Res.* **2006**, *23*, 1687–1695. [CrossRef] [PubMed]

15. Pessina, A.; Bonomi, A.; Coccè, V.; Invernici, G.; Navone, S.; Cavicchini, L.; Sisto, F.; Ferrari, M.; Viganò, L.; Locatelli, A.; et al. Mesenchymal stromal cells primed with paclitaxel provide a new approach for cancer therapy. *PLoS ONE* **2011**, *6*, e28321. [CrossRef]

16. Pessina, A.; Leonetti, C.; Artuso, S.; Benetti, A.; Dessy, E.; Pascucci, L.; Passeri, D.; Orlandi, A.; Berenzi, A.; Bonomi, A.; et al. Drug-releasing mesenchymal cells strongly suppress B16 lung metastasis in a syngeneic murine model. *J. Exp. Clin. Cancer Res.* **2015**, *34*, 82. [CrossRef] [PubMed]

17. Coccè, V.; Farronato, D.; Brini, A.T.; Masia, C.; Giannì, A.B.; Piovani, G.; Sisto, F.; Alessandri, G.; Angiero, F.; Pessina, A. Drug Loaded Gingival Mesenchymal Stromal Cells (GinPaMSCs) Inhibit In Vitro Proliferation of Oral Squamous Cell Carcinoma. *Sci. Rep.* **2017**, *7*, 9376. [CrossRef] [PubMed]

18. Salehi, H.; Al-Arag, S.; Middendorp, E.; Gergely, C.; Cuisinier, F.; Orti, V. Dental pulp stem cells used to deliver the anticancer drug paclitaxel. *Stem Cell Res. Ther.* **2018**, *9*, 103. [CrossRef] [PubMed]

19. Crivelli, B.; Chlapanidas, T.; Perteghella, S.; Lucarelli, E.; Pascucci, L.; Brini, A.T.; Ferrero, I.; Marazzi, M.; Pessina, A.; Torre, M.L. Italian Mesenchymal Stem Cell Group (GISM). Mesenchymal stem/stromal cell extracellular vesicles: From active principle to next generation drug delivery system. *J. Control. Release* **2017**, *262*, 104–117. [CrossRef]

20. Pascucci, L.; Coccè, V.; Bonomi, A.; Ami, D.; Ceccarelli, P.; Ciusani, E.; Viganò, L.; Locatelli, A.; Sisto, F.; Doglia, S.M.; et al. Paclitaxel is incorporated by mesenchymal stromal cells and released in exosomes that inhibit in vitro tumor growth: A new approach for drug delivery. *J. Control. Release* **2014**, *192*, 262–270. [CrossRef]

21. Franzé, S.; Marengo, A.; Stella, B.; Minghetti, P.; Arpicco, S.; Cilurzo, F. Hyaluronan-decorated liposomes as drug delivery systems for cutaneous administration. *Int. J. Pharm.* **2018**, *535*, 333–339. [CrossRef] [PubMed]

22. Hayat, M.F. *Principles and Techniques of Electron Microscopy: Biological Applications*, 4th ed.; Cambridge University Press: Cambridge, UK, 2000.

23. McIntosh, J.C.; Schoumacher, R.A.; Tiller, R.E. Pancreatic adenocarcinoma in a patient with cystic fibrosis. *Am. J. Med.* **1988**, *85*, 592. [CrossRef]

24. Schoumacher, R.A.; Ram, J.; Iannuzzi, M.C.; Bradbury, N.A.; Wallace, R.W.; Hon, C.T.; Kelly, D.R.; Schmid, S.M.; Gelder, F.B.; Rado, T.A. A cystic fibrosis pancreatic adenocarcinoma cell line. *Proc. Natl. Acad. Sci. USA* **1990**, *87*, 4012–4016. [CrossRef] [PubMed]

25. Stein, G.H.T. 98G: An anchorage-independent human tumor cell line that exhibits stationary phase G1 arrest in vitro. *J. Cell. Physiol.* **1979**, *99*, 43–54. [CrossRef] [PubMed]

26. Treves, A.J.; Halperin, M.; Barak, V.; Bar-Tana, R.; Halimi, M.; Fibach, E.; Gamliel, H.; Leizerowitz, R.; Polliack, A. A new myelomonoblastic cell line (M20): Analysis of properties, differentiation, and comparison with other established lines of similar origin. *Exp. Hematol.* **1985**, *13*, 281–288. [PubMed]

27. Martin, C.L.; Reshmi, S.C.; Ried, T.; Gottberg, W.; Wilson, J.W.; Reddy, J.K.; Gollin, S.M. Chromosomal imbalances in oral squamous cell carcinoma. Examination of 31 cell lines and review of the literature. *Oral Oncol.* **2008**, *44*, 369–382. [CrossRef] [PubMed]

28. Reed, L.J.; Muench, H. A simple method of estimating fifty percent endpoints. *Am. J. Hyg.* **1938**, *27*, 493–497.

29. Aizawa, S.; Hojo, H.; Tsuda, A.; Sai, M.; Toyama, K. Rosette formation between stromal and hemopoietic cells: A simple assay for the supportive activity of stromal cells. *Leukemia* **1991**, *5*, 273–276. [PubMed]

30. Pessina, A.; Coccè, V.; Pascucci, L.; Bonomi, A.; Cavicchini, L.; Sisto, F.; Ferrari, M.; Ciusani, E.; Crovace, A.; Falchetti, M.L.; et al. Mesenchymal stromal cells primed with Paclitaxel attract and kill leukaemia cells, inhibit angiogenesis and improve survival of leukaemia-bearing mice. *Br. J. Haematol.* **2013**, *160*, 766–778. [CrossRef] [PubMed]

31. Van Dommelen, S.M.; Vader, P.; Lakhal, S.; Kooijmans, S.A.; van Solinge, W.W.; Wood, M.J.; Schiffelers, R.M. Microvesicles and exosomes: Opportunities for cell-derived membrane vesicles in drug delivery. *J. Control. Release* **2012**, *161*, 635–644. [CrossRef] [PubMed]

32. Bosco, D.B.; Kenworthy, R.; Zorio, D.A.R.; Sang, Q.-X.A. Human Mesenchymal Stem Cells Are Resistant to Paclitaxel by Adopting a Non-Proliferative Fibroblastic State. *PLoS ONE* **2015**, *10*, e0128511. [CrossRef] [PubMed]

33. Münz, F.; Perez, R.L.; Trinh, T.; Sisombath, S.; Weber, K.-J.; Wuchter, P.; Debus, J.; Saffrich, R.; Huber, P.E.; Nicolay, N.H. Human mesenchymal stem cellslose their functional properties after paclitaxel treatment. *Sci. Rep.* **2018**, *8*, 312.

34. Bruno, A.; Pagani, A.; Pulze, L.; Albini, A.; Dallaglio, K.; Noonan, D.M.; Mortara, L. Orchestration of angiogenesis by immune cells. *Front. Oncol.* **2014**, *4*, 131. [CrossRef]

35. Fatima, F.; Navaz, M. Stem cell-derived exosomes: Roles in stromal remodeling, tumor progression, and cancer immunotherapy. *Chin. J. Cancer* **2015**, *34*, 541–553. [CrossRef] [PubMed]

36. Lai, R.C.; Yeo, R.W.; Tan, K.H.; Lim, S.K. Exosomes for drug delivery—A novel application for the mesenchymal stem cell. *Biotechnol. Adv.* **2013**, *31*, 543–551. [CrossRef] [PubMed]

37. Li, Q.; Wijesekera, O.; Salas, S.J.; Wang, J.Y.; Zhu, M.; Aprhys, C.; Chaichana, K.L.; Chesler, D.A.; Zhang, H.; Smith, C.L.; et al. Mesenchymal stem cells from human fat engineered to secrete BMP4 are nononcogenic, suppress brain cancer, and prolong survival. *Clin. Cancer Res.* **2014**, *20*, 2375–2387. [CrossRef] [PubMed]

38. Kalimuthu, S.; Gangadaran, P.; Rajendran, R.L.; Zhu, L.; Oh, J.M.; Lee, H.W.; Gopal, A.; Baek, S.H.; Jeong, S.Y.; Lee, S.W.; et al. A New Approach for Loading Anticancer Drugs Into Mesenchymal Stem Cell-Derived Exosome Mimetics for Cancer Therapy. *Front. Pharmacol.* **2018**, *9*, 1116. [CrossRef]

39. Saari, H.; Lázaro-Ibáñez, E.; Viitala, T.; Vuorimaa-Laukkanen, E.; Siljander, P.; Yliperttula, M. Microvesicle- and exosome-mediated drug delivery enhances the cytotoxicity of Paclitaxel in autologous prostate cancer cells. *J. Control. Release* **2015**, *220*, 727–737. [CrossRef] [PubMed]
40. Akyurekli, C.; Le, Y.; Richardson, R.B.; Fergusson, D.; Tay, J.; Allan, D.S. A systematic review of preclinical studies on the therapeutic potential of mesenchymal stromal cell-derived microvesicles. *Stem Cell Rev* **2015**, *11*, 150–160. [CrossRef] [PubMed]
41. Rani, S.; Ryan, A.E.; Griffin, M.D.; Ritter, T. Mesenchymal Stem Cell-derived Extracellular Vesicles: Toward Cell-free Therapeutic Applications. *Mol. Ther.* **2015**, *23*, 812–823. [CrossRef] [PubMed]

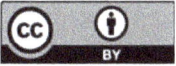

pharmaceutics

MDPI

Article

Protein Corona Fingerprints of Liposomes: New Opportunities for Targeted Drug Delivery and Early Detection in Pancreatic Cancer

Sara Palchetti [1], **Damiano Caputo** [2], **Luca Digiacomo** [1], **Anna Laura Capriotti** [3], **Roberto Coppola** [2], **Daniela Pozzi** [1,4,*] and **Giulio Caracciolo** [1,*]

[1] Department of Molecular Medicine, Sapienza University of Rome, Viale Regina Elena 291, 00161 Rome, Italy; sara.palchetti@uniroma1.it (S.P.); luca.digiacomo@uniroma1.it (L.D.)
[2] Department of General Surgery, University Campus-Biomedico di Roma, Via Alvaro del Portillo 200, 00128 Rome, Italy; d.caputo@unicampus.it (D.C.); r.coppola@unicampus.it (R.C.)
[3] Department of Chemistry, Sapienza University of Rome, P.le Aldo Moro 5, 00185 Rome, Italy; annalaura.capriotti@uniroma1.it
[4] Istituti Fisioterapici Ospitalieri, Istituto Regina Elena, Via Elio Chianesi 53, 00144 Rome, Italy
* Correspondence: daniela.pozzi@uniroma1.it (D.P.); giulio.caracciolo@uniroma1.it (G.C.); Tel.: +39-064-991-3641 (D.P.)

Received: 22 November 2018; Accepted: 8 January 2019; Published: 15 January 2019

Abstract: Pancreatic ductal adenocarcinoma (PDAC) is the fourth cause of cancer-related mortality in the Western world and is envisaged to become the second cause by 2030. Although our knowledge about the molecular biology of PDAC is continuously increasing, this progress has not been translated into better patients' outcome. Liposomes have been used to circumvent concerns associated with the low efficiency of anticancer drugs such as severe side effects and damage of healthy tissues, but they have not resulted in improved efficacy as yet. Recently, the concept is emerging that the limited success of liposomal drugs in clinical practice is due to our poor knowledge of the nano–bio interactions experienced by liposomes in vivo. After systemic administration, lipid vesicles are covered by plasma proteins forming a biomolecular coating, referred to as the protein corona (PC). Recent studies have clarified that just a minor fraction of the hundreds of bound plasma proteins, referred to as "PC fingerprints" (PCFs), enhance liposome association with cancer cells, triggering efficient particle internalization. In this study, we synthesized a library of 10 liposomal formulations with systematic changes in lipid composition and exposed them to human plasma (HP). Size, zeta-potential, and corona composition of the resulting liposome–protein complexes were thoroughly characterized by dynamic light scattering (DLS), micro-electrophoresis, and nano-liquid chromatography tandem mass spectrometry (nano-LC MS/MS). According to the recent literature, enrichment in PCFs was used to predict the targeting ability of synthesized liposomal formulations. Here we show that the predicted targeting capability of liposome–protein complexes clearly correlate with cellular uptake in pancreatic adenocarcinoma (PANC-1) and insulinoma (INS-1) cells as quantified by flow-assisted cell sorting (FACS). Of note, cellular uptake of the liposomal formulation with the highest abundance of PCFs was much larger than that of Onivyde®, an Irinotecan liposomal drug approved by the Food and Drug Administration in 2015 for the treatment of metastatic PDAC. Given the urgent need of efficient nanocarriers for the treatment of PDAC, we envision that our results will pave the way for the development of more efficient PC-based targeted nanomaterials. Here we also show that some BCs are enriched with plasma proteins that are associated with the onset and progression of PDAC (e.g., sex hormone-binding globulin, Ficolin-3, plasma protease C1 inhibitor, etc.). This could open the intriguing possibility to identify novel biomarkers.

Keywords: pancreatic ductal adenocarcinoma; liposomes; protein corona

1. Introduction

With a one-year survival rate of 12% that declines to 1% at five years, pancreatic ductal adenocarcinoma (PDAC) is one of the most lethal tumors worldwide [1]. It is currently the fourth leading cause of cancer-associated mortality and it is predicted to become the second leading cause in the next decade in Western countries [2]. When PDAC is diagnosed, surgery remains the only treatment chance, while chemotherapeutic agents are often inefficacious. To tackle this issue, numerous drugs have been tested. Gemcitabine (GEM) was the first drug to be approved for pancreatic cancer, but it is currently used only as a palliative agent [3]. Cisplatin and 5-Fluorouracile can extend life for a few months but both have collateral toxic properties [4]. Irinotecan is an antitumor drug belonging to the camptothecin family that targets DNA topoisomerase-1, a nuclear enzyme able to prevent torsional stress during DNA replication and transcription [5]. Nanotechnology has recently gained attention for its ability to treat numerous tumors, with nanocarriers being used to circumvent the problems associated with anticancer drugs, including high toxicity and irreversible damage of normal cells [6]. Recently, Onivyde®, an Irinotecan liposomal formulation, has been approved by the Food and Drug Administration (FDA) for the treatment of metastatic pancreatic cancer resistant to gemcitabine chemotherapy [7]. As a matter of fact, encapsulated liposomal drugs exhibit better pharmacokinetics and therapeutic index, as well as reduce the collateral toxic effects of free drugs. However, the adsorption of plasma opsonins (e.g., complement proteins, immunoglobulins, etc.) to the liposomal surface results in the clearance of liposomes from the blood circulation [8]. For a couple of decades, researchers have tried to prevent protein binding by grafting polymers to the liposome surface and, in this regard, polyethylene glycol (PEG) has been the gold standard for stealth polymers in drug delivery [9]. Conjugating PEG terminals to tissue-recognition ligands (e.g., peptides, antibodies, etc.) has long been supposed to provide such "long-circulating" liposomes with selective targeting ability [10]. However, recent findings have demonstrated that grafting polymers to a liposome surface can only reduce protein binding, but cannot fully prevent it [11]. Moreover, Schöttler et al. showed that PEG promotes the recruitment of specific plasma proteins [12], thus contributing to explain the accelerated blood clearance ("ABC phenomenon") of PEGylated nanosystems [13]. The main implication is that active targeting usually fails in vivo with the result that no targeted liposomal drug has been approved so far. While protein binding to a liposome surface is a well-established paradigm in drug delivery [14–16], the emerging field of nano–bio interactions between nanosized objects and biological systems is putting earlier findings in context, providing the liposome field with new perspectives [17–20].

When liposomes are introduced into a biological fluid, they are covered by a dynamic layer of biomolecules, in particular proteins, forming the so-called "protein corona" (PC) [21,22]. This complex interface is formed in seconds and, over time, it changes prevalently in the amount of bound protein and slightly in protein composition [23]. With respect to other kinds of nanoparticles, the liposome–PC evolves significantly during the first hour of exposure to biological fluids [24] and is the reason why exposure time is typically fixed at 1 h [24–26]. As a consequence of PC formation, liposomes lose their synthetic identity and attain a new one that is usually referred to as their "biological identity". It is this newly acquired biological identity that controls undesirable side effects of liposomal drug delivery, such as off-target interactions, toxicity, size-dependent particle recognition by immune cells [27], and clearance from the bloodstream [28,29]. On the other side, it is increasingly accepted that even particle accumulation at the target site is controlled by the biological identity acquired in biological environments [17]. For instance, non-specific interactions between liposomes and target cells are controlled by physical-chemical properties (i.e., size and zeta-potential) of liposome–protein complexes and not by those of pristine liposomes. Moreover, the PC may act as an endogenous trigger, promoting association with receptors of target cells and leading to efficient internalization. In a couple of recent investigations [26,30], we demonstrated that liposomes possessing specific size and zeta-potential are efficiently internalized within cancer cells [26,30]. Moreover, a minor fraction of identified "corona proteins" (typically 1–2%), referred to as "protein corona fingerprints" (PCFs), promote favorable cellular association. Globally, liposome physical-chemical properties, PC composition, and cellular uptake can be combined in a general strategy to predict the interaction of liposomes with cancer cells (Figure 1).

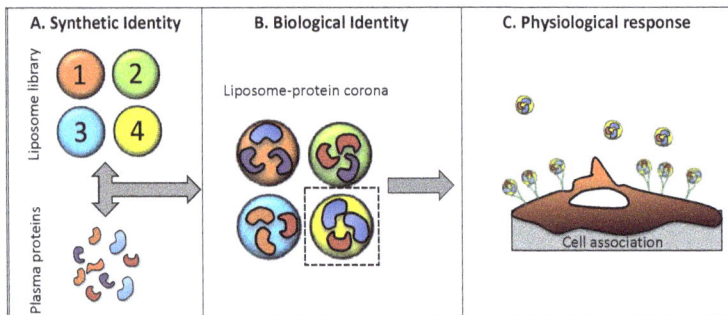

Figure 1. Schematic illustrating the protein corona fingerprinting strategy. (**A**) A library of liposomes is mixed with plasma proteins; (**B**) plasma proteins adsorb to the particle surface, forming liposome–protein complexes that are ranked for enrichment in protein corona 'fingerprints', i.e., plasma proteins that promote association with cancer cells; (**C**) selected formulations are incubated with cells in culture and cell association is measured by flow-assisted flow cytometry.

This work was therefore aimed at exploiting the liposome–PC to target human pancreatic carcinoma (PANC-1) cells. To this end, a library of 10 liposomal formulations was synthesized and liposome–protein complexes were thoroughly characterized by dynamic light scattering (DLS), micro-electrophoresis (ME), and nano-liquid chromatography tandem mass spectrometry (nano-LC MS/MS). Next, liposomes were screened for their particle properties and corona composition. Of note, cellular uptake by PANC-1 cells was found to correlate with physical-chemical properties of liposome–protein complexes and enrichment in PCFs. A second aim of the study was the complete identification of the protein patterns adsorbed to synthesized liposomes. Indeed, the recently introduced concept of the "disease-specific PC" [31] states that the PC composition is affected by changes in human proteome as those induced by numerous diseases such as cancer. Thus, identifying proteins that are related to pancreatic tumor onset and progression could pave the way to identify cancer in the early stages by differential analysis of the PC.

2. Materials and Methods

2.1. Liposomes Preparation

Cationic lipids 1,2-dioleoyl-3-trimethylammonium-propane (DOTAP) and (3β-[N-(N',N'-dimethylaminoethane)carbamoyl])cholesterol; neutral lipids dioleoylphosphatidylethanolamine (DOPE), 1,2-dipalmitoyl-*sn*-glycero-3-phosphocholine (DPPC), and 1,2-diarachidoyl-*sn*-glycero-3-phosphocholine (20:0 PC); the zwitterionic lipid dioleoylphosphocholine (DOPC); and the anionic lipid 1,2-dioleoyl-*sn*-glycero-3-phospho-(1'-rac-glycerol) (DOPG) were purchased from Avanti Polar Lipids (Alabaster, AL, USA), while sphingosine and cholesterol were from Sigma-Aldrich (St. Louis, MO, USA). All lipids were used without further refinement and were prepared at desired molar ratios. Each lipid was dissolved in chloroform and the solvent was evaporated under a vacuum for at least 2 h. Lipid films were hydrated in ultrapure water to obtain a final lipid concentration of 1 mg/mL. The obtained liposome solutions were extruded 20 times through a 0.1-μm polycarbonate carbonate filter with the Avanti Mini-Extruder (Avanti Polar Lipids, Alabaster, AL, USA). Liposomes were incubated with human plasma (HP) (1:1 *v*/*v*) for 1 h at 37 °C. Incubation time was chosen according to previous findings as it represents a typical plateau of the temporal evolution of the liposome–PC [24].

2.2. Size and Zeta-Potential Experiments

For size and zeta-potential experiments, bare liposomes and liposome–HP complexes were diluted 1:100 with ddH$_2$O. All the measurements were performed using a Zetasizer Nano ZS90 (Malvern, UK) at room temperature. Experiments were made in triplicate and the results are given as means ± standard deviation.

2.3. Proteomics Experiments

Lipid films were hydrated with a dissolving buffer (Tris-HCl, pH 7.4, 10 mmol L^{-1}; NaCl, 150 mmol L^{-1}; EDTA, 1 mmol L^{-1}). The obtained solutions were extruded 20 times through a 0.1-μm polycarbonate carbonate filter with the Avanti Mini-Extruder (Avanti Polar Lipids, Alabaster, AL, USA) and stored at 4 °C until use. Liposomes were incubated with HP (1:1 *v/v*) and then incubated at 37 °C for 1 h. After incubation, samples were centrifuged for 15 min at 14,000 rpm. Pellet was robustly washed with phosphate-buffered saline (PBS) and resuspended. This procedure was repeated three times to wash the sample and remove loosely bound proteins. Protein denaturation, digestion, and desalting were carried out by a robust methodology that is commonly used to separate liposome–PC complexes from unbound and loosely bound proteins [11]. In brief, samples were lyophilized by a Speed-Vac apparatus (mod. SC 250 Express; Thermo Savant, Holbrook, NY, USA). Samples were reconstituted with 0.1% HCOOH solution (final concentration 0.32 mg/mL) and stored at −80 °C until LC MS/MS was carried out. Tryptic peptides were investigated by a nano-LC system (Dionex Ultimate 3000, Sunnyvale, CA, USA) connected to a hybrid mass spectrometer (Thermo Fisher Scientific, Bremen, Germany), equipped with a nanoelectrospray ion source. Xcalibur (v.2.07, Thermo Fisher Scientific) raw data files were submitted to Proteome Discover (1.2 version, Thermo Scientific) for a database search using Mascot (version 2.3.2 Matrix Science). Data was searched against the SwissProt database (v 57.15, 20,266 sequences) using the decoy search option of Mascot and protein quantification was made by Scaffold software. For each identified protein, the mean value of the normalized spectral countings (NSCs) was normalized to the protein molecular weight (MWNSC) to obtain the relative protein abundance (RPA) [32]. For each identified protein, the reported RPA is the mean of three independent replicates ± standard deviation.

2.4. Cell Culture

Human pancreatic carcinoma cell line (PANC-1) was purchased from Sigma Aldrich (St. Louis, MO, USA) and maintained in DMEM medium. Rat insulinoma cell line (INS-1) was purchased from Thermo Fisher (Waltham, MA, USA) and was maintained in RPMI. Both mediums were supplemented with 2 mM L-glutamine, 100 IU/mL penicillin-streptomycin, 1 mM sodium pyruvate, 10 mM Hepes, 1.5 mg/L sodium bicarbonate, and 10% fetal bovine serum. Cell lines were cultured at 37 °C in a humidified atmosphere with 5% CO$_2$.

2.5. Flow-Assisted Cell Sorting Experiments

For cellular uptake experiments, Lip-1 and Lip-5 liposomes were synthesized using Texas Red® 1,2-dihexadecanoyl-*sn*-glycero-3-phosphoethanolamine, triethylammonium salt (TX-DHPE) (Thermo Fisher, Waltham, MA, USA). Onyvide-like liposomes were prepared using DSPC, Chol, MPEG-2000-DSPE, and TX-DHPE at the molar ratios 215:143:1:1. Cells were seeded on 12-well plates (150,000 cells/well) in complete medium and, after 2 h, cells were treated with liposomes incubated with human plasma for 1 h using Optimem medium. After 3 h, cells were detached with trypsine/EDTA, washed two times with cold PBS, and run on a BD LSR Fortessa™ (BD Bioscience, San Jose, CA, USA).

3. Results and Discussion

First, we synthesized a combinatorial library of 10 liposomal formulations. According to previous findings [33,34], liposomes were prepared by mixing cholesterol, DC-Chol, DOPC, DOPE, DOTAP, DPPC, PC (20:0), and sphingosine in specific molar ratios (Table 1).

Table 1. The molar ratios of lipids used for synthesized a library of 10 liposomal formulations.

Samples	CHOLESTEROL	DC-CHOL	DOPC	DOPE	DOTAP	DPPC	PC (20:0)	SPHINGOSINE
Lip-1	0	0	0	0.5	0.5	0	0	0
Lip-2	0	0.5	0	0.5	0	0	0	0
Lip-3	0	0.25	0.25	0.25	0.25	0	0	0
Lip-4	0	1	0	0	0	0	0	0
Lip-5	0.2	0	0	0	0	0	0.8	0
Lip-6	0.25	0	0	0	0.5	0	0.25	0
Lip-7	0.25	0	0	0	0.5	0.25	0	0
Lip-8	0.33	0	0	0	0	0	0.33	0.33
Lip-9	0.5	0	0	0	0.5	0	0	0
Lip-10	0.5	0.5	0	0	0	0	0	0

Next, the synthetic identity of liposomes (i.e., size, zeta-potential, and aggregation state post-synthesis) was characterized by DLS and ME (Figure 2). Pristine vesicles were small in size with a hydrodynamic diameter (D_H) ranging from ~100 nm to 150 nm (Figure 2A, blue points). Moreover, the polydispersity index (PDI) indicated that all liposomal formulations were monodisperse (Table 2).

Zeta-potential of liposomes varied between ~0 mV (Lip-5) and ~65 mV (Lip-10) depending on liposomal lipid composition (Figure 2B, blue points). One-hour exposure to HP lead to the formation of liposome–protein complexes that were characterized in terms of size, zeta-potential, and homogeneity of dispersion. The size of liposome–protein complexes (Figure 2A, red points) was larger than that of pristine vesicles and varied appreciably among formulations. This is in full agreement with previous findings showing that lipid composition plays a key role in protein binding to a lipid surface [35]. According to the literature [22], a size increase of a few nanometers is likely due to the formation of a PC on the liposome surface, while an enlargement of a few tenths of a nanometer reflects the clustering of single liposomes coated by plasma proteins [25,32].

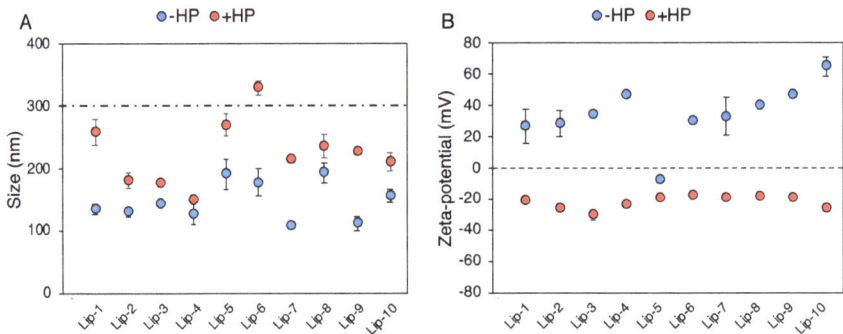

Figure 2. (**A**) Hydrodynamic diameter of liposomes before (blue points, "– human plasma (HP)") and after (red points, "+ HP") 1-h incubation with human plasma (HP) of pancreatic cancer patients. Values are means ± standard deviation from three independent experiments. The dashed line indicates a typical size threshold for particle removal from bloodstream by macrophages. (**B**) Zeta-potential of liposomes before (blue points, "– HP") and after (red points, "+ HP") 1-h incubation with human plasma (HP) of pancreatic cancer patients.

Table 2. Polydispersity index (PDI) of bare liposomal formulations and after 1-h incubation with HP.

Samples	PDI	
	−HP	+HP
Lip-1	0.14 ± 0.04	0.12 ± 0.04
Lip-2	0.11 ± 0.01	0.17 ± 0.05
Lip-3	0.08 ± 0.01	0.13 ± 0.01
Lip-4	0.12 ± 0.02	0.14 ± 0.01
Lip-5	0.10 ± 0.02	0.16 ± 0.05
Lip-6	0.10 ± 0.02	0.17 ± 0.01
Lip-7	0.12 ± 0.02	0.20 ± 0.04
Lip-8	0.11 ± 0.02	0.18 ± 0.03
Lip-9	0.15 ± 0.01	0.22 ± 0.02
Lip-10	0.14 ± 0.01	0.20 ± 0.01

Liposome aggregation is confirmed by an increase in PDI values (Table 2). On the other side, "normalization" in zeta-potential around −20 mV (Figure 2B, red points), regardless of pristine surface charge, has been reported for many classes of nanomaterials and is caused by the fact that most plasma proteins have a negative charge at physiological pH. Besides the size and zeta-potential of liposome–protein complexes, the biological identity of liposomes is also controlled by the composition of the PC. When in the blood, the liposome–PC could hamper the ability of the pristine vesicle to bind to target receptors [36] and may induce activation of the immune system, leading to particle clearance [21,37].

On the other hand, molecular recognition between endogenous plasma proteins (i.e., recruited from the blood) and cancer cell receptors [38] could promote selective accumulation at the tumor site. A crucial step towards the exploitation of the PC for targeted drug delivery is therefore the identification and quantification of corona proteins. Bradford assay results showed that the amount of bound protein is dependent on both the zeta-potential and lipid composition (Table 3).

Table 3. Micrograms of proteins bound to liposomal formulations after 1-h incubation with HP.

Samples	Protein (μg/μL)
	+HP
Lip-1	4.9 ± 0.4
Lip-2	5.3 ± 0.6
Lip-3	4.8 ± 0.5
Lip-4	9.0 ± 0.9
Lip-5	3.1 ± 0.4
Lip-6	4.6 ± 0.3
Lip-7	4.1 ± 0.4
Lip-8	3.7 ± 0.4
Lip-9	9.5 ± 0.9
Lip-10	6.6 ± 0.5

Generally, it was observed that cationic liposomes adsorb more proteins than neutrally charged vesicles. Likewise, nano-LC MS/MS showed that the liposome–PCs were highly complex entities containing between 140 and 222 proteins (Table 4).

The identified number of proteins in Table 4 is larger than that accommodated on the liposome surface. This apparent discrepancy was clarified by recent models that describe the corona as a coating made of several layers held together by protein–protein interactions [39,40]. To facilitate their rational identification, corona proteins were grouped according to physiological functions of the blood system. The relative protein abundance (RPA) of biologically relevant proteins such as complement proteins, coagulation proteins, immunoglobulins, acute phase proteins, tissue leakage, and lipoproteins are displayed in Figure 3.

Table 4. Number of proteins adsorbed on liposomal formulations after 1-h incubation with HP.

Samples	#Identified Proteins
Lip-1	220
Lip-2	140
Lip-3	205
Lip-4	170
Lip-5	174
Lip-6	202
Lip-7	206
Lip-8	180
Lip-9	222
Lip-10	190

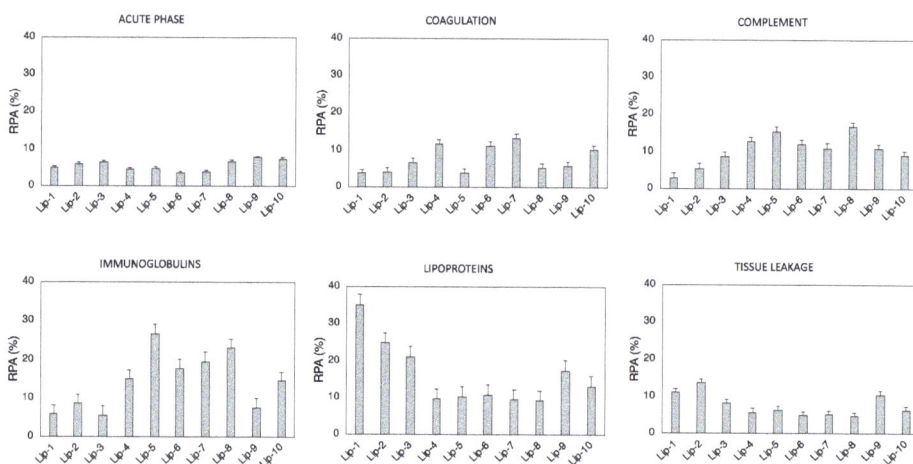

Figure 3. Bioinformatic classification of proteins identified in the corona of Lip-1–Lip-10 after 1-h exposure to HP. The relative protein abundances (RPAs) of total proteins are shown.

Our findings confirmed that each liposome exhibits a specific protein pattern dictated by its specific lipid composition. Over the last decade, numerous studies have tried to relate the cellular uptake of nanoparticle–protein complexes to PC composition by an oversimplified picture of particle–cell interaction; the more abundant a corona protein, the more probable the molecular recognition by cell receptors and, in turn, the more significant its role in promoting nanoparticle–cell association. However, to understand the link between a nanoparticle–corona complex and specific uptake pathways, mapping the exact location of protein binding sites is a necessary step [41,42]. To date, mapping protein epitopes at the liposome surface is challenging. To overcome this issue, computational methods such as quantitative structure–activity relation (QSAR) allow the identification of the most appropriate set of descriptors to predict the interactions between liposomes and cells at the nano–bio interface [43,44]. Correlations between the RPA of individual proteins and cellular uptake allowed us to identify eight "protein fingerprints" (Vitronectin, APOA1, APOA2, APOB, APOC2, Ig heavy chain V-III region BRO, vitamin K-dependent protein, and Integrin beta3) that promote the association of liposomes with cancer cells [26,30]. Among PCFs, a key role is played by Vitronectin, a glycoprotein of the hemopexin family containing an RGD motif (Arg-Gly-Asp) in the Somatomedin B domain (20−63 region) that is specifically recognized by $\alpha_v\beta_3$ integrins [38]. This class of integrins is overexpressed on many solid tumors and in tumor neovasculature [45,46]. This could be extremely relevant in pancreatic cancer, where roughly half of patients show elevated expression of αvβ3, and this is positively correlated with lymph node metastasis [47]. Most chemotherapeutics given in the clinic today damage healthy tissues, leading to unwanted side effects. According to our present understanding, this could likely be related to off-target interactions between corona proteins and cell receptors of healthy cells. This means that receptors targeted by corona proteins should be overexpressed in cancer but not in normal cells. In this regard, it is known that $\alpha_v\beta_3$ integrin is expressed by normal (i.e., not-cancer) cells in a latent state characterized by its inability to stimulate cell adhesion to extra-cellular matrix ligands [48]. We also observed that, of eight PCFs, four are Apolipoproteins. It is well known that Apolipoproteins bind certain receptors such as scavenger receptor class B, type I (SR-BI), and low-density lipoprotein receptors (LDLR) that are overexpressed in several diseases. Recent studies showed that SR-BI and LDLR are overexpressed in pancreatic cancer, thus representing good targets of Apolipoprotein-enriched coronas [49,50]. Liposomal formulations were ranked for their PC-based targeting ability by calculating the total abundance of PCFs [51].

According to Figure 4, Lip-1 was identified as the most promising formulation to promote cellular association within PANC-1 and INS-1 cells. On the other side, Lip-5, being highly defective in PCFs, was expected to promote low cellular internalization. To support our conclusions, we treated PANC-1 cells with fluorescently labeled Lip-1- and Lip-5-protein complexes. Onivyde®, the liposomal formulation approved by the FDA for the treatment of metastatic pancreatic cancer [7,52], was used as a control. In order to obtain a quantitative view on this process, we performed FACS analysis. Figure 5A shows that about 95% of PANC-1 and INS-1 cells treated with Lip-1-protein complexes were fluorescence-positive. On the other hand, Lip-5-protein complexes were poorly internalized by PANC-1 cells, as demonstrated by the fact that less than 20% were positive for the fluorescence signal. This percentage was slightly higher in INS-1 cells (<30%). FACS results also show that the internalization of Onivyde® in both PANC-1 and INS-1 cells is extremely low, with only 10% and 20% of fluorescence-positive cells, respectively. The mean fluorescence intensity reported in Figure 5B shows the same trends as those observed for cellular uptake.

Lastly, our MS/MS results indicate that the composition of the PC (in terms of types and amounts of the constituent proteins) depends strongly on the physical-chemical properties of the liposomes. In particular, we observed that the coronas of Lip-1 and Lip-5 were particularly enriched with plasma proteins and were associated with the onset and progression of pancreatic cancer (e.g., sex hormone-binding globulin, Ficolin-3, plasma protease C1 inhibitor, etc.). Recently, some authors introduced the concept of the disease-specific PC [31], wherein alterations in human proteome of patients with various diseases produce appreciable changes in the PC protein pattern. Consequently, we envision that the manipulation of liposome surface chemistry can dictate the selective binding of plasma proteins with the possibility of identifying cancer at the early stages.

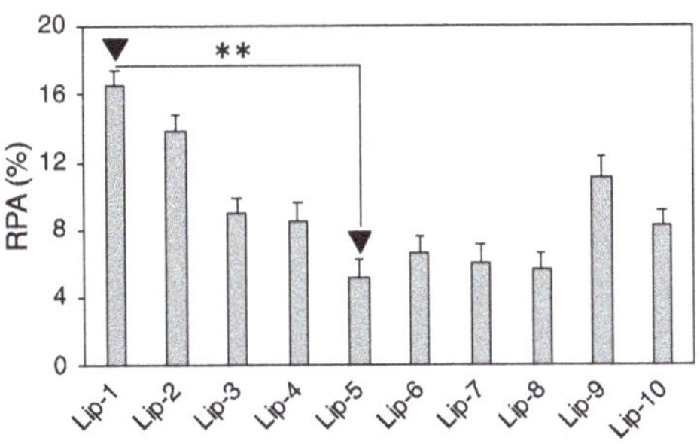

Figure 4. Relative protein abundance of biomolecular corona fingerprints. Lip-1 and Lip-5 were the liposomal formulations with the highest and lowest enrichment in PCFs (Vitronectin, APOA1, APOA2, APOB, APOC2, Ig heavy chain V-III region BRO, vitamin K-dependent protein, and Integrin beta3). Significance was statistically evaluated by Student's *t*-test (** $p < 0.05$).

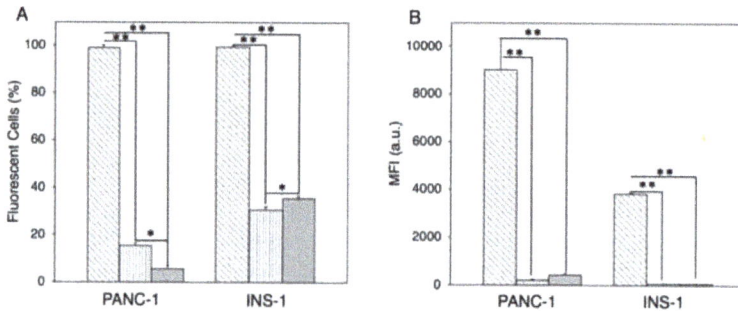

Figure 5. (**A**) Cellular uptake of Lip-1 (grey diagonal hatched lines), Lip-5 (grey vertical hatched lines), and Onivyde® (grey bar) in PANC-1 and INS-1 cells after 1-h incubation with human plasma (HP). (**B**) Mean fluorescence intensity of Lip-1 (grey diagonal hatched lines), Lip-5 (grey vertical hatched lines), and Onivyde® (grey bar) in PANC-1 and INS-1 cells after 1-h incubation with human plasma (HP). Statistical significance was evaluated using Student's *t*-test: * $p < 0.01$; ** $p < 0.005$ (no asterisk means lack of significance).

4. Conclusions

In conclusion, we have synthesized a library of 10 liposomal formulations that exhibit peculiar biological identities when exposed to HP. We found that the formulation exhibiting the highest levels of targeting fingerprints also had major cellular uptake in PANC-1 and INS-1 cells. Our results indicate that the exploitation of PCs could be a valuable means to develop targeted nanomedicine for PDAC treatment. Moreover, we found that the PCs of some liposome formulations were enriched with plasma proteins that are related to PDAC onset and progression. This possibility could pave the way for the identification of novel biomarkers and will be explored in future investigations.

Author Contributions: Conceptualization, D.C., R.C., G.C., and D.P.; methodology, G.C and D.P.; software, L.D.; validation, S.P., formal analysis, L.D.; investigation, S.P., L.D., and A.L.C.; resources, D.C., R.C., G.C., and D.P.; data curation, L.D.; writing—original draft preparation, G.C.; writing—review and editing, S.P, D.C., R.C., G.C., and D.P.; visualization, S.P. and L.D.; supervision, D.C., R.C., G.C., and D.P.; project administration, G.C. and D.P.; funding acquisition, D.C., G.C., and D.P.

Funding: This research was funded by Italian Minister of Health, Progetto Giovani Ricercatori 2011–2012, grant number: GR-2011-02350094. S.P. is recipient of a fellowship (ID 19319) granted from AIRC (Italian Association for Cancer Research). The research leading to these results received funding from AIRC under IG 2017—ID. 20327 project—P.I. Caracciolo Giulio.

Conflicts of Interest: The authors declare no conflict of interest.

References

1. Kamisawa, T.; Wood, L.D.; Itoi, T.; Takaori, K. Pancreatic cancer. *Lancet* **2016**, *388*, 73–85. [CrossRef]
2. Rahib, L.; Smith, B.D.; Aizenberg, R.; Rosenzweig, A.B.; Fleshman, J.M.; Matrisian, L.M. Projecting cancer incidence and deaths to 2030: The unexpected burden of thyroid, liver, and pancreas cancers in the united states. *Cancer Res.* **2014**, *74*, 2913–2921. [CrossRef] [PubMed]
3. Hidalgo, M. Pancreatic cancer. *N. Engl. J. Med.* **2010**, *362*, 1605–1617. [CrossRef]
4. Kundranda, M.N.; Niu, J. Albumin-bound paclitaxel in solid tumors: Clinical development and future directions. *Drug Des. Dev. Ther.* **2015**, *9*, 3767–3777. [CrossRef] [PubMed]
5. Pommier, Y. DNA topoisomerase i inhibitors: Chemistry, biology, and interfacial inhibition. *Chem. Rev.* **2009**, *109*, 2894–2902. [CrossRef] [PubMed]
6. Ud Din, F.; Aman, W.; Ullah, I.; Qureshi, O.S.; Mustapha, O.; Shafique, S.; Zeb, A. Effective use of nanocarriers as drug delivery systems for the treatment of selected tumors. *Int. J. Nanomed.* **2017**, *12*, 7291–7309. [CrossRef] [PubMed]

7. DiGiulio, S. FDA approves onivyde combo regimen for advanced pancreatic cancer. *Oncol. Times* **2015**, *37*, 8. [CrossRef]

8. Liu, D.; Liu, F.; Song, Y.K. Recognition and clearance of liposomes containing phosphatidylserine are mediated by serum opsonin. *Biochim. Biophys. Acta (BBA)-Biomembr.* **1995**, *1235*, 140–146. [CrossRef]

9. Knop, K.; Hoogenboom, R.; Fischer, D.; Schubert, U.S. Poly(ethylene glycol) in drug delivery: Pros and cons as well as potential alternatives. *Angew. Chem. Int. Edit.* **2010**, *49*, 6288–6308. [CrossRef]

10. Prencipe, G.; Tabakman, S.M.; Welsher, K.; Liu, Z.; Goodwin, A.P.; Zhang, L.; Henry, J.; Dai, H. Peg branched polymer for functionalization of nanomaterials with ultralong blood circulation. *J. Am. Chem. Soc.* **2009**, *131*, 4783–4787. [CrossRef]

11. Pozzi, D.; Colapicchioni, V.; Caracciolo, G.; Piovesana, S.; Capriotti, A.L.; Palchetti, S.; De Grossi, S.; Riccioli, A.; Amenitsch, H.; Laganà, A. Effect of polyethyleneglycol (PEG) chain length on the bio-nano-interactions between pegylated lipid nanoparticles and biological fluids: From nanostructure to uptake in cancer cells. *Nanoscale* **2014**, *6*, 2782–2792. [CrossRef] [PubMed]

12. Schöttler, S.; Becker, G.; Winzen, S.; Steinbach, T.; Mohr, K.; Landfester, K.; Mailänder, V.; Wurm, F.R. Protein adsorption is required for stealth effect of poly(ethylene glycol)-and poly(phosphoester)-coated nanocarriers. *Nat. Nanotechnol.* **2016**, *11*, 372–377. [CrossRef] [PubMed]

13. Ishida, T.; Harada, M.; Wang, X.Y.; Ichihara, M.; Irimura, K.; Kiwada, H. Accelerated blood clearance of pegylated liposomes following preceding liposome injection: Effects of lipid dose and peg surface-density and chain length of the first-dose liposomes. *J. Control. Release* **2005**, *105*, 305–317. [CrossRef] [PubMed]

14. Moghimi, S.M.; Hunter, A.C. Recognition by macrophages and liver cells of opsonized phospholipid vesicles and phospholipid headgroups. *Pharm. Res.* **2001**, *18*, 1–8. [CrossRef]

15. Moghimi, S.M.; Hunter, A.C.; Murray, J.C. Long-circulating and target-specific nanoparticles: Theory to practice. *Pharmacol. Rev.* **2001**, *53*, 283–318. [PubMed]

16. Moghimi, S.M.; Szebeni, J. Stealth liposomes and long circulating nanoparticles: Critical issues in pharmacokinetics, opsonization and protein-binding properties. *Prog. Lipid Res.* **2003**, *42*, 463–478. [CrossRef]

17. Caracciolo, G. Liposome-protein corona in a physiological environment: Challenges and opportunities for targeted delivery of nanomedicines. *Nanomed. Nanotechnol. Biol. Med.* **2015**, *11*, 543–557. [CrossRef] [PubMed]

18. Caracciolo, G.; Farokhzad, O.C.; Mahmoudi, M. Biological identity of nanoparticles in vivo: Clinical implications of the protein corona. *Trends Biotechnol.* **2017**, *35*, 257–264. [CrossRef] [PubMed]

19. Caracciolo, G. Clinically approved liposomal nanomedicines: Lessons learned from the biomolecular corona. *Nanoscale* **2018**, *10*, 4167–4172. [CrossRef]

20. Caracciolo, G.; Pozzi, D.; Capriotti, A.L.; Cavaliere, C.; Piovesana, S.; La Barbera, G.; Amici, A.; Laganà, A. The liposome-protein corona in mice and humans and its implications for in vivo delivery. *J. Mater. Chem. B* **2014**, *2*, 7419–7428. [CrossRef]

21. Monopoli, M.P.; Aberg, C.; Salvati, A.; Dawson, K.A. Biomolecular coronas provide the biological identity of nanosized materials. *Nat. Nanotechnol.* **2012**, *7*, 779–786. [CrossRef] [PubMed]

22. Walkey, C.D.; Chan, W.C. Understanding and controlling the interaction of nanomaterials with proteins in a physiological environment. *Chem. Soc. Rev.* **2012**, *41*, 2780–2799. [CrossRef] [PubMed]

23. Tenzer, S.; Docter, D.; Kuharev, J.; Musyanovych, A.; Fetz, V.; Hecht, R.; Schlenk, F.; Fischer, D.; Kiouptsi, K.; Reinhardt, C. Rapid formation of plasma protein corona critically affects nanoparticle pathophysiology. *Nat. Nanotechnol.* **2013**, *8*, 772–781. [CrossRef] [PubMed]

24. Barrán-Berdón, A.L.; Pozzi, D.; Caracciolo, G.; Capriotti, A.L.; Caruso, G.; Cavaliere, C.; Riccioli, A.; Palchetti, S.; Laganà, A. Time evolution of nanoparticle-protein corona in human plasma: Relevance for targeted drug delivery. *Langmuir* **2013**, *29*, 6485–6494. [CrossRef] [PubMed]

25. Pozzi, D.; Caracciolo, G.; Digiacomo, L.; Colapicchioni, V.; Palchetti, S.; Capriotti, A.L.; Cavaliere, C.; Zenezini Chiozzi, R.; Puglisi, A.; Laganà, A. The biomolecular corona of nanoparticles in circulating biological media. *Nanoscale* **2015**, *7*, 13958–13966. [CrossRef] [PubMed]

26. Palchetti, S.; Digiacomo, L.; Pozzi, D.; Peruzzi, G.; Micarelli, E.; Mahmoudi, M.; Caracciolo, G. Nanoparticles-cell association predicted by protein corona fingerprints. *Nanoscale* **2016**, *8*, 12755–12763. [CrossRef] [PubMed]

27. Mirshafiee, V.; Mahmoudi, M.; Lou, K.; Cheng, J.; Kraft, M.L. Protein corona significantly reduces active targeting yield. *Chem. Commun.* **2013**, *49*, 2557–2559. [CrossRef]

28. Harashima, H.; Hiraiwa, T.; Ochi, Y.; Kiwada, H. Size dependent liposome degradation in blood: in vivo/in vitro correlation by kinetic modeling. *J. Drug Target.* **1995**, *3*, 253–261. [CrossRef]

29. Jiang, W.; Kim, B.Y.; Rutka, J.T.; Chan, W.C. Nanoparticle-mediated cellular response is size-dependent. *Nat. Nanotechnol.* **2008**, *3*, 145–150. [CrossRef]

30. Bigdeli, A.; Palchetti, S.; Pozzi, D.; Hormozi-Nezhad, M.R.; Baldelli Bombelli, F.; Caracciolo, G.; Mahmoudi, M. Exploring cellular interactions of liposomes using protein corona fingerprints and physicochemical properties. *ACS Nano* **2016**, *10*, 3723–3737. [CrossRef]

31. Hajipour, M.J.; Laurent, S.; Aghaie, A.; Rezaee, F.; Mahmoudi, M. Personalized protein coronas: A "key" factor at the nanobiointerface. *Biomater. Sci.* **2014**, *2*, 1210–1221. [CrossRef]

32. Monopoli, M.P.; Walczyk, D.; Campbell, A.; Elia, G.; Lynch, I.; Baldelli Bombelli, F.; Dawson, K.A. Physical—Chemical aspects of protein corona: Relevance to in vitro and in vivo biological impacts of nanoparticles. *J. Am. Chem. Soc.* **2011**, *133*, 2525–2534. [CrossRef] [PubMed]

33. Caracciolo, G.; Pozzi, D.; Caminiti, R.; Marchini, C.; Montani, M.; Amici, A.; Amenitsch, H. Transfection efficiency boost by designer multicomponent lipoplexes. *Biochim. Biophys. Acta Biomembr.* **2007**, *1768*, 2280–2292. [CrossRef] [PubMed]

34. Pozzi, D.; Marchini, C.; Cardarelli, F.; Rossetta, A.; Colapicchioni, V.; Amici, A.; Montani, M.; Motta, S.; Brocca, P.; Cantù, L.; et al. Mechanistic understanding of gene delivery mediated by highly efficient multicomponent envelope-type nanoparticle systems. *Mol. Pharm.* **2013**, *10*, 4654–4665. [CrossRef]

35. Caracciolo, G.; Pozzi, D.; Capriotti, A.L.; Cavaliere, C.; Piovesana, S.; Amenitsch, H.; Laganà, A. Lipid composition: A "key factor" for the rational manipulation of the liposome-protein corona by liposome design. *RSC Adv.* **2015**, *5*, 5967–5975. [CrossRef]

36. Salvati, A.; Pitek, A.S.; Monopoli, M.P.; Prapainop, K.; Bombelli, F.B.; Hristov, D.R.; Kelly, P.M.; Åberg, C.; Mahon, E.; Dawson, K.A. Transferrin-functionalized nanoparticles lose their targeting capabilities when a biomolecule corona adsorbs on the surface. *Nat. Nanotechnol.* **2013**, *8*, 137–143. [CrossRef] [PubMed]

37. Mahon, E.; Salvati, A.; Baldelli Bombelli, F.; Lynch, I.; Dawson, K.A. Designing the nanoparticle–biomolecule interface for "targeting and therapeutic delivery". *J. Control. Release* **2012**, *161*, 164–174. [CrossRef]

38. Caracciolo, G.; Cardarelli, F.; Pozzi, D.; Salomone, F.; Maccari, G.; Bardi, G.; Capriotti, A.L.; Cavaliere, C.; Papi, M.; Laganà, A. Selective targeting capability acquired with a protein corona adsorbed on the surface of 1,2-dioleoyl-3-trimethylammonium propane/dna nanoparticles. *ACS Appl. Mater. Interfaces* **2013**, *5*, 13171–13179. [CrossRef]

39. Docter, D.; Westmeier, D.; Markiewicz, M.; Stolte, S.; Knauer, S.; Stauber, R. The nanoparticle biomolecule corona: Lessons learned–challenge accepted? *Chem. Soc. Rev.* **2015**, *44*, 6094–6121. [CrossRef]

40. Treuel, L.; Docter, D.; Maskos, M.; Stauber, R.H. Protein corona–from molecular adsorption to physiological complexity. *Beil. J. Nanotechnol.* **2015**, *6*, 857–873. [CrossRef]

41. Kelly, P.M.; Åberg, C.; Polo, E.; O'Connell, A.; Cookman, J.; Fallon, J.; Krpetić, Ž.; Dawson, K.A. Mapping protein binding sites on the biomolecular corona of nanoparticles. *Nat. Nanotechnol.* **2015**, *10*, 472–479. [CrossRef] [PubMed]

42. Giannelli, M.; Polo, E.; Lopez, H.; Castagnola, V.; Aastrup, T.; Dawson, K. Label-free in-flow detection of receptor recognition motifs on the biomolecular corona of nanoparticles. *Nanoscale* **2018**, *10*, 5474–5481. [CrossRef] [PubMed]

43. Walkey, C.D.; Olsen, J.B.; Song, F.; Liu, R.; Guo, H.; Olsen, D.W.H.; Cohen, Y.; Emili, A.; Chan, W.C. Protein corona fingerprinting predicts the cellular interaction of gold and silver nanoparticles. *ACS Nano* **2014**, *8*, 2439–2455. [CrossRef] [PubMed]

44. Liu, R.; Jiang, W.; Walkey, C.D.; Chan, W.C.; Cohen, Y. Prediction of nanoparticles-cell association based on corona proteins and physicochemical properties. *Nanoscale* **2015**, *7*, 9664–9675. [CrossRef] [PubMed]

45. Lorger, M.; Krueger, J.S.; O'Neal, M.; Staflin, K.; Felding-Habermann, B. Activation of tumor cell integrin $\alpha V\beta 3$ controls angiogenesis and metastatic growth in the brain. *Proc. Natl. Acad. Sci. USA* **2009**, *106*, 10666–10671. [CrossRef]

46. Weis, S.M.; Cheresh, D.A. αV integrins in angiogenesis and cancer. *Cold Spring Harb. Perspect. Med.* **2011**, *1*, a006478. [CrossRef]

47. Hosotani, R.; Kawaguchi, M.; Masui, T.; Koshiba, T.; Ida, J.; Fujimoto, K.; Wada, M.; Doi, R.; Imamura, M. Expression of integrin $\alpha v\beta 3$ in pancreatic carcinoma: Relation to MMP-2 activation and lymph node metastasis. *Pancreas* **2002**, *25*, e30–e35. [CrossRef]

48. Trusolino, L.; Serini, G.; Cecchini, G.; Besati, C.; Ambesi-Impiombato, F.S.; Marchisio, P.C.; De Filippi, R. Growth factor–dependent activation of αvβ3 integrin in normal epithelial cells: Implications for tumor invasion. *J. Cell Biol.* **1998**, *142*, 1145–1156. [CrossRef]

49. Neyen, C.; Plüddemann, A.; Mukhopadhyay, S.; Maniati, E.; Bossard, M.; Gordon, S.; Hagemann, T. Macrophage scavenger receptor a promotes tumor progression in murine models of ovarian and pancreatic cancer. *J. Immunol.* **2013**, *190*, 3798–3805. [CrossRef]

50. Vasseur, S.; Guillaumond, F. LDL receptor: An open route to feed pancreatic tumor cells. *Mol. Cell. Oncol.* **2016**, *3*, e1033586. [CrossRef]

51. Arcella, A.; Palchetti, S.; Digiacomo, L.; Pozzi, D.; Capriotti, A.L.; Frati, L.; Oliva, M.A.; Tsaouli, G.; Rota, R.; Screpanti, I. Brain targeting by liposome–biomolecular corona boosts anticancer efficacy of temozolomide in glioblastoma cells. *ACS Chem. Neurosci.* **2018**. [CrossRef] [PubMed]

52. Papi, M.; Caputo, D.; Palmieri, V.; Coppola, R.; Palchetti, S.; Bugli, F.; Martini, C.; Digiacomo, L.; Pozzi, D.; Caracciolo, G. Clinically approved pegylated nanoparticles are covered by a protein corona that boosts the uptake by cancer cells. *Nanoscale* **2017**, *9*, 10327–10334. [CrossRef] [PubMed]

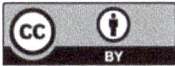

pharmaceutics

MDPI

Article

Long-Lasting, Antinociceptive Effects of pH-Sensitive Niosomes Loaded with Ibuprofen in Acute and Chronic Models of Pain

Francesca Marzoli [1], **Carlotta Marianecci** [2], **Federica Rinaldi** [3], **Daniele Passeri** [4], **Marco Rossi** [4,5], **Paola Minosi** [1], **Maria Carafa** [2] and **Stefano Pieretti** [1,*]

[1] Istituto Superiore di Sanità, National Center for Drug Research and Evaluation, 00161 Rome, Italy; francesca.marzoli@iss.it (F.M.); paola.minosi@iss.it (P.M.)

[2] Department of Drug Chemistry and Technology, Sapienza University of Rome, 00185 Rome, Italy; carlotta.marianecci@uniroma1.it (C.M.); maria.carafa@uniroma1.it (M.C.)

[3] Center for Life Nano Science@Sapienza, Istituto Italiano di Tecnologia (ITT), 00161 Rome, Italy; federica.rinaldi@uniroma1.it

[4] Department of Basic and Applied Sciences for Engineering, Sapienza University of Rome, 00161 Rome, Italy; daniele.passeri@uniroma1.it (D.P.); marco.rossi@uniroma1.it (M.R.)

[5] Research Center for Nanotechnology Applied to Engineering, Sapienza University of Rome (CNIS), 00185 Rome, Italy

* Correspondence: stefano.pieretti@iss.it; Tel.: +39-06-4990-2451

Received: 20 December 2018; Accepted: 28 January 2019; Published: 1 February 2019

Abstract: Ibuprofen is one of the non-steroidal anti-inflammatory drugs (NSAIDs) widely used to treat pain conditions. NSAIDs encounter several obstacles to passing across biological membranes. To overcome these constraints, we decided to study the effects of a new pH-sensitive formulation of niosomes containing Polysorbate 20 derivatized by Glycine and loaded with ibuprofen (NioIbu) in several animal models of pain in mice. We performed two tests commonly used to study acute antinociceptive activity, namely the writhing test and the capsaicin test. Our results demonstrated that NioIbu, administered 2 h before testing, reduced nociception, whereas the free form of ibuprofen was ineffective. In a model of inflammatory pain, hyperalgesia induced by zymosan, NioIbu induced a long-lasting reduction in hyperalgesia in treated mice. In a model of neuropathic pain induced by sciatic nerve chronic constriction, NioIbu reduced both neuropathy-induced allodynia and hyperalgesia. The results obtained in our experiments suggest that pH-sensitive niosomes containing Polysorbate 20 derivatized by Glycine is an effective model for NSAIDs delivery, providing durable antinociceptive effects and reducing the incidence of side effects.

Keywords: Ibuprofen; pH-sensitive niosomes; Pain; Analgesia; NSAIDs

1. Introduction

The non-steroidal anti-inflammatory drug (NSAID) Ibuprofen (α-methyl-4-(2-methylpropyl) benzeneacetic acid, IBU) is commonly used in the treatment of pain, fever, and inflammatory diseases. Ibuprofen was discovered in 1960 for the treatment of some pain conditions and inflammatory autoimmune diseases, such as rheumatoid arthritis [1]. In 1961, Ibuprofen became available in tablet form, and in 1983 was launched as a topical formulation. Ibuprofen is an analgesic drug that inhibits the production of cyclooxygenase (Cox-2) pathway-derived prostaglandins, which increase in inflamed tissues and control inflammatory disorder [2,3]. As is well-known, prostanoids mediate the sensation of peripheral and central pain, increasing membrane excitability and reducing the threshold of nociceptor stimulation [4].

While ibuprofen is completely absorbed after oral administration [5], the plasma level is still low several hours after topical application [6]. Various studies have reported different techniques to increase the permeability of cell membranes and the transdermal transport of ibuprofen and other drugs: preparing colloidal microstructures with lysinate and lecithin [7,8], nanoscaled emulsion with palm olein esters [9], iontophoresis [10], and using surfactants and various vehicles, such as the niosomes [11,12]. Niosomes are unilamellar or multilamellar non-ionic surfactant vesicles similar to liposomes that can be used as therapeutic nanocarriers. The main characteristic of these vesicles is their capability to encapsulate both hydrophilic and lipophilic drugs. Hydrophilic drugs are encapsulated in the inner core where the aqueous compartment is located, while lipophilic drugs are encapsulated into the lipophilic domain of the bilayer [13–15].

The basic components of niosomes are non-ionic surfactants in addition to cholesterol (Chol). The surfactants are mainly composed of two distinct regions and are classified as anionic, cationic, amphoteric, and non-ionic according to the feature of the hydrophilic head, which contains sulfonate or ammonium salts of fatty and zwitterionic acids. Non-ionic surfactants have no charge groups in their hydrophilic heads and are able to form niosomal vesicles that represent an innovative system with better performance compared to conventional drug delivery systems. Indeed, niosomes are more stable than liposomes. They show greater bioavailability compared with conventional dosage forms because they are able to increase the permeation of drugs through the skin [16]. Furthermore, they can be employed for oral and parenteral administration, protecting drugs from biological enzymes and the environment. Moreover, the surfactants employed in the preparation of niosomes are less expensive and more versatile than the phospholipids used for liposomal formulations [17]. To obtain a site-specific drug release, pH-sensitive molecules can be added to the formulation or used to derivatize the surfactants employed. It is well known that some pathological states are associated with pH profiles different from that of normal tissues. Examples include ischemia, infection, inflammation, and cancer, which are often associated with acidosis. Extracellular pH values ranging from 5.5 to 7.0 have been detected in inflamed tissues associated with bacterial infections [18], atherosclerotic plaque, [19], and cancers [20]. This pH gradient is of particular importance since several drugs and drug carriers are taken up by endocytosis and found and/or trapped within endosomes and lysosomes. In this context, niosomes with increased affinity for an acidic pH microenvironment can take advantage of pathological conditions of inflammation for selective targeting. Recently, Rinaldi et al. [21,22] have described the formulation of pH-sensitive niosomes containing Polysorbate 20/Chems (Tween 20, Tw20) or Polysorbate 20 derivatized by Glycine (Tw20-Gly) as an effective strategy for the delivery of anaesthetics and anti-inflammatory drugs. In particular, the preparation steps (panel A) and mechanism of bilayer destabilization (panel B) are shown in Figure 1.

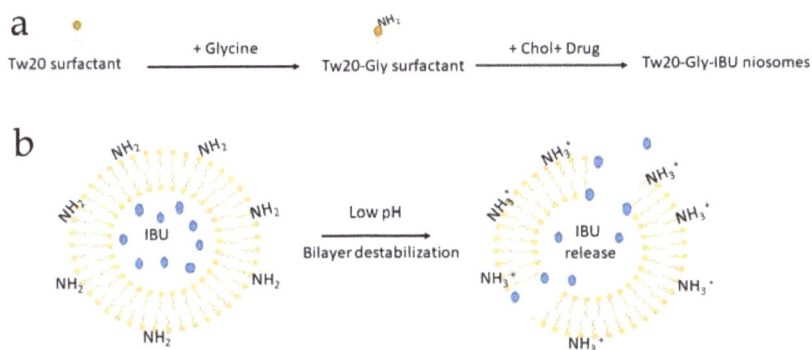

Figure 1. Cartoon describing: (**a**) niosomal preparation by a derivatized surfactant; and (**b**) bilayer destabilization at an acidic pH and consequent drug release. IBU is for Ibuprofen.

In this paper, the well-characterized and selected samples of the previous research study [16,17] were newly prepared to compare the analgesic activity of pH-Tw20Gly niosomes loaded with ibuprofen (NioIbu) to that of free ibuprofen in animal models of acute and chronic pain. We showed that NioIbu strongly increases Ibuprofen's analgesic activity, promoting a longer duration of action of this drug. We suggest that NioIbu is a new and more effective strategy to treat pain arising from chronic inflammatory conditions.

2. Materials and Methods

2.1. Materials

Tween 20 (Tw20), Cholesterol >99% (Chol), *N*-(2-Hydroxyethyl)piperazine-*N*′-(2-ethanesulfonic acid) (HEPES) >99.5%, Sephadex G75, Glycine (Gly), and all other chemicals and solvents of the highest purity and of spectroscopic grade were purchased from Sigma-Aldrich (Sigma-Aldrich S.r.l., Milan, Italy). Water was purified through a Millipore Milli-Q system (Merck S.p.a., Milan, Italy).

2.2. Nanovesicle Formulation and Characterization

Niosomes based on a polysorbate-20 glycine derivative (Tw20Gly) were prepared by the thin film evaporation method at different Ibuprofen loading concentrations (Table 1) and purified by glass chromatography, as previously described [21,22]. A Nano ZS90 Dynamic light scattering LS (Malvern Instruments Ltd., Malvern, UK) at a scattering angle of 90.0° and a LS50B spectrofluorometer (PerkinElmer, MA, USA), were both employed for the physico-chemical characterization of vesicles (hydrodimanic diameter, size distribution, zeta potential, bilayer properties, stability, and in vitro release studies) [21]. Drug entrapment within non-ionic surfactant vesicles was determined using high-performance liquid chromatography (HPLC). HPLC analyses were carried out with a Perkin-Elmer 250 liquid chromatography apparatus (PerkinElmer, MA, USA), equipped with a Perkin-Elmer 235 photo-diode array detector, a 20-μl-loop Rheodyne injector and a computer hardware, as previously described, on purified niosomes after disruption with isopropanol (vesicle dispersion/isopropanol 1:1 *v/v* final ratio) [23].

Table 1. Sample composition (NioIbu 5% has been the analyzed formulation). Nio, pH-Tw20Gly niosomes; NioIbu, pH-Tw20Gly niosomes loaded with different percentages of Ibuprofen Hepes solutions. Tw 20, is for Tween 20; Chol, is for Cholesterol; IBU, is for Ibuprofen.

Sample	Tw20 (mM)	Tw20-Gly (mM)	Chol (mM)	IBU (% *p/v*)
Nio	3.75	11.25	7.5	=
NioIbu 1%	3.75	11.25	7.5	1
NioIbu 3%	3.75	11.25	7.5	3
NioIbu 5%	3.75	11.25	7.5	5
NioIbu 7%	3.75	11.25	7.5	7

Atomic force microscopy (AFM) topographical characterization has been carried out using a standard AFM setup (Dimension Icon, Bruker Inc. in 'soft tapping' mode, Billerica, MA, USA) equipped with standard silicon cantilevers (OTESPA, Bruker Inc., Billerica, MA, USA). Analysis of niosomal dimensions was carried out by means of atomic force microscopy (AFM) by imaging the samples in tapping mode after deposition on a Si substrate. A diameter and height of nine isolated niosomes were measured. These allowed us to determine the surface of the niosomes deposited on the substrate (which obviously lost their original spherical shape) given by the sum of areas of the surface of the spherical cap and of the base circle. Assuming that the flattening of niosomes resulted in the modification of shape and volume without significantly affecting the surface area, the diameter of niosomes in solution was evaluated as that of a sphere having the same surface area.

2.3. Animals and Treatments

We used male CD-1 mice (Harlan, Italy) weighing 25 g in all of the experiments. Mice were housed in colony cages under standard conditions of light, temperature, and relative humidity for at least 1 week before the start of experimental sessions. All experiments were performed according to Legislative Decree 26/14, which implements the European Directive 2010/63/UE on laboratory animal protection in Italy, and were approved by the local ethics committee. Animal studies are reported in accordance with the ARRIVE (Animal Research: Reporting of In Vivo Experiments) guidelines [24].

In all experiments, NioIbu 5%, diluted to obtain the same drug concentration, was compared to: (i) Hepes buffer (HB), (ii) an "unstructured" surfactant formulation (TG), composed of surfactant and cholesterol, and (iii) an "unstructured" surfactant formulation (TG-Ibu), composed of surfactant, cholesterol, and ibuprofen at the same concentrations as the ones present in NioIbu, but not organized in vesicular systems.

2.4. Writhing Test

The procedure was similar to the one previously described [25]. After 1 h of adaptation to transparent cages, mice received a subcutaneous (s.c.) injection of 1500 L of HB, TG, TG-Ibu, and NioIbu into the loose skin over the interscapular area. One hundred and twenty minutes after sample injection, mice received an intraperitoneal (i.p.) injection (10 mL/kg) of 0.6% acetic acid solution. A writhe is characterized by a wave of abdominal muscle contractions accompanied by body elongation and the extension of one or both hind limbs. The number of writhes in a 20-min period was counted, starting 5 min after acetic acid injection.

2.5. Capsaicin-Induced Paw Licking

The method used was similar to the one previously described [26]. Mice were allowed to adapt to transparent cages individually for 1 h before testing. Then, s.c. injections of samples (HB, TG, TG-Ibu, and NioIbu, 40 μL) were performed in the dorsal surface of mice hind paw for 120 min before 1.6 μg of capsaicin (20 μL). A micro syringe with a 26-gauge needle was used to inject capsaicin and samples. The time (in seconds) the animals spent licking the injected paw, for a total period of 5 min, was registered and considered as indicative of pain. Capsaicin was dissolved in DMSO as a stock solution and stored at -20 °C. On the test day, this solution was diluted in order to obtain the final concentration of 1.6 μg/20 μl in DMSO:saline (1:3 *v:v*).

2.6. Zymosan-Induced Hyperalgesia

In these experiments, 20 μL of zymosan A (2.5% *w/v* in saline) were administered s.c. into the dorsal surface of one hind paw. Then, thermal thresholds were determined, as previously reported [27]. Briefly, mice were placed in clear plastic boxes with a glass floor and allowed to acclimatize to their surroundings for at least 1 h in a temperature-controlled (21 °C) experimental room for three consecutive days prior to testing. On the test day, the animals were acclimatized to the experimental room 1 h before paw withdrawal latency (PWL) was measured. Attention was taken to start the test when the animal was not walking, with its hind paw in contact with the glass floor of the apparatus. A radiant heat source was directed at the mouse footpad until an aversive action was observed, such as paw withdrawal, foot drumming, or licking. A timer automatically measured in seconds the paw withdrawal latency. The heat source was set to an intensity of 30 and a cutoff time of 15 s was used to prevent tissue damage. Animals were first tested to determine their baseline PWL; after zymosan injection, the PWL (s) of each animal in response to the plantar test was determined again at 1, 2, 3, 4, 5, 24, and 48 h. In these experiments, HB, TG, TG-Ibu, and NioIbu were injected s.c. in a volume of 40 L in the dorsal surface of mice hind paw, 15 min before zymosan injection.

2.7. Neuropathy-Induced Allodynia and Hyperalgesia

The chronic constriction injury (CCI) model was carried out as previously described [28], with slight modifications [23]. Briefly, mice were anesthetized with chloralium hydrate-xylazine (400 + 10 mg/kg, i.p.). The right sciatic nerve was exposed at the mid-thigh level and, in the vicinity of the sciatic nerve trifurcation, was loosely tied with two ligatures of nylon black monofilament (9–0 non-absorbable, S&T, Neuhausen, Switzerland). Ligatures spaced 1.5–2 mm apart. Then, the muscles and the skin were closed with sutures. These animals were used in two nociceptive tests in the following order: mechanical allodynia followed by thermal hyperalgesia. The threshold for mechanical allodynia was assessed with the dynamic plantar aesthesiometer (Ugo Basile, Italy). Animals were trained on the apparatus, consisting of clear cages with a wire mesh floor, for 3 days before experimental sessions to allow for acclimatization. When the animal was at rest, a straight metal filament exerting an increasing upward force at a constant rate (5 g/s) with a maximum cutoff force of 50 g was placed under the plantar surface of the hind paw. Measurement was stopped when the paw was withdrawn and the results were expressed in grams. The measurement was repeated three times for each paw and averaged.

The development of thermal hyperalgesia was measured by subjecting the injured animals to the plantar test, as described in the "Zymosan-induced hyperalgesia" section.

Behavioural assessments of CCI-induced allodynia and thermal hyperalgesia were carried out 10 days after nerve injury, and behavioural responses compared with the ones measured before surgery. In these experiments, s.c. injection volumes of 40 L of HB, TG, TG-Ibu, and NioIbu were performed in the dorsal surface of mice hind paw.

2.8. Data Analysis and Statistics

Experimental data are presented as mean ± standard error of the mean (s.e.m.). Statistically significant differences between groups were calculated with an analysis of variance (ANOVA) followed by Tukey's post-hoc comparisons. Data were analyzed using the GraphPad Prism 6.03 software. The criterion for significance was set at $P < 0.05$. The data and statistical analysis conformed to the recommendations on experimental design and analysis in pharmacology [29].

3. Results

3.1. Nanovesicle Formulation and Characterization

All in vivo tests were performed by administration of well-characterized (Table 2) and stable (at least 3 months when stored at 4 °C) pH-sensitive vesicles (Nio, NioIbu). AFM characterization indicates that niosomes have a spherical shape (Figure 2). In agreement with DLS, AFM images indicate that NioIbu nanovesicles are smaller and have a less-uniform size than the Nio ones. Sizes deduced from AFM images seem underestimated with respect to the DLS results. In particular, for both the samples, the diameter evaluated by AFM is 70% of that evaluated by DLS, probably due to the approximations assumed in the model. In particular, Ibuprofen-loaded vesicles show the appropriate dimensions and zeta potential to be tested in animal studies. Drug entrapment efficiency is useful to perform in vivo studies, and the bilayer fluidity is quite high to ensure drug release, as reported in Rinaldi et al. [21]. This selection was carried out based on the best in-vitro performance of the sample, in particular in terms of the percentage of released drug [21]; in this previous study, sample characterization in the presence of different pH conditions was carried out, and the pH sensitivity of the selected formulation was confirmed.

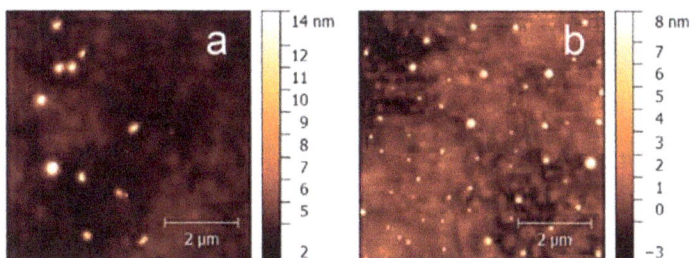

Figure 2. AFM images of Nio (**a**) and NioIbu (**b**) samples.

Table 2. Vesicle characterization. Nio, pH-Tw20Gly niosomes; NioIbu, pH-Tw20Gly niosomes loaded with a 5% Ibuprofen Hepes solution.

Niosomes	Diameter (nm)	AFM Diameter (nm)	ζ Potential (mV)	Polydispersity Index	Fluorescence Anisotropy (AU)	Loaded Drug Conc. (mg/mL)
Nio	215.0 ± 3.0	152 ± 18	−41.0 ± 1.2	0.160 ± 0.08	0.17 ± 0.01	–
NioIbu 5%	122.1 ± 19.6	89 ± 24	−40.2 ± 0.1	0.404 ± 0.05	0.20 ± 0.04	0.37 ± 0.05

3.2. Writing Test

The in vivo antinociceptive activity of NioIbu was first assessed through a writhing test (Figure 2). As detailed in the experimental procedure section, acetic acid was used to induce peripheral pain. Analgesic activity was determined by recording the decrease in the number of writhes after acetic acid injection. The acetic-acid-induced writhing test in mice is the most commonly used method for measuring preliminary antinociceptive activity, since, in this test, both central and peripheral analgesics are detected. In these experiments, tested mice were injected with acetic acid 120 min after drug treatment. Statistical analysis revealed significant differences between treatments [$F_{(3, 28)} = 5.545$, $P = 0.0041$]. In this test, the administration of TG or TG-Ibu did not change the response to acetic acid in mice (Figure 3). Strong inhibition of the number of writhes was instead observed when NioIbu was administered 120 min before the acetic acid (Figure 3). In comparison with the TG group, NioIbu significantly reduced the number of writhes ($P < 0.05$), and the inhibition ratio was 52.5.

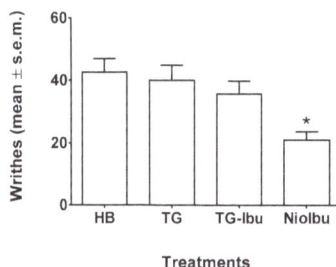

Figure 3. Effects of Hepes buffer (HB), the unstructured surfactant formulation (TG), the unstructured surfactant formulation with the same Ibuprofen (IBU) concentration (TG-Ibu), and TW20-Gly loaded with IBU (NioIbu) on the number of writhes induced by acetic acid. Samples were subcutaneously injected 120 min before acid acetic injection. * is for $P < 0.05$ versus TG. $N = 8$.

3.3. Capsaicin Test

In order to better evaluate the antinociceptive activity of ibuprofen-loaded vesicles, we also performed the capsaicin test (Figure 4). This test reflects acute pain responses related to neurogenic inflammation. In sensory neurons, capsaicin is an activator of the TRPV1 channels present in C-fibers and, to a lesser extent, Aδ. After injection, capsaicin shows a biphasic effect, i.e., it stimulates TRPV1 located in sensory neurons, producing a rapid phase of burning sensation, and local vascular and extravascular responses, followed by a persistent desensitization with concomitant long-lasting analgesia. Statistical analysis revealed significant differences between treatments, as revealed by ANOVA ($F_{(3, 36)}$ = 10.22, $P < 0.0001$). In this test, neither TG nor TG-Ibu reduced the duration of the licking response as compared with the HB-treated mice (Figure 4). A statistically significant antinociceptive effect was shown for NioIbu (inhibition ratio, 55.4%, $P < 0.001$) versus TG-treated mice.

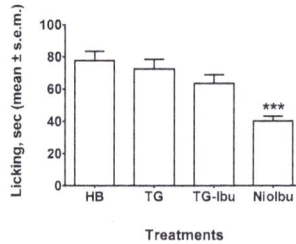

Figure 4. Effects of Hepes buffer (HB), the unstructured surfactant formulation (TG), the unstructured surfactant formulation with the same Ibuprofen (IBU) concentration (TG-Ibu), and TW20-Gly loaded with IBU (NioIbu) on the time spent licking the capsaicin-injected paw. Samples were injected subcutaneously in the dorsal surface of the hind paw 120 min before capsaicin injection. *** is for $P < 0.001$ versus TG. N = 10.

3.4. Zymosan-Induced Hyperalgesia

A s.c. injection of zymosan into mice footpad induces persistent dose- and time-dependent thermal and mechanical hyperalgesia associated with inflammation up to 24 h after treatment (Figure 5). Primary hyperalgesia in the hind paw inflammation model is thought to result from a release of pro-inflammatory mediators that include bradykinin, cytokines, and prostaglandins [30,31]. The reduction in latency response to a thermal stimulus applied to a paw and induced by zymosan was measured as a percentage. In these experiments, samples were injected into the dorsal surface of the right hind paw 15 min before zymonsan injection. As observed in the writhing and capsaicin test, TG and TG-Ibu did not affect the decrease in nociceptive threshold induced by zymosan. On the contrary, the highest increase in pain threshold was observed in NioIbu-treated mice. (Figure 5). Furthermore, the increase in the nociceptive threshold induced by NioIbu was long-lasting, since two-way ANOVA revealed significant differences from 3 to 24 h after NioIbu treatment ($F_{(10, 135)}$ = 3.44, $P = 0.0005$).

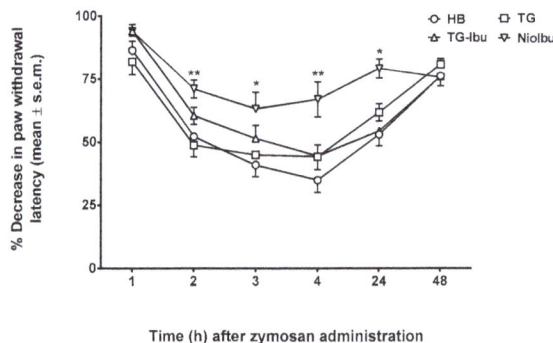

Figure 5. Effects of Hepes buffer (HB), the unstructured surfactant formulation (TG), the unstructured surfactant formulation with the same Ibuprofen (IBU) concentration (TG-Ibu), and TW20-Gly loaded with IBU (NioIbu) on zymosan-induced hyperalgesia. * is for $P < 0.05$ and ** is for $P < 0.01$ versus TG. N = 10.

3.5. Neuropathy-Induced Allodynia and Hyperalgesia

Neuropathic pain is a chronic condition caused by injury to the nervous system. This condition is characterized by spontaneous pain, as well as by exaggerated pain responses to painful stimuli (hyperalgesia) and to normally non-painful stimuli (allodynia). In our experiments, allodynia and hyperalgesia were measured 10 days after nerve injury, because this is when the pain threshold reaches the minimum value. The results obtained in these experiments are shown in Figures 6 and 7. When allodynia was measured (Figure 6), two-way ANOVA showed a significant difference between treatments ($F_{(12, 126)} = 4.453$; $P < 0.0001$). A Tukey's multiple comparison test demonstrated that NioIbu significantly increased paw withdrawal latency from 1 to 3 h after treatment, whereas TG-Ibu induced a transient, not significant increase in the nociceptive threshold (Figure 6).

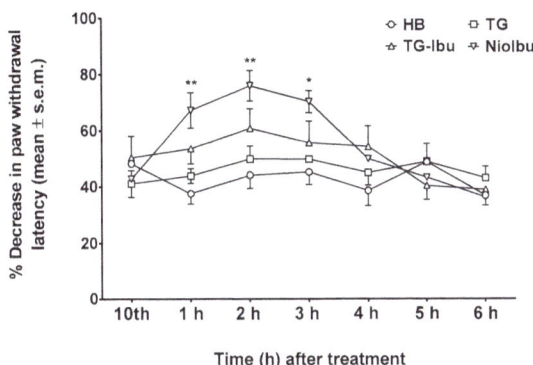

Figure 6. Effects of Hepes buffer (HB), the unstructured surfactant formulation (TG), the unstructured surfactant formulation with the same Ibuprofen (IBU) concentration (TG-Ibu), and TW20-Gly loaded with IBU (NioIbu) on allodynia induced by a chronic constriction injury of the right sciatic nerve. * is for $P < 0.05$ and ** is for $P < 0.01$ versus TG. $N = 8$.

In the same way, two-way ANOVA revealed significant differences in pain threshold when hyperalgesia was measured ($F_{(12, 126)} = 6.811$; $P < 0.0001$) (Figure 7). NioIbu increased the pain threshold from 2 h up to 4 h after treatment, whereas the increase in the pain threshold observed 1 h after TG-Ibu administration was not statistically significant.

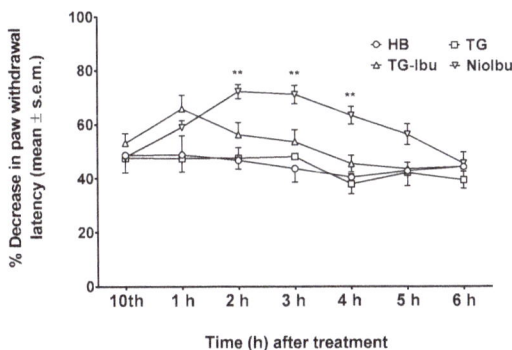

Figure 7. Effects of Hepes buffer (HB), the unstructured surfactant formulation (TG), the unstructured surfactant formulation with the same Ibuprofen (IBU) concentration (TG-Ibu), and TW20-Gly loaded with IBU (NioIbu) on hyperalgesia induced by a chronic constriction injury of the right sciatic nerve. * is for $P < 0.05$ and ** is for $P < 0.01$ versus TG. $N = 8$.

4. Discussion

Several researchers have focused on alternative drug delivery systems to overcome the difficulties associated with the distribution and effectiveness of analgesic drugs. This is mainly due to the low capability of analgesic drugs to pass across biological membranes [32]. One of the strategies adopted to overcome these limitations was loading the drugs into liposomes, which are spherical vesicles composed of phospholipids, such as phosphatidylcholine and phosphatidyl-serine, and possibly other lipids as well [33]. However, liposomes have high production costs due to the phospholipids employed and tend to fuse or aggregate, resulting in an early release of the vesicle payload. Moreover, phospholipids are prone to oxidative degradation. Finally, liposomes have low solubility and stability, and their applicability is limited because they have short half–lives in blood circulation [13,34,35]. To overcome these constraints, we decided to use a new non-toxic drug delivery system, the niosomes. These carriers offer several advantages compared to liposomes: a higher capability to entrap lipophilic, hydrophilic, and amphiphilic drugs; an ability to reach the site of action via oral, parenteral, and topical routes of administration; and a lower cost. [36]. Recently, Di Marzio et al. [13] described specific pH-sensitive, non-ionic surfactant vesicles with polysorbate-20 (Tween-20)/Chems as a good delivery system for analgesic drugs, which increase the stability and affinity in the tissue pH alterations that occur during inflammatory pathologic conditions [37]. These vesicles showed the ability to control and sustain release as well as to protect drugs from catalytic enzymes, thereby increasing drug stability.

Niosomes containing pH-sensitive components, such as TW20Gly, that protonate at lower pH [35] showed bilayer destabilization, leading to localized drug release. This approach could be useful in targeting inflamed tissues. In this study, we evaluated the antinociceptive effects of s.c. injections of Ibuprofen-loaded, pH-sensitive niosomes in comparison with the free form of the drug. To address this issue, we utilized mice under different pain stimuli. This work demonstrates that the use of these nanocarriers enhances the therapeutic efficacy of Ibuprofen, since Ibuprofen-loaded niosomes were effective in reducing pain in laboratory mice. The use of nanovesicles as delivery systems has already been successfully exploited to supply compounds topically and orally. In fact, some studies showed that NSAID-loaded vesicles have better performance in terms of prolonged drug release [38] and improved therapeutic effects [39] compared with the free form of the same compound. Considering that niosomes are a very promising system to administer compounds of different features topically or orally [40–42], we evaluated the capability of niosomes to increase antinociceptive effects of Ibuprofen also in terms of lasting effects after s.c injection. Writhing and capsaicin tests are screening assays commonly used to study peripheral and central antinociceptive activity. Our results showed that, when Ibuprofen-loaded niosomes were administered, there was an increase in the positive response time. In fact, when Ibuprofen was given 120 min earlier, the antinociceptive activity was maintained only in the niosomal form and not in the free form. The capsaicin test confirmed the long-lasting effects of Ibuprofen-loaded niosomes. Similar results were obtained with diclofenac-loaded liposomes administered orally, as reported by Goh et al. [43]. Consistently, in a formalin test, Ibuprofen-loaded niosomes displayed a peripheral antinociceptive activity and were more effective than free Ibuprofen in suppressing inflammatory pain. The niosomal form also had a long-lasting action, while the free form was probably rapidly catabolized [16]. Therefore, the encapsulation of the drug into niosomes significantly enhances drug efficacy and increases the durability of antinociceptive effects. This allows for a reduction in doses and, consequently, might also reduce the drug's side effects.

Some studies reported that nano-formulations reduce hyperalgesic responses to thermal stimuli more efficiently than free drugs [44,45]. Our results on zymosan-induced hyperalgesia are in line with these studies and demonstrate that Ibuprofen-loaded, pH-sensitive niosomes were able to reduce nociception up to 24 h after administration. These results confirm that niosomes release the encapsulated drug efficiently when behavioural experiments were performed. Similarly, Ibuprofen-loaded niosomes decrease neuropathic pain, since the treatment reduced both hyperalgesia and allodynia induced by chronic sciatic nerve constriction.

Pharmaceutics **2019**, *11*, 62

The increase in drug activity when released by niosomes could be explained by the capability of niosomes to transport lipophilic drugs, in this case Ibuprofen, across tissue membranes. This facilitates drug diffusion around the site of application and consequently improves efficacy [13,22].

In conclusion, the present study reveals that Ibuprofen-loaded, pH-sensitive niosomes are able to produce consistent and long-lasting antinociceptive effects. The antinociceptive effects of Ibuprofen-loaded niosomes were observed both in acute and chronic animal models of pain and these results, together with those reported in our previous study [21], suggest that an Ibuprofen pH-sensitive nanocarrier formulation could be further developed and used to treat different pain conditions in humans.

Author Contributions: Conceptualization, S.P. and M.C.; Methodology, S.P., M.C. and M.R.; Formal Analysis, P.M. and D.P.; Investigation, F.M., P.M., F.R. and D.P.; Writing-Original Draft Preparation, F.M., S.P., C.M.; Visualization, P.M. and F.R.

Funding: This research received no external funding.

Acknowledgments: We are grateful to Laura Ciarlo for comments that improved the manuscript. We also thanks Catia Dos Santos for the linguistic revision of the manuscript and Alessandro Paparatti for the graphical abstract.

Conflicts of Interest: The authors declare no conflict of interest.

References

1. Patel, A.; Bell, M.; O'Connor, C.; Inchley, A.; Wibawa, J.; Lane, M.E. Delivery of ibuprofen to the skin. *Int. J. Pharm.* **2013**, *457*, 9–13. [CrossRef] [PubMed]

2. Vane, J.R.; Botting, R.M. Anti-inflammatory drugs and their mechanism of action. *Inflamm. Res.* **1998**, *47*, 78–87. [CrossRef]

3. Doherty, N.S.; Beaver, T.H.; Chan, K.Y.; Coutant, J.E.; Westrich, G.L. The role of prostaglandins in the nociceptive response induced by intraperitoneal injection of zymosan in mice. *Br. J. Pharmacol.* **1987**, *91*, 39–47. [CrossRef] [PubMed]

4. Brunton, L.L.; Chabner, B.A.; Knollman, B.C. *Goodman & Gilman's the Pharmacological Basis of Therapeutics*, 12th ed.; McGraw-Hill Medical: New York, NY, USA, 2011.

5. Moffat, A.C.; Osselton, M.D.; Widdop, B. *Clarke's Analysis of Drugs and Poisons: In Pharmaceuticals, Body Fluids and Postmortem Material*, 2; Pharmaceutical Press and American Pharmacists' Association: London, UK, 2004; p. 1125.

6. Berner, G.; Engels, B.; Vögtle-Junkert, U. Percutaneous ibuprofen therapy with Trauma-Dolgit gel: Bioequivalence studies. *Drugs Exp. Clin. Res.* **2004**, *XV*, 559–564.

7. Pereira-Leite, C.; Nunes, C.; Reis, S. Interaction of nonsteroidal anti-inflammatory drugs with membranes: In vitro assessment and relevance for their biological actions. *Prog. Lipid Res.* **2013**, *52*, 571–584. [CrossRef] [PubMed]

8. Stoye, I.; SchrDer, K.; Müller-Goymann, C.C. Transformation of a liposomal dispersion containing ibuprofen lysinate and phospholipids into mixed micelles—Physico-chemical characterization and influence on drug permeation through excised human stratum corneum. *Eur. J. Pharm. Biopharm.* **1998**, *46*, 191–200. [CrossRef]

9. Abdullah, G.Z.; Abdulkarim, M.F.; Salman, I.M.; Ameer, O.Z.; Yam, M.F.; Mutee, A.F.; Chitneni, M.; Mahdi, E.S.; Basri, M.; Sattar, M.A.; et al. In vitro permeation and in vivo anti-inflammatory and analgesic properties of nanoscaled emulsions containing ibuprofen for topical delivery. *Int. J. Nanomed.* **2011**, *6*, 387–396. [CrossRef] [PubMed]

10. Santi, P.; Nicoli, S.; Colombo, G.; Bettini, R.; Artusi, M.; Rimondi, S.; Padula, C.; Rizzo, P.; Colombo, P. Post-iontophoresis transport of ibuprofen lysine across rabbit ear skin. *Int. J. Pharm.* **2003**, *266*, 69–75. [CrossRef]

11. Park, E.S.; Chang, S.Y.; Hahn, M.; Chi, S.C. Enhancing effect of polyoxyethylene alkyl ethers on the skin permeation of ibuprofen. *Int. J. Pharm.* **2000**, *209*, 109–119. [CrossRef]

12. Brown, M.B.; Hanpanitcharoen, M.; Martin, G.P. An in vitro investigation into the effect of glycosaminoglycans on the skin partitioning and deposition of NSAIDs. *Int. J. Pharm.* **2001**, *225*, 113–121. [CrossRef]

13. Di Marzio, L.; Marianecci, C.; Petrone, M.; Rinaldi, F.; Carafa, M. Novel pH-sensitive non-ionic surfactant vesicles: Comparison between Tween 21 and Tween 20. *Colloids Surf. B Biointerfaces* **2011**, *82*, 18–24. [CrossRef] [PubMed]

14. Dalmoro, A.; Bochicchio, S.; Nasibullin, SF.; Bertoncin, P.; Lamberti, G.; Barba, A.A.; Moustafine, R.I. Polymer-lipid hybrid nanoparticles as enhanced indomethacin delivery systems. *Eur. J. Pharm. Sci.* **2018**, *121*, 16–28. [CrossRef] [PubMed]

15. Rinaldi, F.; Hanieh, P.N.; Chan, L.K.N.; Angeloni, L.; Passeri, D.; Rossi, M.; Wang, J.T.; Imbriano, A.; Carafa, M.; Marianecci, C. Chitosan Glutamate-Coated Niosomes: A Proposal for Nose-to-Brain Delivery. *Pharmaceutics* **2018**, *10*, 38. [CrossRef] [PubMed]

16. Marianecci, C.; Di Marzio, L.; Rinaldi, F.; Celia, C.; Paolino, D.; Alhaique, F.; Esposito, S.; Carafa, M. Niosomes from 80s to present: The state of the art. *Adv. Colloid Interface* **2014**, *205*, 187–206. [CrossRef] [PubMed]

17. Rajera, R.; Nagpal, K.; Singh, S.K.; Mishra, D.N. Niosomes: A controlled and novel drug delivery system. *Biol. Pharm. Bull.* **2011**, *34*, 945–953. [CrossRef]

18. Edlow, D.W.; Sheldon, W.H. The pH of inflammatory exudates. *Proc. Soc. Exp. Biol. Med.* **1971**, *137*, 1328–1332. [CrossRef]

19. Naghavi, M.; John, R.; Naguib, S.; Siadaty, M.S.; Grasu, R.; Kurian, K.C.; van Winkle, W.B.; Soller, B.; Litovsky, S.; Madjid, M.; et al. pH Heterogeneity of human and rabbit atherosclerotic plaques: A new insight into detection of vulnerable plaque. *Atherosclerosis* **2002**, *164*, 27–35. [CrossRef]

20. Gatenby, R.A.; Gillies, R.J. Why do cancers have high aerobic glycolysis? *Nat. Rev. Cancer* **2004**, *4*, 891–899. [CrossRef]

21. Rinaldi, F.; Del Favero, E.; Rondelli, V.; Pieretti, S.; Bogni, A.; Ponti, J.; Rossi, F.; Di Marzio, L.; Paolino, D.; Marianecci, C.; et al. pH-sensitive niosomes: Effects on cytotoxicity and on inflammation and pain in murine models. *J. Enzym. Inhib. Med. Chem.* **2017**, *32*, 538–546. [CrossRef]

22. Marianecci, C.; Rinaldi, F.; Di Marzio, L.; Mastriota, M.; Pieretti, S.; Celia, C.; Paolino, D.; Iannone, M.; Fresta, M.; Carafa, M. Ammonium glycyrrhizinate-loaded niosomes as a potential nanotherapeutic system for anti-inflammatory activity in murine models. *Int. J. Nanomed.* **2014**, *9*, 635–651. [CrossRef]

23. Carafa, M.; Marianecci, C.; Rinaldi, F.; Santucci, E.; Tampucci, S.; Monti, D. Span and Tween neutral and pH-sensitive vesicles: Characterization and in vitro skin permeation. *J. Liposome Res.* **2009**, *19*, 332–334. [CrossRef] [PubMed]

24. Kilkenny, C.; Browne, W.J.; Cuthill, I.C.; Emerson, M.; Altman, D.G. Improving bioscience research reporting: The ARRIVE guidelines for reporting animal research. *PLoS Biol.* **2010**, *8*, 1000412. [CrossRef] [PubMed]

25. Pieretti, S.; Di Giannuario, A.; Capasso, A.; Sorrentino, L.; Loizzo, A. Effects induced by cysteamine on chemically-induced nociception in mice. *Life Sci.* **1994**, *54*, 1091–1099. [CrossRef]

26. Sakurada, T.; Katsumata, K.; Tan-No, K.; Sakurada, S.; Kisara, K. The capsaicin test in mice for evaluating tachykinin antagonists in the spinal cord. *Neuropharmacology* **1992**, *31*, 1279–1285. [CrossRef]

27. Colucci, M.; Maione, F.; Bonito, M.C.; Piscopo, A.; Di Giannuario, A.; Pieretti, S. New insights of dimethyl sulphoxide effects (DMSO) on experimental in vivo models of nociception and inflammation. *Pharmacol. Res.* **2008**, *57*, 419–425. [CrossRef] [PubMed]

28. Bennett, G.J.; Xie, Y.K. A peripheral mononeuropathy in rat that produces disorders of pain sensation like those seen in man. *Pain* **1988**, *33*, 87–107. [CrossRef]

29. Curtis, M.J.; Bond, R.A.; Spina, D.; Ahluwalia, A.; Alexander, S.P.; Giembycz, M.A.; Gilchrist, A.; Hoyer, D.; Insel, P.A.; Izzo, A.A.; et al. Experimental design and analysis and their reporting: New guidance for publication in BJP. *Br. J. Pharmacol.* **2015**, *172*, 3461–3471. [CrossRef]

30. Bélichard, P.; Landry, M.; Faye, P.; Bachvarov, D.R.; Bouthillier, J.; Pruneau, D.; Marceau, F. Inflammatory hyperalgesia induced by zymosan in the plantar tissue of the rat: Effect of kinin receptor antagonists. *Immunopharmacology* **2000**, *46*, 139–147. [CrossRef]

31. Ren, K.; Dubner, R. Inflammatory Models of Pain and Hyperalgesia. *ILAR J.* **1999**, *40*, 111–118. [CrossRef]

32. Lucio, M.; Lima, J.L.; Reis, S. Drug-membrane interactions: Significance for medicinal chemistry. *Curr. Med. Chem.* **2010**, *17*, 1795–1809. [CrossRef]

33. Gaur, P.K.; Bajpai, M.; Mishra, S.; Verma, A. Development of ibuprofen nanoliposome for transdermal delivery: Physical characterization, in vitro/in vivo studies, and anti-inflammatory activity. *Artif. Cells Nanomed. Biotechnol.* **2016**, *44*, 370–375. [CrossRef] [PubMed]

34. Bozzuto, G.; Molinari, A. Liposomes as nanomedical devices. *Int. J. Nanomed.* **2015**, *10*, 975–999. [CrossRef] [PubMed]

35. Masotti, A.; Vicennati, P.; Alisi, A.; Marianecci, C.; Rinaldi, F.; Carafa, M.; Ortaggi, G. Novel Tween 20 derivatives enable the formation of efficient pH-sensitive drug delivery vehicles for human hepatoblastoma. *Bioorg. Med. Chem. Lett.* **2010**, *20*, 3021–3025. [CrossRef] [PubMed]

36. Verma, S.; Singh, S.K.; Syan, N.; Mathur, P.; Valecha, V. Nanoparticle vesicular system: A versatile tool for drug delivery. *J. Chem. Pharm. Res.* **2010**, *2*, 496–509.

37. Lehner, R.; Wang, X.; Wolf, M.; Hunziker, P. Designing switchable nanosystems for medical application. *J. Control. Release* **2012**, *161*, 307–316. [CrossRef]

38. Das, M.K.; Palei, N.N. Sorbitan ester niosomes for topical delivery of rofecoxib. *Indian J. Exp. Biol.* **2011**, *49*, 438–445.

39. Naresh, R.A.; Raja, G.K.; Pillai, N.; Udupa, N.; Chandrashekar, G. Anti-inflammatory activity of niosome encapsulated diclofenac sodium in arthritic rats. *Indian J. Pharmacol.* **1994**, *26*, 46–48.

40. Shahiwala, A.; Misra, A. Studies in topical application of niosomally entrapped Nimesulide. *J. Pharm. Pharm. Sci.* **2002**, *5*, 220–225.

41. Goh, J.Z.; Tang, S.N.; Zuraini, A.; Zakaria, Z.A.; Kadir, A.A.; Chiong, H.S. Enhanced anti-inflammatory effects of nanoencapsulated diclofenac. *Eur. J. Inflamm.* **2013**, *11*, 855–861. [CrossRef]

42. Sankhyan, A.; Pawar, P. Recent Trends in Niosome as Vesicular Drug Delivery System. *J. Appl. Pharm. Sci.* **2012**, *2*, 20–32. [CrossRef]

43. Goh, J.Z.; Tang, S.N.; Chiong, H.S.; Yong, Y.K.; Zuraini, A.; Hakim, M.N. Evaluation of antinociceptive activity of nanoliposome-encapsulated and free-form diclofenac in rats and mice. *Nanomedicine* **2014**, *10*, 297–303. [CrossRef]

44. Narasimha Reddy, D.; Udupa, N. Formulation and Evaluation of Oral and Transdermal Preparations of Flurbiprofen and Piroxicam Incorporated with Different Carriers. *Drug Dev. Ind. Pharm.* **2008**, *19*, 843–852. [CrossRef]

45. Joshi, S.K.; Hernandez, G.; Mikusa, J.P.; Zhu, C.Z.; Zhong, C.; Salyers, A.; Wismer, C.T.; Chandran, P.; Decker, M.W.; Honore, P. Comparison of antinociceptive actions of standard analgesics in attenuating capsaicin and nerve-injury-induced mechanical hypersensitivity. *Neuroscience* **2006**, *143*, 587–596. [CrossRef]

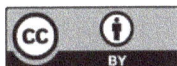

pharmaceutics

MDPI

Article

Development of Multifunctional Liposomes Containing Magnetic/Plasmonic MnFe$_2$O$_4$/Au Core/Shell Nanoparticles

Ana Rita O. Rodrigues [1], Joana O. G. Matos [1], Armando M. Nova Dias [1], Bernardo G. Almeida [1], Ana Pires [2], André M. Pereira [2], João P. Araújo [2], Maria-João R. P. Queiroz [3], Elisabete M. S. Castanheira [1] and Paulo J. G. Coutinho [1,*]

[1] Centro de Física da Universidade do Minho (CFUM), Campus de Gualtar, 4710-057 Braga, Portugal; ritarodrigues@fisica.uminho.pt (A.R.O.R.); pg26303@alunos.uminho.pt (J.O.G.M.); pg36912@alunos.uminho.pt (A.M.N.D.); bernardo@fisica.uminho.pt (B.G.A.); ecoutinho@fisica.uminho.pt (E.M.S.C.)

[2] IFIMUP/IN—Instituto de Nanociência e Nanotecnologia, Universidade do Porto, R. Campo Alegre, 4169-007 Porto, Portugal; ana.pires@fc.up.pt (A.P.); ampereira@fc.up.pt (A.M.P.); jearaujo@fc.up.pt (J.P.A.)

[3] Centro de Química da Universidade do Minho (CQUM), Campus de Gualtar, 4710-057 Braga, Portugal; mjrpq@quimica.uminho.pt

* Correspondence: pcoutinho@fisica.uminho.pt; Tel.: +351-253-604-321

Received: 20 November 2018; Accepted: 24 December 2018; Published: 31 December 2018

Abstract: Multifunctional liposomes containing manganese ferrite/gold core/shell nanoparticles were developed. These magnetic/plasmonic nanoparticles were covered by a lipid bilayer or entrapped in liposomes, which form solid or aqueous magnetoliposomes as nanocarriers for simultaneous chemotherapy and phototherapy. The core/shell nanoparticles were characterized by UV/Visible absorption, X-Ray Diffraction (XRD), Transmission Electron Microscopy (TEM), and Superconducting Quantum Interference Device (SQUID). The magnetoliposomes were characterized by Dynamic Light Scattering (DLS) and TEM. Fluorescence-based techniques (FRET, steady-state emission, and anisotropy) investigated the incorporation of a potential anti-tumor drug (a thienopyridine derivative) in these nanosystems. The core/shell nanoparticles exhibit sizes of 25 ± 2 nm (from TEM), a plasmonic absorption band (λ_{max} = 550 nm), and keep magnetic character. XRD measurements allowed for the estimation of 13.3 nm diameter for manganese ferrite core and 11.7 nm due to the gold shell. Aqueous magnetoliposomes, with hydrodynamic diameters of 152 ± 18 nm, interact with model membranes by fusion and are able to transport the anti-tumor compound in the lipid membrane, with a high encapsulation efficiency (*EE (%)* = 98.4 ± 0.8). Solid magnetoliposomes exhibit hydrodynamic diameters around 140 nm and also carry successfully the anticancer drug (with *EE (%)* = 91.2 ± 5.2), while also being promising as agents for phototherapy. The developed multifunctional liposomes can be promising as therapeutic agents for combined chemo/phototherapy.

Keywords: magnetic/plasmonic nanoparticles; multifunctional liposomes; manganese ferrite; gold shell; anti-tumor drugs; cancer therapy

1. Introduction

In recent years, a revolution in cancer therapy has taken place due to the development of multi-tasked nanostructures or materials for applications in oncology [1,2]. In chemotherapy, the ideal nano-encapsulation system should have biophysical properties that favor the passive accumulation in tumors upon intravenous administration, as well as controlled triggered release of the encapsulated active molecules. In this context, magnetic nano-encapsulation systems are promising since they can enable the magnetic drug targeting by static gradient magnetic fields and magnetic hyperthermia, which produce local heat as a trigger for drug release and a synergistic cytotoxic effect in cancer cells [3–7]. Additionally, systems based on superparamagnetic nanoparticles can generate high-resolution images by T2-weighted magnetic resonance imaging (MRI) for tumor diagnosis [7–9].

Noble metal (Ag, Au) nanoparticles strongly absorb light in the visible region due to coherent oscillations of the metal conduction band electrons in strong resonance with visible frequencies of light. This phenomenon is known as surface plasmon resonance (SPR) [10–13] and is highly dependent on nanoparticles size, shape, surface, and dielectric properties of the surrounding medium [14–16]. Light absorbed by nanoparticles is readily dissipated as heat. Due to their large absorption cross sections, plasmonic nanoparticles can generate a significant amount of heat and increase temperatures in their vicinities [17]. If a sufficient number of nanoparticles are present, the temperature fields overlap and create a substantial global temperature rise [18]. From the point of view of cancer therapeutics, noble metal nanoparticles become very useful as agents for plasmonic photothermal therapy (PTT) on account of their enhanced absorption cross sections, which are four to five orders of magnitude larger than those offered by conventional photo-absorbing dyes [16]. This strong absorption ensures effective laser therapy at relatively lower energies, which render the therapy method minimally invasive. Additionally, metal nanostructures have a higher photo-stability and do not suffer from photo-bleaching [16,19]. Recently, plasmonic nanoparticles have also been used as photoacoustic imaging (PAI) agents to increase tissue penetration, as well as sensitivity and spatial resolution [20].

In nanomedicine, systems with combined magnetic and plasmonic properties are of particular interest for theranostics since they combine simultaneously multiple imaging modalities for diagnosis with complementary synergistic strategies for therapy [21–23]. Gold nanoparticles have been largely used in biomedical applications for their low toxicity, great biocompatibility, easy conjugation with active biomolecules, and their remarkable optical properties, which enable their use as diagnostic and therapeutic agents [19,24]. However, recent works have shown that the conjugation of gold nanoparticles with magnetic ones may decrease the overall magnetization of the nanostructure [25]. Thus, coating magnetic nanoparticles with gold should be carefully considered in order to ensure proper magnetic capabilities for their application. Among all magnetic nanoparticles, those of manganese ferrite have recently received great attention for their high magnetic susceptibility, which suggests that they may be promising as hyperthermia and magnetic drug targeting agents [26,27].

In this study, magnetic/plasmonic nanoparticles possessing a manganese ferrite core and a gold shell were prepared. In order to develop applications in cancer therapy, the prepared nanoparticles were entrapped in liposomes (aqueous magnetoliposomes, AMLs) or covered with a lipid bilayer (solid magnetoliposomes, SMLs). These new nanosystems were tested in this scenario as nanocarriers for a potential anticancer drug, especially active against melanoma, breast adenocarcinoma, and non-small cell lung cancer [28]. In addition, the local heating capability of the developed systems was monitored through the fluorescence quenching of rhodamine B incorporated in the lipid layer when excited with a light source. Considering their potentialities, the new nanosystems developed in this study can be promising for future applications in cancer therapy.

2. Materials and Methods

All the solutions were prepared using spectroscopic grade solvents and ultrapure water of Milli-Q grade (MilliporeSigma, St. Louis, MO, USA).

2.1. Preparation of Manganese Ferrite/Gold Core/Shell Nanoparticles

Manganese ferrite nanoparticles (NPs) were synthesized in 5 mL aqueous solution, by the co-precipitation method, as previously described [26]. First, an aqueous solution containing 612 μL of

50% NaOH solution was heated to 90 °C. Then, a mixture containing 500 µL of 0.5 M MnSO$_4$·H$_2$O solution and 500 µL of 1 M FeCl$_3$·6H$_2$O solution was added, drop by drop, to the previously warmed basic solution under magnetic stirring. After two hours at 90 °C, manganese ferrite nanoparticles were formed. For purification, the obtained sample was washed several times with ethanol, by centrifugation (14,000 *g*) and magnetic decantation.

For growth of the gold shell, a method adapted from a previously described procedure was used [19]. In addition, 5 mL of an aqueous dispersion of the synthesized MnFe$_2$O$_4$ nanoparticles (with concentration of 4 mg/mL) were added to 25 mL of glycerol and heated up to 200 °C, under vigorous stirring. Then, 2 mL of 0.02 M solution of gold(III) chloride hydrate (HAuCl$_4$), from Sigma-Aldrich (St. Louis, MO, USA), were added dropwise. After 15 minutes under continuous stirring at 200 °C, the gold shell was formed around the MnFe$_2$O$_4$ core NPs. To remove glycerol residues, the synthesized NPs were washed by centrifugation (14,000 *g*) with ethanol.

2.2. Preparation of Magnetoliposomes

For magnetoliposomes preparation, the lipids L-α-phosphatidylcholine from egg yolk (Egg-PC), and 1,2-dioleoyl-*sn*-glycero-3-phospho-*rac*-(1-glycerol) sodium salt (DOPG), from Sigma-Aldrich (St. Louis, MO, USA), were used in a final concentration of 1 mM. The ethanol injection method was employed to obtain aqueous magnetoliposomes (AMLs) [29]. Accordingly, a 20 mM lipid solution in ethanol was injected, under vigorous vortexing, to an aqueous dispersion of manganese ferrite/gold nanoparticles (with 4 mg/mL concentration). After encapsulation, the ferrofluid was washed with water and purified by magnetic decantation to remove all the non-encapsulated NPs.

For the preparation of solid magnetoliposomes (SMLs), a method previously described was used [30]. First, 10 µL of a solution of the synthesized MnFe$_2$O$_4$/Au core/shell nanoparticles (0.02 mg/mL) were ultra-sonicated for one minute at 189 W, and 3 mL of chloroform were added to the solution. Then, immediately after vigorous agitation, 150 µL of a 20 mM methanolic solution of the lipid DOPG (1,2-dioleoyl-*sn*-glycero-3-phospho-*rac*-(1-glycerol) sodium salt) were injected under vortexing to form the first lipid layer of the SMLs. To remove the lipid that was not attached to the nanoparticles surface, the particles were washed twice by magnetic decantation with ultrapure water. The lipid bilayer was completed by a new injection of 150 µL of 20 mM lipid methanolic solution, under vortexing, in 3 mL of aqueous dispersion of the particles with the first lipid layer. The SMLs obtained were then washed and purified with ultrapure water by magnetic decantation.

The anti-tumor compound methyl 3-amino-6-(benzo[*d*]thiazol-2-ylamino)thieno[3,2-*b*]pyridine-2-carboxylate was incorporated into aqueous magnetoliposomes by the co-injection method (simultaneous injection of compound and lipid) in a final compound concentration of 2 µM. In solid magnetoliposomes, the compound was incorporated by injection of an ethanolic solution (0.2 mM) immediately before the formation of the second lipid layer.

2.3. Preparation of Giant Unilamellar Vesicles (GUVs)

GUVs of soybean lecithin (L-α-phosphatidylcholine from soybean), from Sigma-Aldrich (St. Louis, MO, USA), were obtained by the thin film hydration method [31,32]. For that, a lipid film of 100 µL of soybean lecithin solution (1 mM) was obtained by solvent evaporation under an argon stream, and 40 µL of water were added, followed by incubation at 45 °C for 30 min. Then, 3 mL of glucose aqueous solution (0.1 M) were added and the resulting solution was again incubated at 37 °C for 2 h. After incubation, the GUVs suspension was centrifuged at 14,000 *g* for 30 minutes at 20 °C, to remove multi-lamellar vesicles and lipid aggregates.

2.4. Spectroscopic Measurements

2.4.1. General Methods

Absorption spectra were performed in a Shimadzu UV-3600 Plus UV-vis-NIR (Shimadzu Corporation, Kyoto, Japan) spectrophotometer. Fluorescence measurements were recorded using a Horiba Fluorolog 3 spectrofluorimeter (HORIBA Jobin Yvon IBH Ltd., Glasgow, UK), equipped with double mono-chromators in both excitation and emission, Glan-Thompson polarizers, and a temperature controlled cuvette holder. Fluorescence spectra were corrected for the instrumental response of the system.

2.4.2. FRET Measurements

Förster Resonance Energy Transfer (FRET) assays were employed to confirm the formation of the lipid bilayer in the solid magnetoliposomes (SMLs). For that purpose, the nitrobenzoxazole labeled lipid NBD-C$_6$-HPC (1-palmitoyl-2-{6-[(7-nitro-2-1,3-benzoxadiazol-4-yl)amino]hexanoyl} -sn-glycero-3-phosphocholine) (from Avanti Polar Lipids, Alabaster, AL, USA) was included in the first lipid layer, while the rhodamine B labeled lipid Rhodamine B-DHPE (1,2-dipalmitoyl-*sn*-glycero-3-phospho-ethanolamine-*N*-lissamine rhodamine B sulfonyl (ammonium salt)) (from Avanti Polar Lipids, Alabaster, AL, USA) was included in the second lipid layer.

FRET efficiency, Φ_{RET}, defined as the proportion of donor molecules that have transferred their excess energy to the acceptor molecules, was calculated through donor emission quenching, by taking the ratio of the donor integrated fluorescence intensities in the presence of acceptor (F_{DA}) and in the absence of acceptor (F_D) (Equation (1)) [33].

$$\Phi_{RET} = 1 - \frac{F_{DA}}{F_D} \tag{1}$$

The distance between the donor and acceptor molecules was determined through the FRET efficiency (Equation (2)).

$$r = R_0 \left[\frac{1 - \Phi_{RET}}{\Phi_{RET}} \right]^{1/6} \tag{2}$$

where R_0 is the Förster radius (critical distance), that can be obtained by the spectral overlap, $J(\lambda)$, between the donor emission and the acceptor absorption, according to Equations (3) and (4) (with R_0 in Å, λ in nm, $\varepsilon_A(\lambda)$ in M^{-1} cm^{-1}) [33].

$$R_0 = 0.2108 \left[k^2 \Phi_D^0 n^{-4} J(\lambda) \right]^{1/6} \tag{3}$$

$$J(\lambda) = \int_0^\infty I_D(\lambda)\, \varepsilon_A(\lambda)\, \lambda^4 d\lambda \tag{4}$$

where $k^2 = \frac{2}{3}$ is the orientational factor assuming random orientation of the dyes, n is the refraction index of the medium, $I_D(\lambda)$ is the fluorescence spectrum of the donor normalized so that $\int_0^\infty I_D(\lambda)d\lambda = 1$, and $\varepsilon_A(\lambda)$ is the molar absorption coefficient of the acceptor. Φ_D^0, the fluorescence quantum yield of the donor in the absence of energy transfer, was determined by the standard method (Equation (5)) [34,35].

$$\Phi_D^0 = \frac{A_r F_D n_D^2}{A_D F_r n_r^2} \Phi_r \tag{5}$$

where A is the absorbance at the excitation wavelength, F is the integrated emission area, and n is the refraction index of the solvents used. Subscripts refer to the reference (r) or donor (D). The absorbance at the excitation wavelength was always lower than 0.1 to avoid the inner filter effects. The NBD-C$_6$-HPC molecule intercalated in lipid membranes was used as a reference, $\Phi_r = 0.32$ at 25 °C, as reported by Invitrogen [36].

The hydrophobic dye Nile Red (energy acceptor) was also incorporated in magnetoliposomes labelled with NBD-C_6-HPC (NBD as energy donor) for monitoring the interaction of magnetoliposomes with GUVs by FRET.

2.4.3. Fluorescence Anisotropy Measurements

The steady-state fluorescence anisotropy, r, is calculated by the equation below.

$$r = \frac{I_{VV} - G I_{VH}}{I_{VV} + 2G I_{VH}} \tag{6}$$

where I_{VV} and I_{VH} are the intensities of the emission spectra obtained with vertical and horizontal polarization, respectively (for vertically polarized excitation light), and $G = I_{HV}/I_{HH}$ is the instrument correction factor, where I_{HV} and I_{HH} are the emission intensities obtained with vertical and horizontal polarization (for horizontally polarized excitation light).

2.4.4. Drug Encapsulation Efficiency

The encapsulation efficiency, EE (%), of the potential anti-tumor drug in magnetoliposomes, was determined through fluorescence emission measurements. Therefore, drug loaded magnetoliposomes were subjected to centrifugation at 11,000 rpm for 60 min using Amicon® Ultra centrifugal filter units 100 kDa (Merck Millipore, Darmstadt, Germany). Then, the filtrate (containing the non-encapsulated drug) was pipetted out, the water was evaporated, and the same amount of ethanol was added. After vigorous agitation, its fluorescence was measured, which allowed it to determine the drug concentration using a calibration curve (fluorescence intensity *vs.* concentration) previously obtained in the same solvent. Three independent measurements were performed for each system and standard deviations (SD) were calculated. The encapsulation efficiency was determined using Equation (7).

$$EE(\%) = \frac{(total\ amount - amount\ of\ non\ encapsulated\ compound)}{total\ amount} \times 100 \tag{7}$$

2.5. Structural Characterization

2.5.1. Transmission Electron Microscopy (TEM)

TEM images of nanoparticles and solid magnetoliposomes were acquired using a Transmission Electron Microscope Leica LEO 906E (Leica Microsystems, Wetzlar, Germany) operating at 120 kV, at UME (Electron Microscopy Unit), University of Trás-os-Montes and Alto Douro (Vila Real, Portugal). For SMLs, a negative staining was employed, using a 2% aqueous solution of ammonium molybdate tetrahydrate. In addition, 20 μL of the sample and 20 μL of the staining solution were mixed and a drop of the mixture was placed onto a Formvar grid (Agar Scientific Ltd., Essex, UK), held by tweezers. After 20 s, almost all the solution was removed with filter paper and left to dry. TEM images were processed using *ImageJ* software (National Institutes of Health (NIH), Bethesda, MD, USA) with the addition of a value to all pixels so that a white background resulted, which was followed by inversion and enhanced local contrast. Subsequently, the ParticleSizer plugin [37] was used and was followed by particle analysis. The area of each particle allowed an estimation of the particle diameter. The resulting histogram was fitted to a bimodal Gaussian distribution.

2.5.2. X-Ray Diffraction (XRD)

X-Ray Diffraction (XRD) analyses were performed using a conventional Philips PW 1710 (Royal Philips, Amsterdam, The Netherlands) diffractometer, operating with CuK$_\alpha$ radiation, in a Bragg-Brentano configuration.

2.5.3. Dynamic Light Scattering (DLS)

The mean diameter and size distribution (polydispersity index) of aqueous and solid magnetoliposomes (1 mM lipid concentration) were measured using Dynamic Light Scattering (DLS) equipment NANO ZS Malvern Zetasizer (Malvern Panalytical Ltd., Malvern, UK) at 25 °C, using an He-Ne laser of λ = 632.8 nm and a detector angle of 173°. The measurements were also carried out for the magnetoliposomes in a solution of human serum albumin (35 mg/mL) in PBS buffer (pH = 7.4). Five independent measurements were performed for each sample.

2.6. Magnetic Measurements

Magnetic measurements of the dry core/shell nanoparticles were performed at room temperature in a Superconducting Quantum Interference Device (SQUID) magnetometer Quantum Design MPMS5XL (Quantum Design Inc., San Diego, CA, USA) using applied magnetic fields up to 5.5 T.

2.7. Measurement of the Photothermal Effect

Solid magnetoliposomes incorporating the labelled lipid Rhodamine B-DHPE were irradiated and Rhodamine B emission was monitored by a function of time, using the detection system of a SPEX Fluorolog 2 spectrofluorimeter (HORIBA Jobin Yvon IBH Ltd., Glasgow, UK). The irradiation setup consisted in a Xenon arc lamp (200 W) and an optical fiber, using a Thorlabs FEL0600 (Thorlabs Inc., Newton, NJ, USA) long pass filter with cut-on wavelength at 600 nm, to ensure the excitation of only the gold nanoparticles (not exciting Rhodamine B dye).

3. Results and Discussion

3.1. Nanoparticles Characterization

3.1.1. Absorption Spectra

Figure 1 displays the UV-Visible absorption spectrum of the synthesized manganese ferrite/gold core/shell nanoparticles. The absorption spectra of net gold nanoparticles and net manganese ferrite nanoparticles are also shown for comparison.

The spectrum of manganese ferrite NPs is typical of an indirect semiconductor, as reported earlier [26], while the spectrum of gold nanoparticles obtained by the standard Turkevish method [38] reveals a characteristic local surface plasmon resonance (LSPR) band, with a maximum around 530 nm. In comparison, the absorption spectrum of manganese ferrite/gold core/shell NPs exhibits a broader and red shifted plasmon band (maximum at 550 nm). The absorption spectrum of gold nanoshells depends on their thickness, as well as on the refraction index of both core and surrounding media [39]. Theoretical studies have shown that, for an air filled core of 10 nm size and a gold shell of 5 nm in water medium, the resonance peak is expected to occur at 538 nm, while, for a 10-nm shell, it should appear at 552 nm [40]. The increase of the core refraction index results in a red shift of the plasmon resonance peak [39]. For a 3-nm gold shell thickness on a 10-nm magnetite core, a resonance peak at 560 nm was found [41].

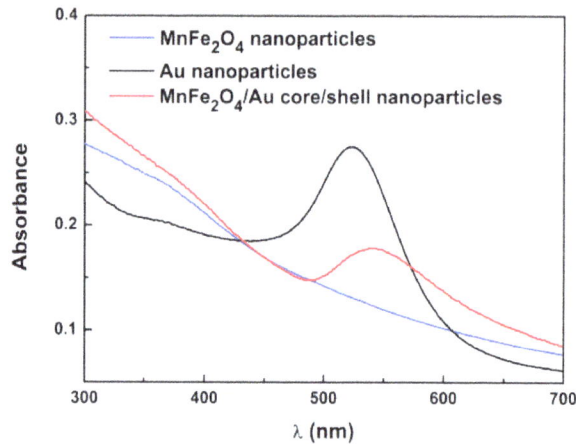

Figure 1. UV-Visible absorption spectra of aqueous dispersions of manganese ferrite nanoparticles, gold nanoparticles, and $MnFe_2O_4$/Au core/shell nanoparticles.

3.1.2. X-Ray Diffraction (XRD) Measurements

XRD analysis confirmed the synthesis of a pure crystalline phase of manganese ferrite/gold nanoparticles, since all their characteristic peaks (CIF 2300618 for manganese ferrite and CIF 9013035 for gold), marked by their indices, were observed (Figure 2b). The percentage amounts obtained for $MnFe_2O_4$ and Au were 59.1% and 40.9%, respectively. Mean sizes of 13.3 nm for manganese ferrite and 11.7 nm for gold, were estimated through a Rietveld analysis using Fullprof software [42]. Table 1 summarizes the main results of the Rietveld analysis. For the net manganese ferrite powdered sample, it resulted in a poor R_F factor of 9.0. It was possible to improve it by optimizing the overall isothermal factor, B_{over}, but an unreasonable value of -2.79 was obtained. A similar improvement was possible by accounting for the effect of sample microstructure (Figure 2a), according to Equation (8) [43], which gives the micro-absorption correction term, P.

$$P = P_0 + C\frac{\tau}{\sin\theta}\left(1 - \frac{\tau}{\sin\theta}\right) \tag{8}$$

where P_0 is the bulk contribution to the micro-absorption effect and τ is the normalized surface roughness parameter [43].

Table 1. Selected Rietveld analysis parameters.

Sample	$O_{x,y,z}$ (*)	i (*)	Micro Absorption Correction	Overall Temperature Factor, B_{over}	Lattice Constant (nm)	Size (nm)	R_f	χ^2
$MnFe_2O_4$	0.251	0.928	No	0 (+)	0.84693	13.8	9.03	1.33
$MnFe_2O_4$	0.251	0.898	No	-2.79	0.84684	13.2	4.45	1.18
$MnFe_2O_4$	0.257	0.60	Yes (#)	0 (+)	0.84685	13.3	3.18	1.18
$MnFe_2O_4$/Au	0.257 (+)	0.60 (+)	Yes (##)	0 (+)	0.84685 (*)	13.3	4.70	1.56
	—	—		0 (+)	0.406945	11.7	0.68	

(#) $P_0 = 0.629$, $C = 1.31$, $\tau = 0.055$. (##) $P_0 = 0.607$, $C = 1.15$, $\tau = 0.084$. (+) fixed values. (*) Values in CIF file 2360018 are $O_{x,y,z} = 0.25053$ and $i = 0.33$.

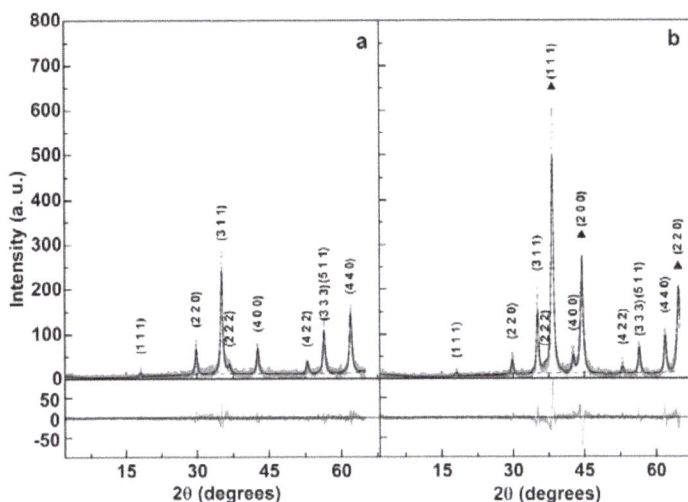

Figure 2. XRD diffractogram of manganese ferrite (**a**) and manganese ferrite/gold core/shell nanoparticles (**b**). Gold diffraction peaks are marked by a filled triangle.

Considering $\mu\bar{l} = 0.01$ (μ is the linear absorption coefficient and $\bar{l}$ is the mean chord length of the powder particle) and the values in Table 1 for Equation (8) parameters, a degree of inversion of $i = 0.60$ is obtained for manganese ferrite. This value is close to the one reported by Chen et al. ($i = 0.67$) [44], using a similar preparation method for $MnFe_2O_4$. The Rietveld analysis of gold phase was not optimal, as the intensity of peak (111) is lower and that of peak (200) is higher than the experimental ones. In addition, the analysis of $MnFe_2O_4$ phase decreased its quality, as the R_F factor increased from 3.18 to 4.70 and the peak (311) got much lower than the experimental one. This could be due to the expected shell morphology of gold in the prepared $MnFe_2O_4/Au$ nanocomposites in which a layer of gold grows on the $MnFe_2O_4$ surface. This morphology, through lattice mismatch induced stress, is predictable to change the intensity of the diffraction peaks [45]. An atomistic modelling of the core/shell nanoparticle is anticipated to yield a better description of the XRD diffractogram [46] and this will be addressed in a future study. The obtained weight fraction of gold was 40.9%, but this is calculated using proportionality factors between diffraction intensity and mass, ATZs [42], that do not take into account the dependence of diffraction intensity on particle size. Since the lattice constant of Au is less than half that of $MnFe_2O_4$, the reduction of diffraction intensity with particle size is much more pronounced for Au than for $MnFe_2O_4$. This means that the value given by Fullprof software is expected to be much lower than the real one. Considering the obtained size of manganese ferrite of 13.3 nm and using the phase densities that resulted from the XRD analysis (5.04 g cm^{-3} for $MnFe_2O_4$ and 19.4 g cm^{-3} for Au), the mass percentage of gold would be 98.7% if the obtained size of gold phase (11.7 nm) corresponds to the shell thickness. This percentage would change to 95.6% if the obtained size value of 11.7 nm corresponds to the double of the shell thickness. This would be true if the effect of the two gold layers in given X-ray crosses contributes equally to the broadening of the diffraction peak. Thus, from XRD data analysis, the thickness of the gold shell is expected to be 5.85 nm. This value is compatible with the observed position of the surface plasmon resonance peak, as discussed in the previous section. Additionally, in magnetite/gold core/shell nanoparticles, reported in Reference [41], the diffraction peak widths were identical for the 10 nm magnetite core and for the 2 nm gold shell (where its dimensions were obtained from HR-TEM measurements). Therefore, the actual value of the gold shell thickness in $MnFe_2O_4/Au$ NPs could be even lower.

A nanostructure consisting of a 5.85 nm gold shell surrounding a cluster of $MnFe_2O_4$ nanoparticles cannot be ruled out. In that case, the calculated mass percentage of gold changes to 91% for a compact over-coating layer of 12 spheres. Nevertheless, in the case of gold shell growth, the magnetic nanoparticles are dispersed in glycerol at a high temperature, before the addition of HAuCl₄ solution. This means the magnetic nanoparticles can effectively be dispersed with their surface well stabilized and passivated by the abundant OH groups of glycerol. Furthermore, the formation of the gold shell occurs through oxidation of glycerol. This process originates in other molecules, such as glyceric acid or tartronic acid, which can act as gold surface stabilizers. This is the case in terms of the citric acid in the Turkevish gold nanoparticles synthesis procedure [38]. Therefore, the prepared MnFe₂O₄/Au core/shell nanoparticles are expected to be surface passivated by hydroxyacids and, as such, well dispersible in aqueous media.

3.1.3. Transmission Electron Microscopy (TEM)

TEM images (Figure 3a) of the MnFe₂O₄/Au prepared nanoparticles and the corresponding image after processing by *ImageJ* (Figure 3b) revealed a generally spherical shape with the presence of some aggregation. These aggregates probably arise from the sample preparation on TEM grids (slow evaporation of a drop of an aqueous dispersion of nanoparticles). The size histogram that results from the area of the highlighted particles was fitted to a bimodal Gaussian distribution in order to better separate the presence of aggregates from the individual nanoparticles (Figure 3c). A bimodal size distribution of 25 ± 2 nm and 32 ± 6 nm was obtained. The former population is in accordance with the size estimated from XRD measurements, which is 25 nm when the gold shell thickness is 5.85 nm.

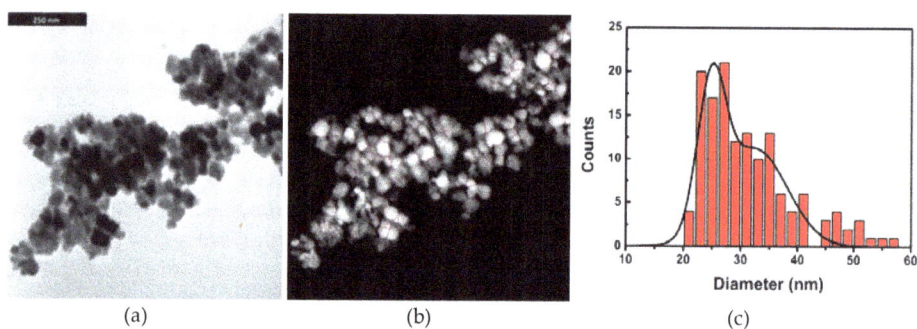

Figure 3. (a) TEM image of the synthesized MnFe₂O₄/Au core/shell nanoparticles. (b) TEM image processed by *ImageJ* (same scale of image a). (c) Particles size histogram and fitting to a bimodal Gaussian distribution (total number of 141 particles).

Below is a critical diameter of 42.9 nm. MnFe₂O₄ nanoparticles possess a superparamagnetic behavior [47,48], losing at least 90% of the magnetization when an applied magnetic field is removed, which is important for biomedical applications. The size of the nanoparticles obtained in this study is within this limit, and, therefore, these NPs are suitable for applications in biomedicine.

3.2. Magnetic Properties

The magnetic properties of MnFe₂O₄/Au core/shell nanoparticles (Figure 4) were characterized by measuring their magnetic hysteresis loop, which shows the relationship between the induced magnetic moment and the applied magnetic field (H). The core/shell nanoparticles present a superparamagnetic behavior since the ratio between remnant magnetization (M_r) and saturation magnetization (M_s) is below 0.1 [49] (Table 2).

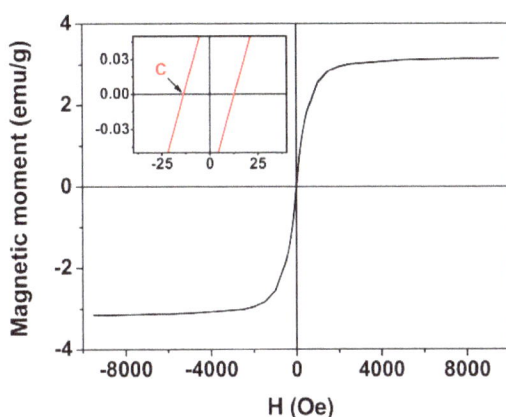

Figure 4. Magnetization hysteresis loop of $MnFe_2O_4$/Au core/shell nanoparticles measured at room temperature. Inset: Enlargement of the loop in the low field region.

Table 2. Coercive field (H_c), saturation magnetization (M_s), remnant magnetization (M_r), and ratio M_r/M_s for $MnFe_2O_4$/Au core/shell nanoparticles at room temperature.

	H_c (Oe)	M_s (emu/g)	M_r (emu/g)	M_r/M_s
$MnFe_2O_4$/Au NPs	13.57	3.15	0.08	0.03

The low saturation magnetization values are due to the presence of a diamagnetic gold layer. The gold shell thickness of $MnFe_2O_4$/Au core/shell nanoparticles was estimated using the magnetic hysteresis cycle. The particles were considered to have a well ordered $MnFe_2O_4$ core covered by a non-magnetic gold shell (with a thickness δ), acting as a "dead layer". Thus, the obtained saturation magnetization, M_s, is proportional to the core volume that possesses a spontaneous magnetization, which is related to the thickness of the dead layer and to the particle diameter, through Equation (9) [49].

$$M_s = M_{s0}\left(1 - \frac{6\delta}{D}\right)$$ (9)

where D is the particle diameter and M_{s0} is the saturation magnetization of $MnFe_2O_4$.

Chen et al. [44] observed that the saturation magnetization of manganese ferrite depends on particle size, which is estimated to be a value of 58 emu/g for $MnFe_2O_4$ nanoparticles of 13.3 nm (also prepared by coprecipitation). Using this value, a gold layer thickness of δ = 4.0 nm is obtained for particles with a diameter of 25 nm (from TEM) and M_s = 3.15 emu/g. This is roughly in accordance with XRD results.

3.3. Magnetoliposomes as Drug Nanocarriers

The obtained magnetic/plasmonic nanoparticles were either entrapped in liposomes (aqueous magnetoliposomes, AMLs) or covered by a lipid bilayer that forms the so-called solid magnetoliposomes (SMLs). The potential of both types of magnetoliposomes as drug carriers was investigated. A potential anti-tumor compound, which is a fluorescent thienopyridine derivative (Figure 5), was incorporated into AMLs and SMLs and its fluorescence emission was studied. This compound can be promising as an anticancer agent in oncological therapy, as it exhibited very low growth inhibitory concentrations (GI$_{50}$), between 3.5 µM (for A375-C5 melanoma cell line) and 6.4 µM (for non-small cell lung cancer, NCI-H460 cell line), when tested in vitro in several human tumor cell lines [28]. Moreover, the same compound has shown a very low affinity for the multi-drug resistance protein (MDR1), which is a protein that promotes drug resistance in cells [50]. This compound exhibits fluorescence in several polar and non-polar media, but not in aqueous solution [50]. Therefore, fluorescence-based methodologies (fluorescence emission, FRET, and fluorescence anisotropy) are advantageous techniques to monitor behavior and location of this compound in magnetoliposomes.

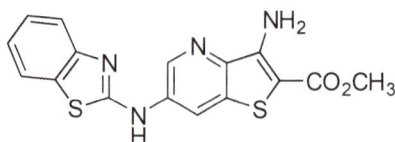

Figure 5. Structure of the potential anti-tumor thienopyridine derivative.

3.3.1. Aqueous Magnetoliposomes

The emission of the thienopyridine derivative in AMLs and liposomes (the latter without nanoparticles and with the same concentration of compound) is shown in Figure 6a. Since this potential drug is not fluorescent in aqueous media [50], the emission observed is indicative of the encapsulation of the compound in magnetoliposomes. A quenching of the compound fluorescence is observed in AMLs relative to the liposomes, which confirms its incorporation in the magnetic nanocarriers since this effect is attributed to the presence of the nanoparticles that absorb in a wide wavelength range [26]. Figure 6b displays the absorption spectra of AMLs containing the core/shell nanoparticles, with and without the anti-tumor drug, which confirms the successful loading of the drug into the magnetoliposomes and shows the overlap of the absorption spectra of nanoparticles with the compound fluorescence emission. This indicates that the nanoparticles can quench, by energy transfer, the compound fluorescence, as already observed [26]. Additionally, the gold shell can also introduce a quenching effect through electron transfer processes.

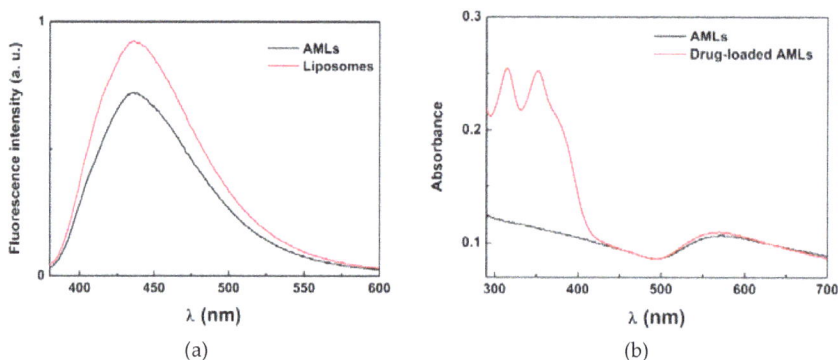

Figure 6. (a) Fluorescence spectra (λ_{exc} = 360 nm) of the anti-tumor compound (2 × 10^{-6} M) in liposomes and AMLs of Egg-PC containing $MnFe_2O_4$/Au core/shell nanoparticles; (b) Absorption spectra of AMLs containing the core/shell nanoparticles with and without the anti-tumor drug.

Moreover, the fluorescence anisotropy measurements (Table 3) confirmed that the anti-tumor compound is located mainly in the lipid bilayer. The anisotropy values were analogous to those previously determined in liposomes of the same lipids [50]. The behavior observed is similar to the one previously reported for magnetoliposomes containing manganese ferrite nanoparticles (without the gold shell) [26], which indicates that gold does not influence compound location in magnetoliposomes.

Table 3. Steady-state fluorescence anisotropy (r) values, at 25 °C, for the anti-tumor compound in magnetoliposomes in comparison with the values in neat liposomes.

	Lipid	r
Liposomes [50]	Egg-PC	0.176
	DOPG	0.181
AMLs	Egg-PC	0.173
	DOPG	0.168
SMLs	DOPG	0.175

The size of DOPG AMLs containing the magnetic/plasmonic nanoparticles were determined by Dynamic Light Scattering (DLS), which exhibit hydrodynamic diameters of 152 ± 18 nm and with a low polydispersity index (PDI = 0.19 ± 0.04). This size is larger than the one reported for Egg-PC aqueous magnetoliposomes containing manganese ferrite nanoparticles [26], but very similar to the one of DOPG solid magnetoliposomes based on $MnFe_2O_4$ [26]. In the presence of human serum albumin (HSA), 35 mg/mL (typical concentration in serum) in PBS buffer, the size of AMLs slightly increases and possesses hydrodynamic diameters of 157 ± 29 nm with a slightly higher polydispersity (PDI = 0.23 ± 0.09). For enhanced permeability and a retention (EPR) effect of loaded drugs, the diameter of (magneto)liposomes must be small. A successful extravasation into tumors has been shown to occur for nanocarriers with sizes below 200 nm [51]. Moreover, an encapsulation efficiency of EE (%) = 98.4 ± 0.8 was obtained for the anti-tumor thienopyridine derivative in these aqueous magnetoliposomes, which anticipate that these systems contain $MnFe_2O_4$/Au NPs as very promising nanocarriers for anti-cancer drugs.

The interaction of AMLs containing $MnFe_2O_4$/Au nanoparticles with Giant Unilamellar Vesicles (GUVs), used as models of biological membranes, was also investigated. The aim of this study was to evaluate the ability of magnetoliposomes to release drugs by fusing with cell membranes, considering future applications in cancer therapy/theranostics. Taking into account the fluorescence quenching caused by the presence of the core/shell nanoparticles, the emission of the anti-tumor compound incorporated in aqueous magnetoliposomes was measured before and after interaction with GUVs (Figure 7a). After interaction with GUVs, the observed unquenching effect indicates the occurrence of membrane fusion between AMLs and the model membranes, with an increase in the distance between the drug and the nanoparticles (decreasing the interaction that leads to emission quenching).

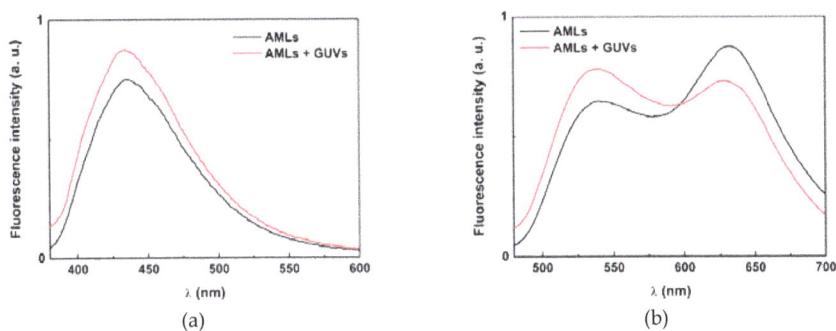

(a)

(b)

Figure 7. (a) Fluorescence spectra (λ_{exc} = 360 nm) of the thienopyridine derivative (2×10^{-6} M) in AMLs of Egg-PC containing $MnFe_2O_4$/Au nanoparticles, before and after interaction with GUVs. (b) Fluorescence spectra (λ_{exc} = 400 nm) of AMLs containing both NBD-C_6-HPC (2×10^{-6} M) and Nile Red (2×10^{-6} M), before and after interaction with GUVs.

To further confirm that this unquenching is, in fact, due to fusion between AMLs and GUVs, the interaction between these two systems was also monitored by FRET (Förster Resonance Energy Transfer). For that purpose, AMLs containing both the labeled lipid NBD-C_6-HPC and the lipid probe Nile Red [52–54] were prepared. In this case, the NBD moiety acted as the energy donor and the dye Nile Red acted as the energy acceptor [55]. Exciting only the donor NBD, a strong band due to Nile Red emission was observed (with maximum around 630 nm), which resulted from energy transfer to Nile Red (Figure 7b). After interaction with GUVs, the donor fluorescence (λ_{max} = 535 nm) increased and the acceptor emission band decreased, which showed the diminution of FRET process efficiency and, consequently, proved the membrane fusion between AMLs and GUVs.

3.3.2. Solid Magnetoliposomes

The preparation of solid magnetoliposomes, where a cluster of nanoparticles is successively covered by two lipid layers, was performed using a methodology previously developed [30]. This method has proven to be successful for solid magnetoliposomes containing magnetic nanoparticles of manganese ferrite [26], nickel ferrite [30], and magnetite [56]. To confirm that the same procedure can be applied to nanoparticles with a gold shell, the formation of the lipid bilayer around $MnFe_2O_4$/Au nanoparticles was confirmed by FRET.

The labeled lipid NBD-C_6-HPC (NBD as energy donor) was included in the first lipid layer of the SMLs and the lipid Rhodamine B-DHPE (rhodamine as the acceptor) was included in the second lipid layer. The emission of SMLs containing only the NBD-labelled lipid and SMLs containing both donor and acceptor labeled lipids were measured (Figure 8a), exciting only the donor NBD.

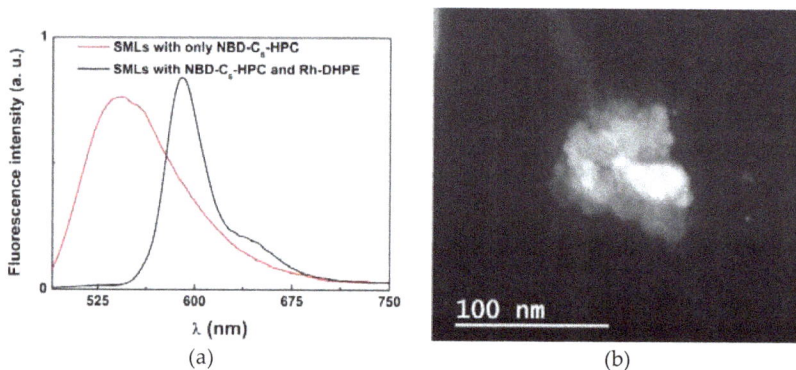

Figure 8. (a) Fluorescence spectra (λ_{exc} = 470 nm, no rhodamine excitation) of SMLs of DOPG containing $MnFe_2O_4$/Au core/shell nanoparticles labeled with only NBD-C_6-HPC and labeled with both NBD-C_6-HPC and rhodamine B-DHPE; (b) TEM image (dark field mode) of SMLs containing core/shell nanoparticles (obtained with a negative staining).

The fluorescence spectrum of SMLs with only the donor shows, as expected, a characteristic NBD emission band (λ_{max} = 535 nm). On the other hand, the fluorescence spectrum of the SMLs containing both donor and acceptor rates reveals a decrease in the NDB emission opposing the strong rise in the rhodamine B emission band, which shows the energy transfer of the excited NBD moiety to rhodamine B. A distance between donor and acceptor of r_{DA} = 3.1 nm was determined, from the calculated FRET efficiency of 0.65 (Equations (2)–(5)). Considering that donor and acceptor are each in one of the lipid layers, the distance between them proves the bilayer formation in SMLs, considering the typical cell membrane thickness (7–9 nm) [57]. TEM images of solid magnetoliposomes (Figure 8b) containing the core/shell nanoparticles point to nanosystems with diameters around 100 nm. DLS measurements revealed that these solid liposomes exhibit hydrodynamic diameters of 138 ± 19 nm and a low value for the polydispersity index (PDI = 0.20 ± 0.07). In the presence of HSA (PBS buffer, pH = 7.4), the size determined by DLS rises to 160 ± 32 nm (PDI = 0.24 ± 0.08), but is still below 200 nm.

The incorporation of the anti-tumor thienopyridine derivative in SMLs and the fusion with model membranes (GUVs) were confirmed in a similar way to the AMLs. As such, the emission of compounds loaded in SMLs was measured, as well as the emission after interaction of the SMLs with GUVs (Figure 9a). It was observed that a quenching effect of the compound fluorescence emission by the presence of magnetic/plasmonic nanoparticles (relative to the observed in liposomes) indicates incorporation of the thienopyridine derivative in the SMLs membrane. This quenching is more pronounced than for AMLs due to the lower distance between the NPs cluster and the drug. Figure 9b shows the absorption spectra of drug loaded and unloaded SMLs. Like in the case of AMLs, SMLs can also absorb (through the core/shell nanoparticles) in the compound emission region.

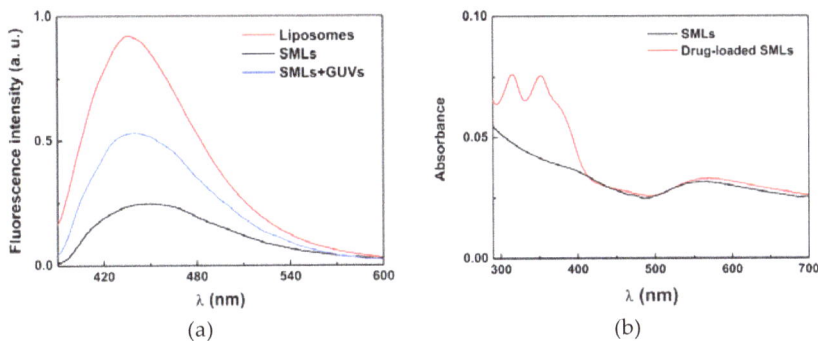

Figure 9. (a) Fluorescence spectra (λ_{exc} = 360 nm) of the thienopyridine derivative (2×10^{-6} M), in SMLs of DOPG containing $MnFe_2O_4$/Au core/shell nanoparticles, before and after interaction with GUVs. (b) Absorption spectra of SMLs containing the core/shell nanoparticles, with and without the anti-tumor drug.

The fluorescence anisotropy value of the anti-tumor drug in these SMLs is also similar to the one in liposomes and AMLs of the same lipid (Table 3). This indicates that the main location of the compound is in the lipid membrane, as reported for liposomes [50]. The drug encapsulation efficiency in SMLs is slightly lower than the one for AMLs, EE (%) = 91.2 ± 5.2, but still quite high.

The unquenching effect detected upon interaction with GUVs proves membrane fusion of SMLs with the model membranes. Again, these results are similar to the ones in magnetoliposomes containing net $MnFe_2O_4$ nanoparticles [26] and, hence, the SMLs containing magnetic/plasmonic nanoparticles are promising nanocarriers for this anti-tumor drug.

3.4. Magnetoliposomes as Agents for Phototherapy

For the study of photo thermal ability, solid magnetoliposomes containing $MnFe_2O_4$/Au core/shell nanoparticles and including the labeled lipid Rhodamine B-DHPE were synthesized and Rhodamine B emission was measured under irradiation (λ > 600 nm) along time (Figure 10). The local heating produced by gold propagates by heat diffusion, resulting in quenching of the rhodamine emission, due to the increase of efficiency of the non-radiative decay pathways. This effect is observed in Figure 10, where a monotonic decrease in Rhodamine fluorescence intensity is detected along the irradiation time, which leads to a local temperature increase. The solution temperature raised only 2 °C during irradiation time, but this increase also occurred in the absence of irradiation. This indicates that the excitation light from the spectrofluorometer, which is always incident in the sample during measurement, has higher intensity than the irradiation light (at λ > 600 nm), so that the effect of the latter is negligible. When only the excitation light hits the sample, the rhodamine emission intensity is approximately constant (Figure 10). On the contrary, upon irradiation at λ > 600 nm, an emission quenching occurs, that can only originate from a local temperature increase. The corresponding heat must, therefore, originate from the photo-thermal effect of the gold nanoshell upon light irradiation with λ > 600 nm. Huang et al. [58] studied local heating produced by laser irradiation of gold nanoparticles in the interior of a cell, both experimentally and theoretically. It was found that, for a 50 mW laser power focused into a 0.1 mm spot, the temperature at the vicinity of gold nanoparticles would increase from 25 °C to approximately 38 °C, after 4 min of irradiation and for an absorption at the plasmon resonance wavelength of 0.1. Using a light power meter (Thorlabs PM100USB with a S140C sensor), the light intensity through the λ > 600 nm filter was ~5 mW. Assuming 50% loss upon the used coupling to an optical fiber with a 1-mm diameter, and considering the final irradiation time of 120 min, the equivalent light power in the conditions of the calculations of Huang et al. [58] would be ~18 mW. According to the reported linear relation between the calculated temperature near gold nanoparticles and irradiation time [58], a local temperature increase of ~5 °C is expected. This temperature increase is compatible with the observed rhodamine fluorescence quenching. A much higher local temperature increase using laser irradiation of the developed magnetic/plasmonic lipid covered systems is then expected.

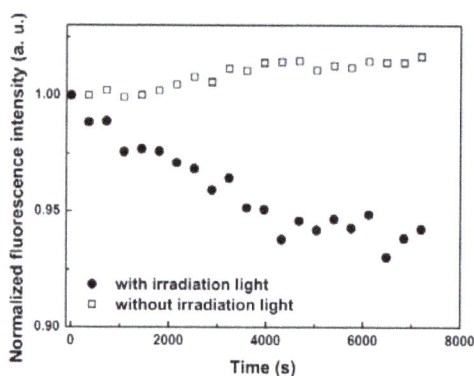

Figure 10. Fluorescence intensity (normalized to initial intensity) of irradiated SMLs with $MnFe_2O_4$/Au core/shell nanoparticles labelled with Rhodamine B-DHPE, as a function of time. For comparison, the behavior without irradiation light is also shown.

Therefore, these results show that solid magnetoliposomes based on manganese ferrite/gold core/shell nanoparticles are promising agents for plasmonic photothermal therapy. The local temperature increase caused by irradiation of the core/shell nanoparticles will also promote an increase in fluidity of the lipid membrane of liposomes, which enhances drug release.

4. Conclusions

In this work, liposomes containing magnetic/plasmonic nanoparticles with manganese ferrite core and a gold shell were prepared. The multifunctional liposomes obtained, with sizes around or below 150 nm, were revealed to be suitable nanocarriers for an anticancer drug (a thienopyridine derivative), exhibiting high encapsulation efficiencies. Drug-loaded aqueous magnetoliposomes (with the nanoparticles entrapped in liposomes) were able to interact with model membranes by fusion. The solid magnetoliposomes (where the core/shell nanoparticles are covered by a lipid bilayer) have shown the ability to be used in photothermia applications. Therefore, the multifunctional liposomes containing $MnFe_2O_4$/Au core/shell nanoparticles were found to be promising agents for combined chemo/phototherapy.

Author Contributions: E.M.S.C. and P.J.G.C. conceived and designed the experiments. A.R.O.R., J.O.G.M., and A.M.N.D. performed the synthesis and structural characterization of magnetic/plasmonic nanoparticles, liposomes, and magnetoliposomes, and the photo physical studies. P.J.G.C. supervised the structural characterization and analysis of the results. A.P., A.M.P., and J.P.A. performed the experimental magnetic measurements. B.G.A. and A.M.P. performed the analysis of the magnetic properties and the corresponding discussion. M.J.R.P.Q. synthesized the anti-tumor compound and contributed to the interpretation of the results. E.M.S.C. supervised the photo physical measurements and the interpretation of the results. A.R.O.R. and E.M.S.C. participated in the draft of the manuscript. P.J.G.C. wrote the final manuscript. All the authors revised and approved the manuscript.

Funding: This research was funded by the Portuguese Foundation for Science and Technology (FCT) in the framework of the Strategic Funding of CF-UM-UP (UID/FIS/04650/2013) and CQUM (UID/QUI/00686/2016) and through the research project PTDC/QUI-QFI/28020/2017 (POCI-01-0145-FEDER-028020), financed by the European Fund of Regional Development (FEDER), COMPETE2020 and Portugal2020. The APC was also funded by FCT. A.R.O.R. acknowledges FCT for a research grant under UID/FIS/04650/2013 funding.

Acknowledgments: The authors acknowledge the Center for Biological Engineering (CEB) of University of Minho for the availability of DLS equipment.

Conflicts of Interest: The authors declare no conflict of interest.

References

1. Piktel, E.; Niemirowicz, K.; Watek, M.; Wollny, T.; Deptula, P.; Bucki, R. Recent insights in nanotechnology-based drugs and formulations designed for effective anti-cancer therapy. *J. Nanobiotechnol.* **2016**, *14*, 1–33. [CrossRef] [PubMed]

2. Su, C.W.; Chiang, C.S.; Li, W.M.; Hu, S.H.; Chen, S.Y. Multifunctional nanocarriers for simultaneous encapsulation of hydrophobic and hydrophilic drugs in cancer treatment. *Nanomedicine* **2014**, *9*, 1499–1515. [CrossRef] [PubMed]

3. Zeng, H.; Sun, S. Synthesis, Properties, and Potential Applications of Multicomponent Magnetic Nanoparticles. *Adv. Funct. Mater.* **2008**, *18*, 391–400. [CrossRef]

4. Silva, S.M.; Tavallaie, R.; Sandiford, L.; Tilley, R.D.; Gooding, J.J. Gold coated magnetic nanoparticles: From preparation to surface modification for analytical and biomedical applications. *Chem. Commun.* **2016**, *52*, 7528–7540. [CrossRef] [PubMed]

5. Stafford, S.; Garcia, R.S.; Gun'ku, Y.K. Multimodal Magnetic-Plasmonic Nanoparticles for Biomedical Applications. *Appl. Sci.* **2018**, *8*, 97. [CrossRef]

6. Espinosa, A.; Di Corato, R.; Kolosnjaj-Tabi, J.; Flaud, P.; Pellegrino, T.; Wilhelm, C. Duality of Iron Oxide Nanoparticles in Cancer Therapy: Amplification of Heating Efficiency by Magnetic Hyperthermia and Photothermal Bimodal Treatment. *ACS Nano* **2016**, *10*, 2436–2446. [CrossRef] [PubMed]

7. Huang, L.; Ao, L.; Hu, D.; Wang, W.; Shend, Z.; Su, W. Magneto-Plasmonic Nanocapsules for Multimodal Imaging and Magnetically Guided Combination Cancer Therapy. *Chem. Mater.* **2016**, *28*, 5896–5904. [CrossRef]

8. Felton, C.; Karmakar, A.; Gartia, Y.; Ramidi, P.; Biris, A.S.; Gosh, A. Magnetic nanoparticles as contrast agents in biomedical imaging: Recent advances in iron- and manganese-based magnetic nanoparticles. *Drug Metab. Rev.* **2014**, *46*, 142–154. [CrossRef]

9. Ahmas, A.; Bae, H.; Rhee, I. Highly stable silica-coated manganese ferrite nanoparticles as high-efficacy T2 contrast agents for magnetic resonance imaging. *AIP Adv.* **2018**, *8*, 55019–55028. [CrossRef]

10. Kerker, M. *The Scattering of Light and Other Electromagnetic Radiation*, 1st ed.; Academic Press: New York, NY, USA, 1969; pp. 27–96. ISBN 978-0-12-404550-7.

11. Papavassiliou, C.G. Optical properties of small inorganic and organic metal particles. *Prog. Solid State Chem.* **1979**, *12*, 185–271. [CrossRef]

12. Bohren, C.F.; Huffman, D.R. *Absorption and Scattering of Light by Small Particles*, 1st ed.; Wiley-VCH: Weinheim, Germany, 1998; pp. 286–324. ISBN 978-0-47-129340-8.

13. Kreibig, U.; Vollmer, M. *Optical Properties of Metal Clusters*, 1st ed.; Springer: Heidelberg, Germany, 1995; pp. 30–68. ISBN 978-3-642-08191-0.

14. Ozbay, E. Plasmonics: Merging photonics and electronics at nanoscale dimensions. *Science* **2006**, *13*, 189–193. [CrossRef] [PubMed]

15. Noguez, C. Surface Plasmons on Metal Nanoparticles: The Influence of Shape and Physical Environment. *J. Phys. Chem. C* **2007**, *111*, 3806–3819. [CrossRef]

16. Huang, X.; Jain, P.K.; El-Sayed, I.; El-Sayed, M.A. Plasmonic photothermal therapy (PPTT) using gold nanoparticles. *Lasers Med. Sci.* **2008**, *23*, 217–228. [CrossRef] [PubMed]

17. Govorov, A.O.; Richardson, H.H. Generating Heat with Metal Nanoparticles. *Nano Today* **2007**, *2*, 30–38. [CrossRef]

18. Keblinski, P.; Cahill, D.G.; Bodapati, A.; Sullivan, C.R.; Taton, T.A. Limits of Localized Heating by Eletromagnetically Excited Nanoparticles. *J. Appl. Phys.* **2006**, *100*, 54301–54305. [CrossRef]

19. Elsherbini, A.A.M.; Saber, M.; Aggag, M.; El-Shahawy, A.; Shokier, H.A.A. Laser and radiofrequency-induced hyperthermia. *Int. J. Nanomed.* **2011**, *6*, 2155–2165. [CrossRef] [PubMed]

20. Kim, C.; Favazza, C.; Wang, L.V. In Vivo Photoacoustic Tomography of Chemicals: High-Resolution Functional and Molecular Optical Imaging at New Depths. *Chem. Rev.* **2010**, *110*, 2756–2782. [CrossRef]

21. Perez-Lorenzo, M.; Vaz, B.; Salgueirin, V.; Correa-Duarte, M.A. Hollow-Shelled Nanoreactors Endowed with High Catalytic Activity. *Chem. Eur. J.* **2013**, *19*, 12196–12211. [CrossRef]

22. He, Q.; Guo, S.; Qian, Z.; Chen, X. Development of Individualized Anti-Metastasis Strategies by Engineering Nanomedicines. *Chem. Soc. Rev.* **2015**, *44*, 6258–6286. [CrossRef]

23. Li, Z.; Yi, S.; Cheng, L.; Yang, K.; Li, Y.; Liu, Z. Magnetic Targeting Enhanced Theranostic Strategy Based on Multimodal Imaging for Selective Ablation of Cancer. *Adv. Funct. Mater.* **2014**, *24*, 2312–2321. [CrossRef]

24. Larsen, G.K.; Farr, W.; Murph, S.E.H. Multifunctional Fe_2O_3-Au Nanoparticles with different shapes: Enhanced catalysis, photothermal effects, and magnetic recyclability. *J. Phys. Chem. C* **2016**, *120*, 15162–15172. [CrossRef]

25. Sood, A.; Arora, V.; Shah, J.; Kotnala, R.K.; Jain, T.K. Multifunctional gold coated iron oxide core-shell nanoparticles stabilizedusing thiolated sodium alginate for biomedical applications. *Mater. Sci. Eng. C* **2017**, *80*, 274–281. [CrossRef] [PubMed]

26. Rodrigues, A.R.O.; Ramos, J.M.F.; Gomes, I.T.; Almeida, B.G.; Araújo, J.P.; Queiroz, M.-J.R.P.; Coutinho, P.J.G.; Castanheira, E.M.S. Magnetoliposomes based on manganese ferrite nanoparticles as nanocarriers for anti-tumor drugs. *RSC Adv.* **2016**, *6*, 17302–17313. [CrossRef]

27. Pereira, C.; Pereira, A.M.; Fernandes, C.; Rocha, M.; Mendes, R.; Garcia, M.P.F.; Guedes, A.; Tavares, P.B.; Grenèche, J.-M.; Araújo, J.P.; et al. Superparamagnetic MFe_2O_4 (M = Fe, Co, Mn) Nanoparticles: Tuning the Particle Size and Magnetic Properties through a Novel One-Step Coprecipitation Route. *Chem. Mater.* **2012**, *24*, 1496–1504. [CrossRef]

28. Queiroz, M.-J.R.P.; Calhelha, R.C.; Vale-Silva, L.; Pinto, E.; Nascimento, M.S.-J. Novel [6-(hetero)arylamino]thieno[3,2-*b*]pyridines: Synthesis and anti-tumoral activities. *Eur. J. Med. Chem.* **2010**, *45*, 5732–5738. [CrossRef] [PubMed]

29. Kremer, J.M.H.; Esker, M.W.J.V.D.; Pathmamanoharan, C.; Wiersema, P.H. Vesicles of variable diameter prepared by a modified injection method. *Biochemistry* **1977**, *16*, 3932–3935. [CrossRef] [PubMed]

30. Rodrigues, A.R.O.; Gomes, I.T.; Almeida, B.G.; Araújo, J.P.; Castanheira, E.M.S.; Coutinho, P.J.G. Magnetoliposomes based on nickel ferrite nanoparticles for biomedical applications. *Phys. Chem. Chem. Phys.* **2015**, *17*, 18011–18021. [CrossRef]

31. Tamba, Y.; Terashima, H.; Yamazaki, M. A membrane filtering method for the purification of giant unilamellar vesicles. *Chem. Phys. Lipids* **2011**, *164*, 351–358. [CrossRef]

32. Tanaka, T.; Tamba, Y.; Masum, S.M.; Yamashita, Y.; Yamazaki, M. La^{3+} and Gd^{3+} induce shape change of giant unilamellar vesicles of phosphatidylcholine. *Biochim. Biophys. Acta* **2002**, *1564*, 173–182. [CrossRef]

33. Valeur, B. *Molecular Fluorescence—Principles and Applications*, 1st ed.; Wiley-VCH: Weinheim, Germany, 2001; pp. 247–261. ISBN 3-527-29919-X.

34. Demas, J.N.; Crosby, G.A. The measurement of photoluminescence quantum yields—Review. *J. Phys. Chem.* **1971**, *75*, 991–1024. [CrossRef]

35. Fery-Forgues, S.; Lavabre, D. Are fluorescence quantum yields so tricky to measure? A demonstration using familiar stationery products. *J. Chem. Educ.* **1999**, *76*, 1260–1264. [CrossRef]

36. Johnson, I.; Spence, M.T.Z. *Molecular Probes Handbook: A Guide to Fluorescent Probes and Labeling Technologies*, 11th ed.; Life Technologies: Carlsbad, CA, USA, 2010; pp. 545–587. ISBN 978-0982927915.

37. Wagner, T.; Eglinger, J. Thorstenwagner/Ij-Particlesizer: v1.0.9 Snapshot Release (Version v1.0.9-SNAPSHOT). Zenodo: Genève, Switzerland, June 2017. [CrossRef]

38. Kimling, J.; Maier, M.; Okenve, B.; Kotaidis, V.; Ballot, H.; Plech, A. Turkevich method for gold nanoparticle synthesis revisited. *J. Phys. Chem. B* **2006**, *110*, 15700–15707. [CrossRef] [PubMed]

39. Wu, D.; Xu, X.; Liu, X. Influence of dielectric core, embedding medium and size on the optical properties of gold nanoshells. *Solid State Commun.* **2008**, *146*, 7–11. [CrossRef]

40. Qian, X.; Bai, J. Theoretical Studies of the Optical Properties of Hollow Spherical Metallic Nanoshells. *J. Comput. Theor. Nanosci.* **2013**, *10*, 2354–2360. [CrossRef]

41. Xu, Z.; Hou, Y.; Sun, S. Magnetic Core/Shell Fe_3O_4/Au and Fe_3O_4/Au/Ag Nanoparticles with Tunable Plasmonic Properties. *J. Am. Chem. Soc.* **2007**, *129*, 8698–8699. [CrossRef] [PubMed]

42. Rodriguez-Carvajal, J. Recent advances in magnetic structure determination by neutron powder diffraction. *Phys. B* **1993**, *192*, 55–69. [CrossRef]

43. Pitschke, W.; Hermann, H.; Mattern, N. The influence of surface roughness on diffracted X-ray intensities in Bragg–Brentano geometry and its effect on the structure determination by means of Rietveld analysis. *Powder Diffr.* **1993**, *8*, 74–83. [CrossRef]

44. Chen, J.P.; Sorensen, C.M.; Klabunde, K.J.; Hadjipanayis, G.C.; Devlin, E.; Kostikas, A. Size-dependent magnetic properties of $MnFe_2O_4$ fine particles synthesized by coprecipitation. *Phys. Rev. B* **1996**, *54*, 9288–9296. [CrossRef]

45. Yeh, J.-W.; Chang, S.-Y.; Hong, Y.-D.; Chen, S.-K.; Lin, S.-J. Anomalous decrease in X-ray diffraction intensities of Cu-Ni-Al-Co-Cr-Fe-Si alloy systems with multi-principal elements. *Mat. Chem. Phys.* **2007**, *103*, 41–46. [CrossRef]

46. Neder, R.B.; Korsunskiy, V.I.; Chory, C.; Müller, G.; Hofmann, A.; Dembski, S.; Graf, C.; Rühl, E. Structural characterization of II-VI semiconductor nanoparticles. *Phys. Status Solidi C* **2007**, *4*, 3221–3233. [CrossRef]

47. Rafique, M.Y.; Li-Qing, P.; Javed, Q.; Iqbal, M.Z.; Hong-Mei, Q.; Farooq, M.H.; Zhen-Gang, G.; Tanveer, M. Growth of monodisperse nanospheres of $MnFe_2O_4$ with enhanced magnetic and optical properties. *Chin. Phys. B* **2013**, *22*, 107101–107107. [CrossRef]

48. Huang, J.-R.; Cheng, C. Cation and magnetic orders in $MnFe_2O_4$ from density functional calculations. *J. Appl. Phys.* **2013**, *113*, 33912–33918. [CrossRef]

49. Smit, J. *Magnetic Properties of Materials*; McGraw Hill: New York, NY, USA, 1971; p. 89. ISBN 978-0070584457.

50. Costa, C.N.C.; Hortelão, A.C.L.; Ramos, J.M.F.; Oliveira, A.D.S.; Calhelha, R.C.; Queiroz, M.-J.R.P.; Coutinho, P.J.G.; Castanheira, E.M.S. A new anti-tumoral heteroarylaminothieno[3,2-*b*]pyridine derivative: Its incorporation into liposomes and interaction with proteins monitored by fluorescence. *Photochem. Photobiol. Sci.* **2014**, *13*, 1730–1740. [CrossRef] [PubMed]

51. Sawant, R.R.; Torchilin, V.P. Challenges in development of targeted liposomal therapeutics. *AAPS J.* **2012**, *14*, 303–315. [CrossRef]

52. Greenspan, P.; Mayer, E.P.; Fowler, S.D. Nile red: A selective fluorescent stain for intracellular lipid droplets. *J. Cell Biol.* **1985**, *100*, 965–973. [CrossRef]

53. Coutinho, P.J.G.; Castanheira, E.M.S.; Rei, M.C.; Real Oliveira, M.E.C.D. Nile Red and DCM fluorescence anisotropy studies in $C_{12}E_7$/DPPC mixed systems. *J. Phys. Chem. B* **2002**, *106*, 12841–12846. [CrossRef]

54. Feitosa, E.; Alves, F.R.; Niemiec, A.; Oliveira, M.E.C.D.R.; Castanheira, E.M.S.; Baptista, A.L.F. Cationic liposomes in mixed didodecyldimethylammonium bromide and dioctadecyldimethylammonium bromide aqueous dispersions studied by differential scanning calorimetry, Nile Red fluorescence, and turbidity. *Langmuir* **2006**, *22*, 3579–3585. [CrossRef]

55. Rodrigues, A.R.O.; Gomes, I.T.; Almeida, B.G.; Araújo, J.P.; Castanheira, E.M.S.; Coutinho, P.J.G. Magnetoliposomes based on nickel/silica core/shell nanoparticles: Synthesis and characterization. *Mater. Chem. Phys.* **2014**, *148*, 978–987. [CrossRef]

56. Rodrigues, A.R.O.; Mendes, P.M.F.; Silva, P.M.L.; Machado, V.A.; Almeida, B.G.; Araújo, J.P.; Queiroz, M.J.R.P.; Castanheira, E.M.S.; Coutinho, P.J.G. Solid and aqueous magnetoliposomes as nanocarriers for a new potential drug active against breast cancer. *Colloids Surf. B Biointerfaces* **2017**, *158*, 460–468. [CrossRef]

57. Curtis, H.; Barnes, N.S. *Biology*, 5th ed.; Worth Publishers: New York, NY, USA, 1989; Part 1; ISBN 978-0879013943.

58. Huang, X.; Jain, P.K.; El-Sayed, I.H.; El-Sayed, M.A. Determination of the minimum temperature required for selective photothermal destruction of cancer cells with the use of immunotargeted gold nanoparticles. *Photochem. Photobiol.* **2006**, *82*, 412–417. [CrossRef]

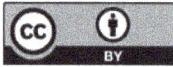

pharmaceutics

MDPI

Article

Buspirone Nanovesicular Nasal System for Non-Hormonal Hot Flushes Treatment

Elka Touitou *, Hiba Natsheh and Shaher Duchi

The Institute for Drug Research, School of Pharmacy, Faculty of Medicine, The Hebrew University of Jerusalem, P.O. Box 12065, Jerusalem 91120, Israel; hiba.natsheh@mail.huji.ac.il (H.N.); shaherd75@gmail.com (S.D.)
* Correspondence: elka.touitou@mail.huji.ac.il; Tel.: +972-54-638-0819

Received: 6 June 2018; Accepted: 2 July 2018; Published: 3 July 2018

Abstract: The aim of this work was to design and characterize a new nanovesicular nasal delivery system (NDS) containing buspirone, and investigate its efficiency in an animal model for the treatment of hot flushes. The presence of multilamellar vesicles with a mean size distribution of 370 nm was evidenced by transition electron microscopy (TEM), cryo-scanning electron microscopy (Cryo-SEM), and dynamic light scattering (DLS) tests. Pharmacodynamic evaluation of the nasal treatment efficacy with the new system was carried out in ovariectomized (OVX) rat—an animal model for hot flushes—and compared with other treatments. We found that the nasal administration of a buspirone NDS resulted in a significant reduction in tail skin temperature (TST). This effect was not observed in the control buspirone-treated groups. Buspirone levels in the plasma and brain of nasally-treated normal rats were quantified and compared with those of rats that had received oral administration by a LC-MS/MS assay. A significantly higher bioavailability was achieved with the new treatment relative to an oral administration of the same drug dose. No pathological changes in the nasal cavity were observed following sub-chronic nasal administration of buspirone NDS. In conclusion, the data of our investigation show that buspirone in the new nanovesicular nasal carrier could be considered for further studies for the development of a treatment for the hot flushes ailment.

Keywords: nanovesicular nasal carrier; nasal delivery system; buspirone; hot flushes; ovariectomized rat

1. Introduction

Currently, most of therapeutic products for hot flushes are based on hormone therapy (HT), involving the administration of estrogen alone or in combination with progesterone. There is a growing demand for a safer treatment alternative to HT for hot flushes [1].

Drugs affecting serotonin levels were investigated for non-hormonal therapies for hot flushes. In a previous study, we reported that buspirone administrated in a transdermal system has efficiently treated hot flushes in an animal model [2]. Buspirone—a 5-HT1A agonist—is currently administered orally and indicated for the treatment of generalized anxiety disorder (GAD). Buspirone HCl belongs to biopharmaceutics classification system (BCS) class I, being highly soluble and highly permeable. However, oral administration of this drug is associated with low bioavailability: ~4% due to an extensive first-pass metabolism [3]. In addition, this centrally acting drug lacks the ability to penetrate the blood–brain barrier (BBB).

Nasal administration, being able to circumvent the first pass metabolism and bypass the BBB, could be a promising alternative for the oral administration of buspirone. Despite this, the nasal delivery of many molecules is poor, due to the low permeability of the nasal mucosa [4,5].

Touitou and Illum emphasized the role of the carrier in the design of an efficient nasal product [4]. To overcome the above drawbacks, we propose here the nasal administration of buspirone incorporated in a new nanovesicular delivery system (NDS) to be tested in a hot flushes animal model. We have shown that the new vesicular nasal carrier enhanced the pharmacodynamic effect of a number of other drugs [6–8].

Various aspects of nasal delivery of buspirone were previously studied [9–12]. Khan et al. investigated the nasal clearance, bioavailability, and delivery to brain of buspirone in chitosan mucoadhesive nasal formulation in vivo [9–11]. Mathure et al. studied the ex vivo permeation of buspirone niosomes gel through sheep nasal mucosa [12].

In this work, we designed and characterized buspirone NDS, tested its pharmacodynamic effect in an ovariectomized (OVX) animal model for hot flushes, and measured the drug levels in brain and plasma. The safety of the local application of the nanovesicular system on the animal nasal cavity was also examined.

To our knowledge, this pharmacodynamic effect of nasally administrated buspirone in a nanovesicular carrier has not been previously investigated.

2. Materials and Methods

2.1. Materials

Buspirone HCl was a gift from Unipharm, Israel. Ethinylestradiol (EE) was purchased from Sigma (Jerusalem, Israel). Phosphatidylcholine phospholipid, Phospholipon 90 G, was bought from Lipoid GmbH (Berlin, Germany). Propylene glycol and Vitamin E (Tocopheryl acetate) were acquired from Tamar (Rishon Lezion, Israel). Ethanol absolute (Gadot, Netanya, Israel) was acquired from the Hebrew University warehouse. All of the other materials used in this work were of analytical or pharmaceutical grade.

2.2. Animals

All of the procedures performed on animals were conducted according to The National Institutes of Health regulations and approved by the Committee for Animal Care and Experimental Use of the Hebrew University of Jerusalem, Ethics No. MD-11-12833-3 (2011–2015).

Sprague–Dawley female rats (weighing 250–360 g) were purchased from Harlan (Rehovot, Israel). The rats were housed in separate cages and were maintained on a 12 h light, 12 h dark cycle, with lights on from 07:00 to 19:00 daily with free access to food and water.

The administration of buspirone from all of the systems was carried out under short anesthesia with isoflurane, including the animals in the control groups. This was sufficient to keep the rats sedated for a short period of 1–2 min during the instillation of nasal formulations to prevent sneezing.

2.3. Preparation and Characterization of Buspirone NDS

The new carrier was composed of phospholipid: propylene glycol: ethanol at the ratio 1:4:3 per weight. Additional components were vitamin E and water [6].

Buspirone NDS was prepared by a simple mixing method using an overhead Heidolph® stirrer (Heidolph Digital 200 RZR-2000, Schwabach, Germany). Briefly, phospholipid was dissolved in ethanol; then, propylene glycol and vitamin E were added. Buspirone HCl aqueous solution was then added slowly with continuous mixing; the nanovesicles were generated at this stage.

In this work, we present the results obtained with 3% *w/w* buspirone NDS. The system was tested for drug chemical content, the presence of nanovesicles, the size distribution of vesicles, viscosity, pH, and three months' stability.

2.3.1. Drug Chemical Content

The concentration of buspirone in the system was quantified by HPLC (Merck-Hitachi D-7000 equipped with an L-7400 variable UV detector, L-7300 column oven, L-7200 auto-sampler, L-7100 pump, and an Hardware Security Module (HSM) computerized analysis program, Tokyo, Japan). The drug concertation in the samples was determined using a modified method described by

Foroutan et al. [13]. The chromatographic conditions were set as follows: UV detection 240 nm, a Nucleosil C18 125 mm × 4 mm 5 micron column with a mobile phase of acetonitrile: phosphate buffer 0.01 M pH 3.5 (40:60, *v/v*) at a flow of 1 mL/min.

2.3.2. Visualization of Vesicles by Transition Electron Microscopy (TEM) and Cryo-Scanning Electron Microscopy (Cryo-SEM)

For transition electron microscopy (TEM) visualization, one day before the examination, the system was diluted 1:10 with suitable diluent and stained with 1% aqueous solution of phosphotungstic acid (PTA), dried at room temperature for 20 min, and viewed under the microscope (Philips TECHNAI CM 120 electron microscope, Eindhoven, The Netherlands) at 26.5–110 k-fold enlargement.

For cryo-scanning electron microscopy (cryo-SEM) visualization, specimen preparation was performed with a BAF-060 system (BalTec AG, Balzers, Liechtenstein). A small drop of the buspirone NDS was placed on an electron microscopy copper grid and sandwiched between two gold planchettes. The "sandwich" was plunged into liquid ethane at its freezing point, transferred into liquid nitrogen, and inserted into a sample fracture block that had been pre-cooled by liquid nitrogen. The block was split open to fracture the frozen sample drop. A Pt–C conductive thin film of 4 nm was deposited on the surfaces (at a 90° angle). The coated specimens were transferred under vacuum by a BalTec VCT100 shuttle that had been pre-cooled with liquid nitrogen into a Zeiss Ultra Plus High-Resolution Scanning Electron Microscope (HR-SEM) (Oberkochen, Germany), and maintained at −150 °C. The microscopic examination was performed under 3000-fold enlargement.

2.3.3. Vesicles Size Distribution by Dynamic Light Scattering (DLS)

Buspirone NDS was analyzed using a Malvern Zetasizer-nano, ZEN 3600, Malvern Instruments, Malvern, UK. The system was diluted 1:500 with suitable diluent one hour prior to measurement. Three batches of each system were tested. Each batch was analyzed by intensity, three times, at 25 °C. The duration and the set position of each measurement were fixed automatically by the apparatus.

2.3.4. Viscosity and pH of the System

The viscosity of the nanovesicular system was measured by Brookfield DV III Rheometer -LV (Brookfield engineering labs, Stoughton, MA, USA), spindle 18 and a small sample adaptor, at a rotation speed of 30 rpm.

The pH measurements were performed by a Fisher pH meter (Fisher Instruments, Pittsburgh, PA, USA). The system was diluted with double distilled water 1:5. All of the measurements were duplicated.

2.3.5. Stability Test for Buspirone NDS

Changes in drug chemical content, structure, and size distribution of the nanovesicles, viscosity, and pH of the system were measured and compared to zero time values following three months storage at room temperature (RT).

2.4. Pharmacodynamic Effect Evaluation in Animal Model

2.4.1. Animal Model

The protocol for the animal model and the experiments was conducted according to The National Institutes of Health regulations and approved by the Committee for Animal Care and Experimental Use of the Hebrew University of Jerusalem, as above in Section 2.2.

The effect of nasal administration of buspirone NDS on a hot flushes animal model was tested in bilateral ovariectomized rats (OVX). This is a model for estrogen deficiency-associated thermoregulatory dysfunction. The treatment effect was evaluated by monitoring the changes in tail skin temperature (TST) [2].

A total of 71 rats weighing 250–330 g underwent bilateral ovariectomies (OVX) (*n* = 63) or sham surgeries (*n* = 8) (which left their ovaries intact) at Harlan Biotech (Rehovot, Israel) followed by a recovery period of two weeks. No surgical or medical complications were observed.

Sixteen rats were used to test the animal model (including the eight sham and eight OVX), and 55 OVX rats were used for testing various treatments.

To test the reliability of the OVX animal model, the increase in the TST in OVX rats was assessed as compared with sham animals. The TST values for sham animals were considered the normal values [14].

2.4.2. Treatments and TST Measurements

For testing various treatments, 48 OVX animals were divided into six groups (*n* = 8/group) as follows: single administration of 3 mg/kg buspirone from NDS as compared to nasal aqueous solution (NAQ), oral aqueous solution (PO), and subcutaneous injection (SC). In addition, the effect of buspirone NDS was evaluated compared to the positive control, ethinylestradiol (EE), which was administrated subcutaneously to OVX rats at a dose of 0.3 mg/kg once daily for seven days. Untreated OVX rats served as control. A 3% *w/w* buspirone aqueous solution was used as the nasal or oral control system, while a 0.3% *w/w* buspirone solution in normal saline was used for SC administration. The 0.03% *w/w* ethinylestradiol SC solution was prepared in sesame oil. The administrated volumes were calculated to achieve a dose of 3 mg/kg buspirone and 0.3 mg/kg EE to each animal.

The experiments were carried out in two replicates; each replicate included four rats for each treatment group. The intra and interobserver variations were ≤4.6% and 3.9%, respectively. The drug dose was chosen following the evaluation of the dose- effect relationship (data is not shown).

TST was measured using Thermalert TH-5 (Physitemp Instruments Inc., Clifton, NJ, USA). A thermocouple skin sensor probe SST-1 (Physitemp Instruments Inc., Clifton, NJ, USA) was fixed on the dorsal surface of the tail approximately one cm away from the base, and the animals were retained in a flat-bottomed restraint during the 30–60 s sampling period. All of the measurements were performed from 10:00 to 15:00 and at 21.5 ± 0.1 °C.

On the day of the experiment, the rats were acclimatized in the experiment room for two hours. TST values were recorded before treatment (baseline) and 30 min, 60 min, 120 min, 180 min, and 240 min after treatment.

The following parameters were used to evaluate the effect of the various treatments: the average TST value (TSTave, °C) for each time point was the average of the readings recorded in the two experimental replicates for animals in the same treatment group [15]. The ΔTST value for each treatment at a certain time point was obtained by subtracting TSTave at baseline from the value at that time point. The duration of effect is the time period (min) in which TSTave is statistically different from the TST at baseline [16].

As a next step, we determined the onset of the action of buspirone NDS by measuring the TST values of OVX rats each minute following the treatment (*n* = 7).

2.5. Determination of Buspirone Levels in Rat Plasma and Brain

The concentration of buspirone in the plasma and brain tissue of normal animals at various time points was measured post-dose of 3 mg/kg drug nasal administration in NDS and oral administration (PO).

2.5.1. Drug Concentration in Plasma Measurement

Ten rats were randomly divided equally into two groups of five animals. Blood samples of 400–500 µL were collected from tail 5 min before treatment (zero-time point) and 5 min, 10 min, 20 min, 30 min, 60 min, 120 min, and 240 min after drug administration.

Briefly, blood samples were centrifuged at 3000 rpm for 10 min at room temperature, and plasma was transferred and stored at −20 °C until assayed. On the day of analysis, the samples were thawed, and buspirone was extracted from plasma by a modified protein precipitation method described by

Foroutan et al. [13]. One hundred microliters of plasma samples were extracted with 125 µL acetonitrile and diluted with 275 µL of water. Samples were centrifuged at 14,000 rpm for 5 min at room temperature. Supernatants were filtered and injected into LC-MS/MS (Thermo Scientific, San Jose, CA, USA).

2.5.2. Drug Concentration in Brain Tissue Measurement

Sixteen rats were randomly divided into four equal groups for testing two time points and two treatments. Animals were sacrificed 10 min or 30 min after administration. Brains were collected, immediately weighed, and kept at −70 °C until analysis. Brain tissues were purified by a modified liquid–liquid extraction method described by Lai et al. [17]. On the day of analysis, the brain tissues were thawed and homogenized with 2 mL of water/g brain tissue. The homogenates were alkalinized with 10% *w/v* NaOH solution. Buspirone was extracted with 5 mL a mixture (4:1) of hexane and ethyl acetate. Samples were then centrifuged at 4000 rpm for 45 min at 4 °C. Supernatants were collected and evaporated at room temperature. Dried residues were reconstituted with mobile phase, and centrifuged at 14,000 rpm for 10 min at room temperature. Final supernatants were filtered and injected into LC-MS/MS.

2.5.3. Buspirone LC-MS/MS Assay

Buspirone content in plasma and brain was quantified by a specific validated LC-MS/MS method according to the FDA regulation guidelines of bioanalytical validation. A Kinetex™ column (2.6 µm Minibore C18 50 × 2.1 mm, Phenomenex®, Torrance, CA, USA) was used. Flow rate and injection volume were 400 µL/min and 5 µL, respectively. At these defined conditions, the retention time of buspirone was 1.33 min. Buspirone plasma levels were expressed in ng/mL, and in ng/g in brain tissue. Standard calibration curves of buspirone hydrochloride were prepared with plasma and brain homogenates spiked with known amounts of drug (1–1000 ng/mL and 100–500 ng/g, respectively). For the standard calibration curve, each concentration was injected five times, and the experiment was duplicated. The inter-coefficients and intra-coefficients of variation were <2.2% and 4.0%, respectively. The sensitivity of the method was 1 ng/mL, and the recovery was 78% and 96.3% for plasma and brain, respectively.

The following parameters were used to evaluate the concentration profile in plasma: C_{max}, T_{max}, and AUC0-240 (from zero to 240 min). The AUC0−240 $_{[NDS]}$ and AUC0-240 $_{[PO]}$ represent the means of individual AUC0-240 from nasal and oral experimental groups, respectively. The area under the curve of plasma concentration was calculated using the linear trapezoidal rule. All of the pharmacokinetic parameters were calculated using a windows-based program for noncompartmental analysis of pharmacokinetic data, NCOMP; version 3.1 11-SEP-97 in (c) 1996-7 Fox Chase Cancer Center (Philadelphia, PA, USA).

The relative bioavailability (F %) was calculated according to the following equation:

$$F \% = [(AUC0 - 240 \,_{[NDS]} \times DOSE_{PO})]/[(AUC0 - 240 \,_{[PO]} \times DOSE \,_{NDS})] \times 100$$

2.6. Local Safety Assessment

In this experiment, we evaluated the effect of buspirone NDS on the nasal cavity in rats by a method previously described by Duchi et al. [7,8]. In brief, six rats were divided into three equal groups. Rats in the nasal administration groups received 15 µL of buspirone NDS or saline into both nostrils twice a day for seven days. Two rats were untreated and served as a negative control. At the end of the experiment, animals were sacrificed, and their nasal cavities were removed and fixed in 3.8% buffered formaldehyde, pH 7.4. Sections of the nasal cavity were cut serially at 7-µm thickness and stained with hematoxylin and eosin. The sections were examined by a professional histopathologist (Authority for Animal Facilities, Hebrew University of Jerusalem, Israel) by Zeiss Axioskop 2 plus (Oberkochen, Germany). Local toxicity was assessed by evaluating the histopathological alterations in different regions of the nasal cavity (cartilage and turbinate bone, lamina propria and submucosa, mucosal epithelium and lumen).

2.7. Statistical Analysis

Data is reported as mean ± SD and analyzed by one-way ANOVA with the Tukey–Kramer multiple comparisons post-test or by unpaired two-tailed *t*-test. $p < 0.05$ is considered significant in all cases.

3. Results

3.1. Buspirone NDS Characterization

The TE and cryo-SE micrographs presented in Figures 1 and 2 indicate the presence of nanovesicles in the tested samples.

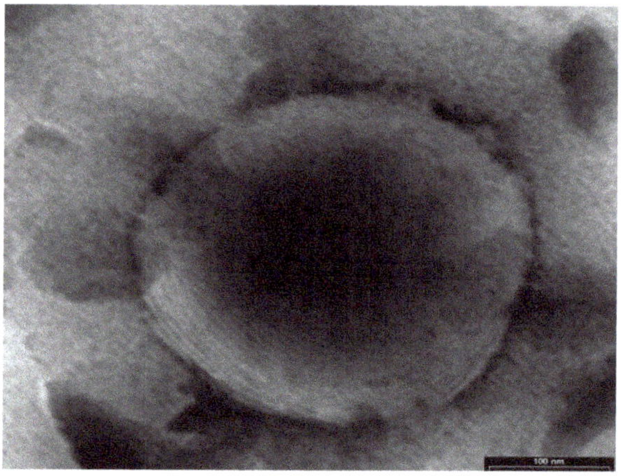

Figure 1. A multilamellar vesicle apparent in the transition electron (TE) micrograph of a buspirone nanovesicular delivery system (NDS) (110 k, Philips TEM CM 120 electron microscope).

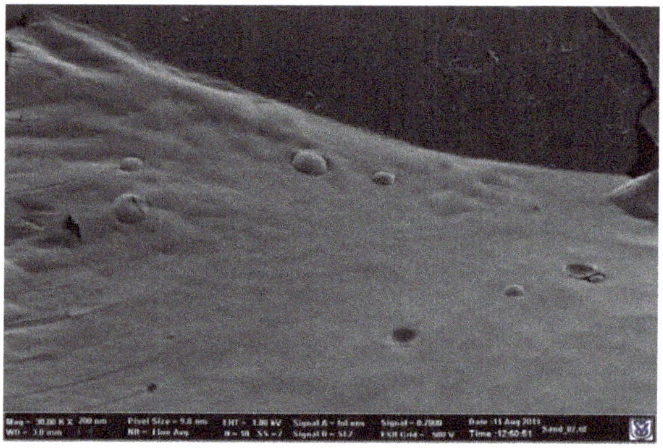

Figure 2. Cryo-scanning electron (cryo-SE) micrograph of a buspirone NDS (Zeiss Ultra Plus HR-SEM) showing multiple nanovesicles.

The micrograph in Figure 1 shows a spherical multilamellar nanovesicle.

The mean size distribution of the vesicles obtained by DLS measurements was 370.0 ± 68.8 nm. Other important system characteristics were viscosity 72.7 ± 8.1 cP and pH 5.8 ± 0.2.

Stability tests results for samples kept three months at room temperature are given in Table 1 and Figure 3.

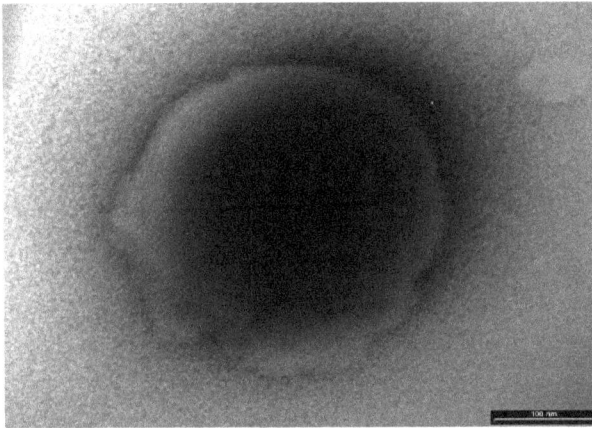

Figure 3. TE micrographs of buspirone NDS after three months of storage at room temperature (RT).

Table 1. Stability parameters for buspirone nasal nanovesicular delivery system (NDS) at zero time and after three months of storage at RT (mean ± SD).

Time	0 Time	Three Months	% of Initial after Three Months *
Drug Content, % w/w	3.13 ± 0.05	2.88 ± 0.02	92.0
Vesicles Mean Size Distribution, nm	395.1 ± 162.9	332.6 ± 111.1	84.0
Viscosity, cP	87.0 ± 3.1	91.0 ± 4.3	104.6
pH	5.73 ± 0.10	5.85 ± 0.05	102.1

* Calculated by the following equation: (value after three months/value at 0 time) × 100%.

As shown in Table 1, the percentage of change in drug content, viscosity, and pH after three months' storage at RT were less than 10% compared to the values at the initial time (zero time) storage. It is noteworthy that although the mean size distribution of vesicles decreased by 16%, the values remained in the initial nanosized range. No changes in the appearance of the vesicles were observed; the vesicles kept their spherical shape and multilamellar arrangement (Figure 3). These results suggest that the nanovesicular buspirone NDS preserved its characteristics and structure during the tested storage period.

3.2. Effect of Buspirone Nasal Administration on TST Values in Animal Model

The effect of buspirone NDS on TST values was tested in OVX animals.

The first step was to validate the OVX animal model by comparing the TST values in untreated OVX rats versus intact rats (sham-operated). The TSTave (°C) values in OVX rats at all of the tested time points were significantly higher than the values obtained in sham rats with an overall mean TST of 28.8 ± 0.3 °C vs. 26.1 ± 0.3 °C, respectively ($p < 0.001$) (Figure 4).

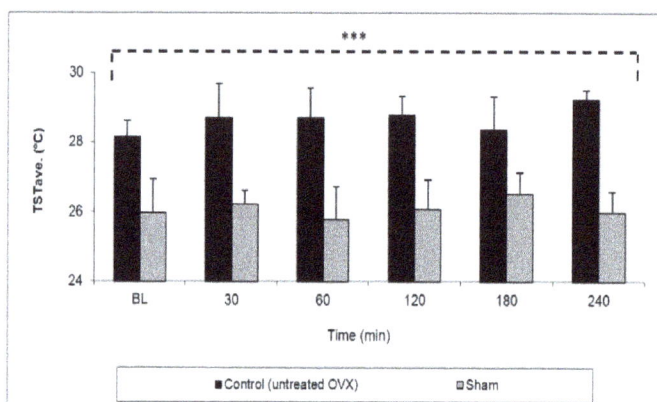

Figure 4. Tail skin temperature (TST) average values in untreated ovariectomized (OVX) Sprague–Dawley female rats and an untreated sham group. Data represent the mean ± SD, $n = 8$ for each group. *** $p < 0.001$ extremely significant by unpaired two-tailed t-test.

Buspirone was administrated at a dose of 3 m/kg as follows: in NDS, nasal aqueous solution, subcutaneous injection, and oral solution, and compared with results in untreated OVX rats. The TST baseline values were ≥ 28.5 °C in all of the OVX animal groups. The results in Figure 5 show that the nasal drug administration of buspirone NDS leads to a rapid and significant reduction in TST 30 min after treatment, achieving TSTave and ΔTST values of 26.26 ± 0.86 and -2.40 ± 0.48 °C, respectively. The treatment resulted in a statistically significant decrease in TST over the four hours of tested time as compared with PO, NAQ, or untreated OVX animals.

TST values reduction at 30 min was seen only in the treatment with buspirone NDS. At this time point, the TST values for all of the other controls were comparable to those of untreated OVX animals. At 60 min, low changes in TST were measured for the NAQ and PO groups. Further, the first significant reduction for the SC-treated group was at 60 min, indicating a relatively slow onset of action (Figure 5 and Table 2).

Table 2. Pharmacodynamic parameters of buspirone NDS administration to OVX rats as compared with controls ($n = 8$ for each group), mean ± SD.

System	Mean ΔTST, °C	Duration *, (min)	Max ΔTST, °C (Time, min)
NDS **	-2.61 ± 1.07	210	-3.88 ± 0.95 (120)
NAQ **	-0.46 ± 0.75	60	-1.16 ± 0.88 (60)
PO **	-0.39 ± 1.05	60	-0.58 ± 0.91 (120)
SC **	-1.86 ± 1.78	180	-3.71 ± 1.15 (180)
EE ***	-2.71 ± 0.47	240	-3.55 ± 0.20 (30)

TST, tail skin temperature; NDS, nasal nanovesicular delivery system; PO, oral administration; NAQ, nasal aqueous solution; SC, subcutaneous injection; EE, subcutaneous ethinylestradiol injection. * Duration of effect is the time at which the average TST is statistically different from the TST at baseline by one-way ANOVA, with the Tukey–Kramer multiple comparisons post-test. ** Buspirone administrated from systems at a single dose of 3 mg/kg. *** Subcutaneous ethinylestradiol administrated at a dose 0.3 mg/kg once daily for 7 days.

The calculated pharmacodynamic parameters of the above described experiments are presented in Table 2. The duration of a statistical significant effect on TST was 210 min for buspirone NDS administration and only 180 min and 60 min for SC and NAQ or PO, respectively. In addition, the absolute values of mean and maximum ΔTST were significantly higher in OVX rats treated with buspirone NDS than in the three control groups.

Further, it was interesting to compare the effect of one buspirone NDS treatment with one week of repeated subcutaneous EE.

The mean ΔTST values obtained were −2.61 ± 1.07 and −2.71 ± 0.47 for the nasal administration and the end of one week EE administration, respectively (Table 2). The TST values were near the baseline in the normal rat model.

Another important parameter is the onset of action of buspirone NDS. The evaluation was carried out by measuring the TST values of OVX rats each minute for the first 30 min following the treatment. The baseline TST value was 28.3 ± 0.5 °C; a slight increase was observed in the first five minutes following treatment, which could be a result of stress from anesthesia and administration procedures. At 10 min, a temperature reduction was measured followed by significant decrease at 15 min ($p < 0.05$) lasting to the end of experiment.

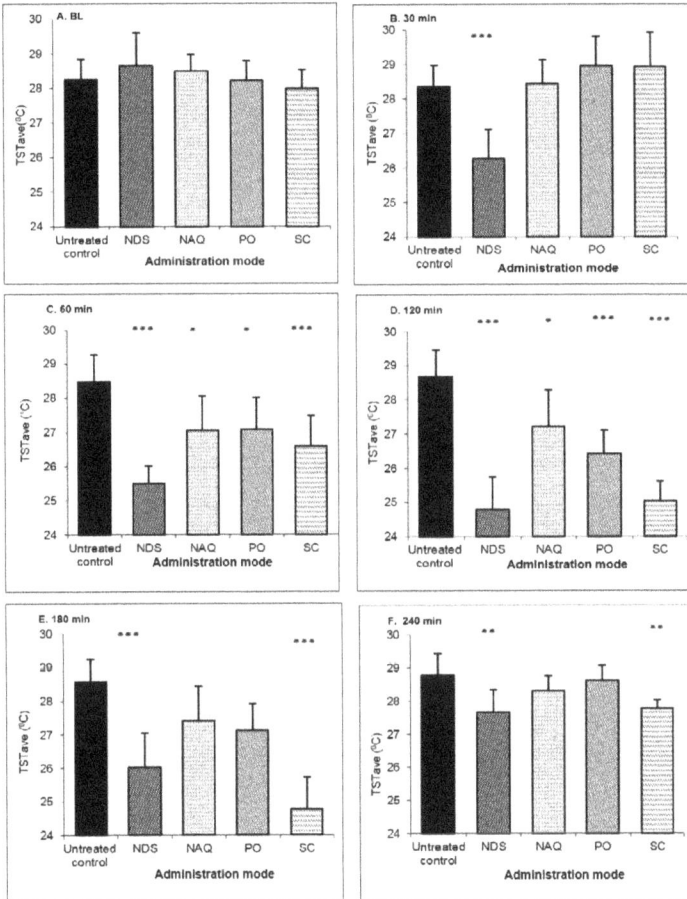

Figure 5. TST average values after buspirone NDS administration to OVX rats at dose 3 mg/kg compared to nasal aqueous solution (NAQ), oral administration (PO) and subcutaneous injection (SC) and in untreated control at: (**A**) baseline (BL); (**B**) 30 min; (**C**) 60 min; (**D**) 120 min; (**E**) 180 min; and (**F**) 240 min time points. Data represent the mean ± SD, $n = 8$ for each group. * $p < 0.05$, significant, ** $p < 0.01$ very significant, *** $p < 0.001$ extremely significant; compared to control (untreated OVX) by one-way ANOVA, with the Tukey–Kramer multiple comparisons post-test.

3.3. Buspirone Levels in Plasma and in Brain

Plasma and brain drug concentration as a function of time were measured following a single dose of 3 mg/kg buspirone nasal administration to normal rats from NDS and compared with a PO administration of a similar dose.

The results show that nasal drug administration produced a rapid increase in the drug plasma levels reaching concentrations of 764.2 ± 420.0 ng/mL and 478.2 ± 253.8 ng/mL at 5 min and 10 min post-administration, respectively. Then, the drug concentration decreased gradually 240 min after administration. Following oral administration, a relatively slow and mild increase in buspirone concentration was measured, 109.7 ± 74.9 ng/mL, 141.7 ± 95.3 ng/mL and 157.1 ± 102.9 ng/mL at 5 min, 10 min, and 20 min, respectively. A slow decrease occurred after 20 min, and the drug levels reached zero 240 min post-administration. The calculated parameters indicated that the drug nasal administration allowed for a four times higher C_{max} value than oral administration (764.2 ± 420.0 ng/mL and 181.5 ± 106.5 ng/mL, respectively) with a three times shorter T_{max} value (5.0 ± 0.0 min and 15.0 ± 7.1 min, respectively). The calculated AUC0−240 [NDS] and AUC0−240 [PO] values were 27515.3 ± 9104.4 and 12089.3 ± 8826.3, respectively, indicating a relative plasma bioavailability of 212.7% (Figure 6, Table 3).

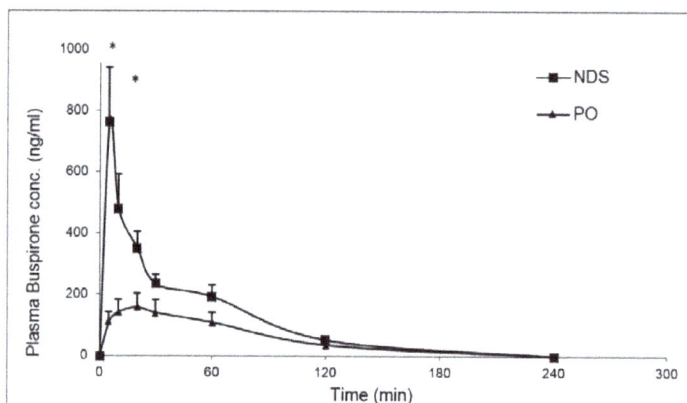

Figure 6. Plasma buspirone concentration-time profile after the administration of buspirone NDS to rat at a dose of 3 mg/kg compared with oral administration (PO). Data given as mean ± SD, $n = 5$ for each group. * $p < 0.05$ significant by an unpaired two-tailed *t*-test.

Table 3. Pharmacokinetic parameters following the administration of 3 mg/kg buspirone in NDS and PO to rat at a similar dose ($n = 5$, for each group), mean ± SD.

Pharmacokinetic Parameter	Administration Mode	
	NDS	PO
T_{max} (min)	5.0 ± 0.0	15.0 ± 7.1
C_{max} (ng/mL)	764.2 ± 420.0	181.5 ± 106.5
AUC0−240 (ng × min/mL)	25,715.3 ± 9104.4	12,089.3 ± 8826.3

NDS: nasal nanovesicular delivery system; PO: oral administration. C_{max}: maximum plasma concentrations; T_{max}: time at which C_{max} is achieved; AUC0−240: area under the curve from zero time to 240 min.

Drug quantities measured in the brain tissue at 10 min and 30 min post-buspirone NDS administration were 688.4 ± 204.7 ng/g and 511.1 ± 149.4 ng/g, respectively. It is noteworthy that the drug concentrations that were detected in the brain tissue following PO administration were lower by five and two times (179.6 ± 58.8 ng/g and 258.9 ± 91.7 ng/g at 10 min and 30 min, respectively) (Figure 7).

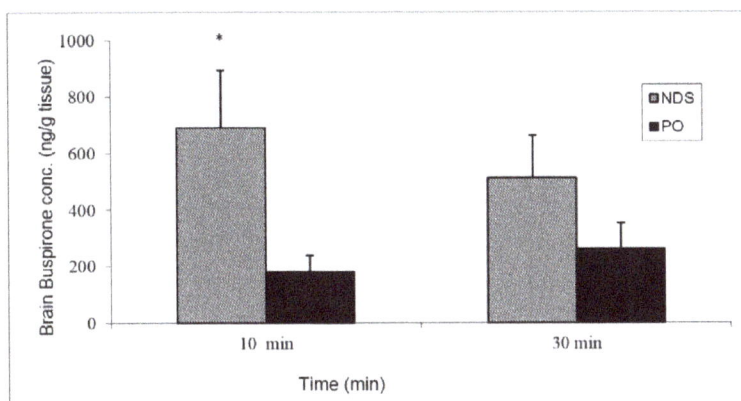

Figure 7. Brain buspirone concentrations after administration of buspirone NDS to rat at a dose of 3 mg/kg compared with oral administration (PO). Data represent the mean ± SD, $n = 5$ for each group. * $p < 0.05$ significant by unpaired two-tail *t*-test.

3.4. Local Safety

Histopathological analysis of the cavity and nasal tissue following sub-chronic buspirone NDS administration was assessed by comparing the nasal cavities treated with the new system or with saline and untreated rats.

No pathological findings were observed in the histopathological analysis of the nasal cavities excised from rats in the buspirone NDS and saline groups (images not shown). The results show intact mucosal epithelium, empty lumen, and no infiltration of inflammatory cells. Overall, there was no evidence of inflammation. Turbinate bone integrity was preserved. Epithelium was normal with no evidence of erosion or ulceration, and ciliated epithelium was intact. These findings are sustained by previous results obtained with tramadol NDS [7].

4. Discussion

Nasal administration is a nice alternative to improve the bioavailability of drugs that are poorly absorbed by the oral route. This mode of administration is generally associated with good patient compliance [4]. However, the nasal administration of some drugs may also result in low absorption due to their insufficient permeation across the nasal mucosa [18]. In previous publications, we proposed a new effective and safe nasal nanovesicular carrier for various drugs and treatments. The enhanced effect of drugs in pain and Multiple Sclerosis animal models was achieved following nasal administration using this delivery system [6–8].

In this work, we designed and characterized buspirone NDS, which is the nanovesicular carrier containing the drug. The effect of this system on hot flushes was evaluated in OVX rats. The OVX rat model used in the present study for pharmacodynamic evaluation is an acceptable model for estrogen deficiency-associated thermoregulatory dysfunction [2,14]. Subsequently, the elevation in TST is considered similar to menopausal hot flushes in women [19,20].

The ability of the new nasal nanovesicular system to enhance the systemic and brain delivery of buspirone was also investigated.

We found that the system is composed of spherical nanosized multilamellar vesicles, as evidenced by electron microscopy and DLS measurements. The pH of buspirone NDS was shown to be within the suitable range for nasal administration. Moreover, the system was stable for three months of storage at RT.

Treating OVX rats nasally with buspirone NDS lead to a significant reduction in TST. The effect was higher and over a longer time period than oral or nasal aqueous solutions, or subcutaneous injection.

The improved systemic and brain delivery of buspirone were proven by higher drug levels achieved in plasma and the brain (C_{max}), in addition to shorter T_{max} values following administration in the nanovesicular system compared with oral administration. The efficient delivery of buspirone to the brain via the nanovesicular NDS points toward the ability of the system to target the drug to the animal brain.

It is notable that other non-hormonal drugs including serotonin/norepinephrine reuptake inhibitors, gabapentinoids, and clonidine have been considered for the management of vasomotor symptoms (VMS) to overcome the side effects of HT [21]. These drugs are usually administered via the oral route.

The treatment we suggest here presents a new approach to be further investigated for hot flushes management in cases where women experience symptoms hourly, or suffer from night sweats and sleep disturbances. It is also suggested to be helpful in menopause women suffering from VMS associated with anxiety, owing to the approved anxiolytic effect of buspirone [22]. In addition, the nasal administration of buspirone could avoid drugs interaction in the gastrointestinal tract when the oral administration of other drugs is required.

5. Conclusions

Buspirone that was incorporated in the new nanovesicular carrier delivered nasally to the OXV animal model for hot flushes was more efficient than the administration of the same drug dose in nasal or oral aqueous solutions and subcutaneous injection. Buspirone levels in the brain and plasma of rats following nasal administration of the drug in the new carrier were superior to those measured in oral administration. Sub-chronic nasal administration of the buspirone nanosystem has shown no pathological changes in the mucosa for the tested period.

The feasibility data generated in this investigation point toward the possibility of considering buspirone NDS for further studies, and the development of a non-hormonal treatment of hot flushes.

6. Patents

Touitou, E.; Godin, B.; Duchi, S. Compositions for nasal delivery. 2014. US patent 8,911,751 B2.

Author Contributions: E.T. conceptualization, design, supervision, experimental design, writing, review editing, editing the final version. H.N. experimental, draft writing, contribution to the final version. S.D. experimental, draft preparation, assay validation, quantitative assay development.

Funding: This research received no external funding.

Acknowledgments: We would like to thank Unipharm, Israel for kindly providing us buspirone hydrochloride.

Conflicts of Interest: The authors declare no conflict of interest.

References

1. Krause, M.S.; Nakajima, S.T. Hormonal and nonhormonal treatment of vasomotor symptoms. *Obstet. Gynecol. Clin. N. Am.* **2015**, *42*, 163–179. [CrossRef] [PubMed]
2. Shumilov, M.; Touitou, E. Buspirone transdermal administration for menopausal syndromes, in vitro and in animal model studies. *Int. J. Pharm.* **2010**, *387*, 26–33. [CrossRef] [PubMed]
3. Mahmood, I.; Sahajwalla, C. Clinical pharmacokinetics and pharmacodynamics of buspirone, an anxiolytic drug. *Clin. Pharmacokinet.* **1999**, *36*, 277–287. [CrossRef] [PubMed]
4. Touitou, E.; Illum, L. Nasal drug delivery. *Drug Deliv. Transl. Res.* **2013**, *3*, 1–3. [CrossRef] [PubMed]
5. Lim, S.T.; Forbes, B.; Brown, M.B.; Martin, G.P. Physiological factors affecting nasal drug delivery. In *Enhancement in Drug Delivery*; Touitou, E., Barry, B.W., Eds.; CRC Press: Boca Raton, FL, USA, 2007; pp. 355–372. ISBN 0-8493-3203-6.
6. Touitou, E.; Godin, B.; Duchi, S. Compositions for Nasal Delivery. U.S. Patent 8,911,751 B2, 16 December 2014.

7.   Duchi, S.; Touitou, E.; Pradella, L.; Marchini, F.; Ainbinder, D. Nasal tramadol delivery system: A new approach for improved pain therapy. *Eur. J. Pain Suppl.* **2011**, *5*, 449–452. [CrossRef]

8.   Duchi, S.; Ovadia, H.; Touitou, E. Nasal administration of drugs as a new non-invasive strategy for efficient treatment of multiple sclerosis. *J. Neuroimmunol.* **2013**, *258*, 32–40. [CrossRef] [PubMed]

9.   Khan, S.; Patil, K.; Yeole, P.; Gaikwad, R. Brain targeting studies on buspirone hydrochloride after intranasal administration of mucoadhesive formulation in rats. *J. Pharm. Pharmacol.* **2009**, *61*, 669–675. [CrossRef] [PubMed]

10.   Khan, S.A.; Patil, K.S.; Yeole, P.G. Intranasal mucoadhesive buspirone formulation: In vitro characterization and nasal clearance studies. *Pharmazie* **2008**, *5*, 348–351.

11.   Mittal, D.; Ali, A.; Md, S.; Baboota, S.; Sahni, J.K.; Ali, J. Insights into direct nose to brain delivery: Current status and future perspective. *Drug Deliv.* **2014**, *2*, 75–86. [CrossRef] [PubMed]

12.   Mathure, D.; Madan, J.R.; Gujar, N.K.; Tupsamundre, A.; Ranpise, A.H.; Dua, K. Formulation and evaluation of niosomal in situ nasal gel of a serotonin receptor agonist, buspirone hydrochloride for the brain delivery via intranasal route. *Pharm. Nanotechnol.* **2018**, *1*, 69–78. [CrossRef] [PubMed]

13.   Foroutan, S.M.; Zarghi, A.; Shafaati, A.R.; Khoddam, A. Simple high-performance liquid chromatographic determination of buspirone in human plasma. *Farmaco* **2004**, *59*, 739–742. [CrossRef] [PubMed]

14.   Kobayashi, T.; Tamura, M.; Hayashi, M.; Katsuura, Y.; Tanabe, H.; Ohta, T.; Komoriya, K. Elevation of tail skin temperature in ovariectomized rats in relation to menopausal hot flushes. *Am. J. Physiol. Regul. Integr. Comp. Physiol.* **2000**, *278*, 863–869. [CrossRef] [PubMed]

15.   Opas, E.E.; Rutledge, S.J.; Vogel, R.L.; Rodan, G.A.; Schmidt, A. Rat tail skin temperature regulation by estrogen, phytoestrogens and tamoxifen. *Maturitas* **2004**, *48*, 463–471. [CrossRef] [PubMed]

16.   Sipe, K.; Leventhal, L.; Burroughs, K.; Cosmi, S.; Johnston, G.H.; Deecher, D.C. Serotonin 2A receptors modulate tail-skin temperature in two rodent models of estrogen deficiency-related thermoregulatory dysfunction. *Brain Res.* **2004**, *1028*, 191–202. [CrossRef] [PubMed]

17.   Lai, C.T.; Tanay, V.A.; Rauw, G.A.; Bateson, A.N.; Martin, I.L.; Baker, G.B. Rapid, sensitive procedure to determine buspirone levels in rat brains using gas chromatography with nitrogen–phosphorus detection. *J. Chromatogr. B Biomed. Sci.* **1997**, *704*, 175–179. [CrossRef]

18.   Arora, P.; Sharma, S.; Garg, S. Permeability issues in nasal drug delivery. *Drug Discov. Today* **2002**, *7*, 967–975. [CrossRef]

19.   Holinka, C.F.; Brincat, M.; Coelingh Bennink, H.J. Preventive effect of oral estetrol in a menopausal hot flush model. *Climacteric* **2008**, *11* (Suppl. 1), 15–21. [CrossRef] [PubMed]

20.   Bowe, J.; Li, X.F.; Kinsey-Jones, J.; Heyerick, A.; Brain, S.; Milligan, S.; O'Byrne, K. The hop phytoestrogen, 8-prenylnaringenin, reverses the ovariectomy-induced rise in skin temperature in an animal model of menopausal hot flushes. *J. Endocrinol.* **2006**, *191*, 399–405. [CrossRef] [PubMed]

21.   Sicat, B.L.; Brokaw, D.K. Nonhormonal alternatives for the treatment of hot flashes. *Pharmacotherapy* **2004**, *24*, 79–93. [CrossRef] [PubMed]

22.   Morrow, P.K.; Mattair, D.N.; Hortobagyi, G.N. Hot flashes: A review of pathophysiology and treatment modalities. *Oncologist* **2011**, *16*, 1658–1664. [CrossRef] [PubMed]

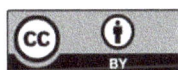

pharmaceutics

MDPI

Review

Mesoporous Silica Nanoparticles: A Comprehensive Review on Synthesis and Recent Advances

Reema Narayan [1], Usha Y. Nayak [1,*] , Ashok M. Raichur [2] and Sanjay Garg [3]

[1] Department of Pharmaceutics, Manipal College of Pharmaceutical Sciences,
    Manipal Academy of Higher Education, Manipal 576104, India; nsreema@gmail.com
[2] Department of Materials Engineering, Indian Institute of Science, Bengaluru 560012, India; amr@iisc.ac.in
[3] School of Pharmacy and Medical Science, University of South Australia, Adelaide, SA 5000, Australia;
    Sanjay.Garg@unisa.edu.au
*   Correspondence: usha.nayak@manipal.edu; Tel.: +91-820-2922482

Received: 30 June 2018; Accepted: 31 July 2018; Published: 6 August 2018

Abstract: Recent advancements in drug delivery technologies utilizing a variety of carriers have resulted in a path-breaking revolution in the approach towards diagnosis and therapy alike in the current times. Need for materials with high thermal, chemical and mechanical properties have led to the development of mesoporous silica nanoparticles (MSNs). These ordered porous materials have garnered immense attention as drug carriers owing to their distinctive features over the others. They can be synthesized using a relatively simple process, thus making it cost effective. Moreover, by controlling the parameters during the synthesis; the morphology, pore size and volume and particle size can be transformed accordingly. Over the last few years, a rapid increase in research on MSNs as drug carriers for the treatment of various diseases has been observed indicating its potential benefits in drug delivery. Their widespread application for the loading of small molecules as well as macromolecules such as proteins, siRNA and so forth, has made it a versatile carrier. In the recent times, researchers have sorted to several modifications in the framework of MSNs to explore its potential in drug resistant chemotherapy, antimicrobial therapy. In this review, we have discussed the synthesis of these multitalented nanoparticles and the factors influencing the size and morphology of this wonder carrier. The second part of this review emphasizes on the applications and the advances made in the MSNs to broaden the spectrum of its use especially in the field of biomedicine. We have also touched upon the lacunae in the thorough understanding of its interaction with a biological system which poses a major hurdle in the passage of this carrier to the clinical level. In the final part of this review, we have discussed some of the major patents filed in the field of MSNs for therapeutic purpose.

Keywords: mesoporous silica nanoparticles; MCM-41; protocells; SBA-15; Stober's synthesis; tetraethyl orthosilicate

1. Introduction

Modern nanotechnology has evolved as the principal component of science in the current century. Over the years, diagnosis of diseases and its therapy is constantly leaping milestones due to the application of nanotechnology in the field of biomedicine. The evolution of nanomedicine and green technology for its production have been a great boon and have shifted paradigms in therapy and tissue engineering, owing to the advantages of nanocarriers such as a high surface area to volume ratio, unique features of surface modification and engineering to obtain particles of various sizes, shapes and different chemical characteristics. These have proven to be biocompatible, biodegradable and non-toxic which adds to its advantages [1–5]. Lipid-based nanocarriers [6–8], polymeric nanoparticles [9–11], dendrimers [12] have revolutionized the therapy for various conditions especially cancer and infectious diseases. Many of these products have been approved and are commercially available. Table 1 enlists some of the marketed nanomedicines.

Table 1. List of some marketed products containing nanoparticles.

Marketed Product	Formulation	Drug	Use	References
AmBisome®	Liposome	Amphotericin B	Antifungal	[13]
DaunoXome®	Liposome	Daunorubicin	Kaposi's sarcoma associated with HIV	[14]
Doxil®	Liposome	Doxorubicin	Kaposi's sarcoma associated with HIV, breast cancer, ovarian cancer	[15]
Myocet®	Liposome	Doxorubicin	Breast cancer	[16]
Emend®	Nanocrystals	Aprepitant	Antiemetic	[17]
Megace ES®	Nanocrystals	Megestrol acetate	Anorexia	[17]
Tricor®	Nanocrystals	Fenofibrate	In hypercholesterolemia	[17]

Apart from the above mentioned organic nanoparticles, inorganic nanoparticles have also been widely explored for their application in biomedicine. Out of them, quantum dots, iron oxide nanoparticles have been approved and are commercially available. Carbon dots, nanoparticles of gold, silver, various other metal oxides, layered double hydroxide nanoparticles and silica nanoparticles have been widely used for various diagnostic and therapeutic purposes [2,18–20]. Of these, silica nanoparticles comprising of organic dyes and radioactive iodide known as Cornell dots (C dots) has successfully attained an important benchmark of safety by its approval for Phase I human trials which is vital for any substance requiring Investigational New Drug (IND) approval. C dots are core-shell silica nanoparticles containing fluorescent molecules within the silica core surrounded with silica shell which is further coated with polyethylene glycol (PEG). C dots were first developed by the Spencer T. Olin Professor of Engineering, Ulrich Wiesner from Department of Materials Science and Engineering at Cornell University [21,22].

Silica nanoparticles with mesopores–referred to as mesoporous silica nanoparticles (MSNs)–have gained wide popularity over the recent years. Its advantages of uniform and tunable pore size, easy independent functionalization of the surface, internal and external pores and the gating mechanism of the pore opening make it a distinctive and promising drug carrier. Scientists have successfully worked on the utilization of these carriers for loading variety of cargo ranging from drugs to macromolecules such as proteins [23,24], DNA [25,26] and RNA [27,28]. An exhaustive set of literatures are available and research is still underway in evaluating new avenues for the use of MSNs in drug delivery. Several reviews pertaining to MSNs in improving the solubility of the drug [29,30], as controlled/sustained drug delivery system [31], applications in biomedicine [32,33] have been published. The present review focuses on literatures published on a broad perspective of MSNs ranging from synthesis to the patents filed. In doing so, we realize that all the reported papers in each of the areas could not be discussed in detail. We have detailed and overviewed the recent research and patents applied for MSNs specifically on Mobil Crystalline Materials (MCM-41) and Santa Barbara Amorphous type material (SBA-15). An overview of the synthesis and theory behind the formation of MSNs is provided to discuss the factors affecting the shape and size of MSNs. The major research in the field of MSNs related to the biomedical applications for therapy based on small molecules and the related patents literature are included.

2. Origin of Mesoporous Silica Materials

Although the synthesis of mesoscopic materials dates back to 1970s, Mobil Research and Development Corporation was the first to synthesize mesoporous solids from aluminosilicate gels using liquid crystal template mechanism in the year 1992. They designated it as (Mobil Crystalline Materials or Mobil Composition of Matter) MCM-41. As per IUPAC, mesoporous materials are defined as the one having a pore size in the range of 2–50 nm and an ordered arrangement of pores giving an ordered structure to it [34–36]. The pore size of these could be varied and tuned through the choice of surfactants used. Generally, MCM-41 is hexagonal with a pore diameter of 2.5 to 6 nm wherein cationic surfactants were used as templates. MCM-41 is one of the most widely explored materials for drug delivery. Apart from this, various other materials of mesoporous nature have also been synthesized by varying the starting precursors and reaction conditions. These may vary in their structural arrangement or the pore size. MCM-48 has a cubic arrangement whereas MCM-50 has a lamella-like arrangement [37]. Non-ionic triblock copolymers like alkyl poly(ethylene oxide) (PEO) oligomeric surfactants and poly(alkylene oxide) block copolymers have also been used as a template which has been designated as SBA-11 (cubic), SBA-12 (3-*d* hexagonal), SBA-15 (hexagonal) and SBA-16 (cubic cage-structured) based on the symmetry of the mesoporous structure and the triblock polymers used. The ratio of ethylene oxide to propylene oxide was varied to achieve the desired symmetry of mesoporous materials. Highly ordered mesoporous structure of SBA-15 has also been widely used for the biomedical purpose. This was first synthesized by University of California, Santa Barbara and hence named Santa Barbara Amorphous type material (SBA). This is different from MCM in that they possess larger pores of 4.6–30 nm and thicker silica walls [38]. FSM-16, that is, folded sheets of mesoporous materials are another type of mesoporous materials, which are synthesized using quaternary ammonium surfactant as a template and layered polysilicate kanemite. Tozuka et al. demonstrated that FSM-16 could be used for pharmaceutical applications other than as an adsorbent and for catalysis [39]. Various other MSNs coined Technical Delft University (TUD-1), Hiroshima Mesoporous Material-33 (HMM-33), Centrum voor Oppervlaktechemie en Katalyse/Centre for Research Chemistry and Catalysis (COK-12) have been synthesized which vary in their pore symmetry and shape [40,41]. The structural characteristics of some mesoporous materials have been listed in Table 2. Figure 1 shows the representation of some MSNs. Of these, MCM-41, MCM-48, SBA-15, SBA-16 are widely employed for drug delivery. In addition, they have also been explored as adsorbents, catalysis and as biosensors. MCM-50, SBA-11 and SBA-12 have been reported to behave as excellent adsorbents and in catalysis.

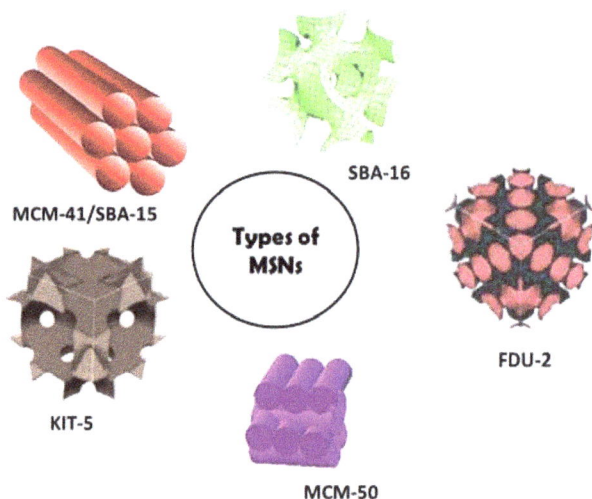

Figure 1. Representation of different types of mesoporous silica nanoparticles (MSNs).

Table 2. List of some of the types of mesoporous silica nanoparticles (MSNs) and their characteristics.

MSN Family	MSN Type	Pore Symmetry	Pore Size (nm)	Pore Volume (cm³/g)	References
M41S	MCM-41	2D hexagonal *P6mm*	1.5–8	>1.0	[42,43]
	MCM-48	3D cubic Ia3d	2–5	>1.0	[42,43]
	MCM-50	Lamellar *p2*	2–5	>1.0	[44,45]
SBA	SBA-11	3D cubic *Pm3m*	2.1–3.6	0.68	[45–47]
	SBA-12	3D hexagonal *P6₃/mmc*	3.1	0.83	[48–50]
	SBA-15	2D hexagonal *p6mm*	6–0	1.17	[43,51]
	SBA-16	Cubic Im3m	5–15	0.91	[43,52]
KIT	KIT-5	Cubic Fm3m	9.3	0.45	[53,54]
COK	COK-12	Hexagonal *P6m*	5.8	0.45	[55,56]

MCM-Mobil Crystalline Materials; SBA- Santa Barbara Amorphous; KIT- Korea Advanced Institute of Science and Technology, COK- Centre for Research Chemistry and Catalysis.

3. Synthesis of MSNs

Stober was the pioneer in developing a system of chemical reactions for the synthesis of spherical monodisperse micron size silica particles [57]. From then on, the method is known as Stober synthesis. Many modifications have constantly been made to the Stober's synthesis to yield monodisperse, ordered, nanosized silica particles. The synthesis of MSNs can be accomplished in basic, acidic and neutral conditions. Manipulating the reaction parameters resulted in particles with different shapes and sizes. The Stober's method of synthesis was first modified by Grun et al. where they introduced a cationic surfactant as a template to yield a spherical rather than a hexagonal MCM-41 structure. They were successful in generating spherical MCM-41 with similar properties as that generated by other methods [58]. Constant research has led to a lot of variations in the synthesis conditions and methods to yield stable, monodisperse MSNs.

For MSNs to be an ideal carrier for drug delivery the particle size needs to be uniform; pore volume has to be large to enhance loading capacity. These parameters can be controlled during the synthesis by varying the pH of the reaction mixture, temperature, concentration of surfactant and silica source. The synthesis of MSNs occurs by liquid crystal template mechanism wherein hydrolysis and condensation of silica on the surface of surfactant micelles takes place. The liquid silica (tetraethyl orthosilicate) transforms to solid silica [59–61].

3.1. Mechanism of Formation of MSNs

A thorough understanding of the mechanism of formation of MSNs is essential to obtain particles with desired properties for drug delivery. The early reports on the mechanism suggested that the silica network gets built throughout the liquid–crystalline phases of non-ionic surfactants. This is particularly true for materials prepared from a dilute solution of surfactants as no evidence of regular mesostructured materials was observed [62]. The literature has shown that either the hydrolysed silica gets adsorbed around the micelles or in the case of SBA-15, the surfactant and the silica interact at the initial stage and form a core shell-like structure [63]. The mechanism for the formation of MCM-41 is represented in Figure 2. Efforts have been on since then by research groups to unveil the exact mechanism behind the formation of MSNs.

The in-situ usage of time-resolved small-angle neutron scattering (SANS) has been used to study the formation of MSNs. Using this method, they were able to predict the changes happening concurrently with the formation process. It was observed that during the early hydrolysis (~40 s) of silica source tetramethyl orthosilicate (TMOS), the silicate ions tend to adsorb around the surfactant micelles during the growth phase. As the charge around the surfactant reduces due to the initial hydrolysis and the condensation of the silica precursor, the intermicellar repulsion reduces, allowing the further formation of small aggregates of silica. After ~400 s, the reaction mixture contained sufficiently discrete hexagonally ordered mesopores of silica which was confirmed by transmission electron microscopy (TEM) studies. This is in accordance with the previously proposed 'current bun model' for the mechanism of formation of MSNs [64,65].

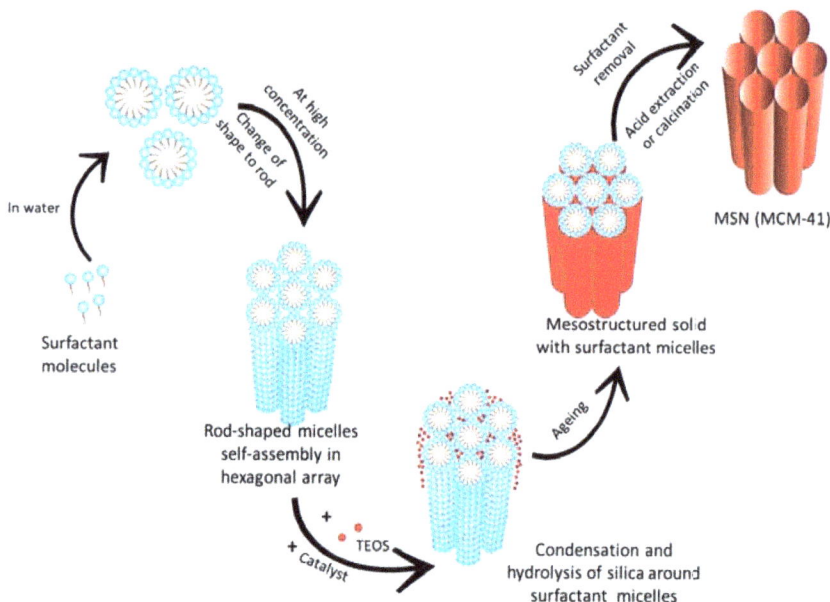

Figure 2. Mechanism of formation of Mobil Crystalline Materials No.41 (MCM-41).

Another mechanism named 'swelling-shrinking mechanism' was proposed for the formation of MSNs utilizing the technique of time-resolved synchrotron small-angle X-ray scattering (SAXS). This mechanism holds well when tetraethyl orthosilicate (TEOS) alone is used as the precursor in the absence of any other solvent like ethanol. TEOS being oil-like monomer showed phase separation under static condition, whereas, under vigorous stirring, an emulsion-like system was obtained. Initially, cetyltrimethylammonium bromide (CTAB) forms ellipsoidal micelles with an inner core consisting of the hydrophobic tail. When TEOS is added, it gets solubilized in the hydrophobic core, thus enlarging the micelles and resulting in the transformation of micelle shape from ellipsoidal to spherical. On hydrolysis of TEOS, the monomers become hydrophilic and are released into the aqueous surroundings. The negatively charged hydrolysed monomers of TEOS get adsorbed onto positively charged CTAB micelles via electrostatic attraction. On complete consumption of the TEOS within the hydrophobic core, the micelles shrink and become smaller in size. As this process of hydrolysis and condensation occurs simultaneously, the micelles shrink continuously until all the TEOS gets hydrolysed and form silica shell around the micelles. The neighbouring micelles aggregate, resulting in particle growth forming a mesoporous structure [66].

3.2. Approaches for the Synthesis of MSNs

Majority of the MSNs are fabricated by modified Stober's method otherwise popularly known as a sol-gel process. Sol-gel chemistry is a widely explored process for the synthesis of many inorganic materials. It involves the hydrolysis and condensation of the alkoxide monomers into a colloidal solution (sol), which acts as a precursor to form an ordered network (gel) of polymer or discrete particles. A typical sol-gel process takes place in the presence of an acid or a base catalyst. Depending on the reaction conditions and the molar ratio of Si/H_2O, the alkoxide group gets hydrolysed. The rate of hydrolysis proceeds faster in basic conditions compared to acidic. Condensation succeeds the hydrolysis step and the effective condensation depends on the hydrolysis step. Multiple condensation results in a chain-like structure in the sol and network-like structure in gel form [67]. The schematic representation of the reaction is shown in Equation (1).

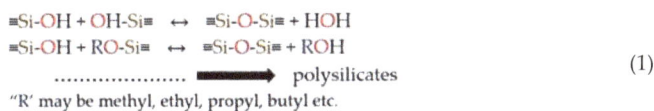

$$\equiv\text{Si-OH} + \text{OH-Si}\equiv \;\;\leftrightarrow\;\; \equiv\text{Si-O-Si}\equiv + \text{HOH}$$
$$\equiv\text{Si-OH} + \text{RO-Si}\equiv \;\;\leftrightarrow\;\; \equiv\text{Si-O-Si}\equiv + \text{ROH}$$

$$\cdots\cdots\cdots\cdots \longrightarrow \text{polysilicates} \tag{1}$$

"R' may be methyl, ethyl, propyl, butyl etc.

To yield particles of the desired size and to enhance the properties of MSNs, the sol-gel process has been modified. Some of the approaches are discussed below:

A simple quenching approach was adopted by Mann et al. to synthesize small sized and ordered MSNs. The reaction was quenched after 40 s by the addition of an excess of water followed by neutralization to pH 7 with dilute hydrochloric acid after a delay time ranging from 60 s to 220 s. The rest of the experimental condition and reagents were maintained the same as in the routine procedure. It was observed that dilution reduces coalescence, and neutralization reduces the rate of silica condensation. The results showed that greater the delay in the neutralization, larger the particle size [68,69]. Similar results were observed by Moller group. The colloidal suspension obtained was found to be stable for long periods of time. However, the MSNs produced by this technique were found to be less ordered in a structure which could be due to scale-up issues during dilution [70].

Evaporation-induced self-assembly (EISA) is another approach for the synthesis of MSNs. In this technique, all the reactants undergo concentration changes during evaporation throughout the process. This results in the organization of a liquid-crystal like template of the silica precursor. In this method, the required concentration of precursor formulations was prepared in ethanol/water solvent with a surfactant. This was converted to monodisperse droplets via injection into an aerosol generator. The droplet size can be controlled by altering its orifice. The alcohol evaporation during drying induces micelle formation and the co-assembly of silica-surfactant into liquid-crystal mesophases [71]. Fontecave et al. modified the EISA method by incorporating different amphiphilic drugs (stearoyl choline, sophorolipid and glucosyl-resveratrol) which behave both as a structure directing agent as well as an active cargo. Sol compositions containing TEOS, drug, water, ethanol and HCl were prepared and injected into an aerosol apparatus. A spray dryer with sufficient air flow and pressure was provided to convert the droplets into solid particles. Characterization of the particles for its pore size and structure using TEM revealed similar results to those with CTAB as surfactant template. Even though the mesostructure formation was not that good, the drug loading was found to be high in all the three cases with complete elimination of burst release. This method would be an ideal strategy for hydrophilic drugs functionalized with hydrophobic tails. Due to the absence of the surfactant template, intrinsic toxicity can be reduced [72].

A recent widely used modification to the synthesis of parent MSNs is encapsulating drugs in hollow mesoporous silica nanoparticles (HMSNs). Their large hollow cavity inside each MSN has garnered tremendous attention. These hollow cavities are capable of holding a high amount of drug compared to its non-hollow counterparts. This unique property of HMSNs makes it widely useful in cancer therapy and imaging [73,74]. Shi et al. were one of the first groups to report the synthesis of HMSNs [75,76]. Preliminary studies to ascertain its enhanced loading capacity was performed using ibuprofen as the model drug wherein, HMSNs showed an enhanced drug loading of 744.5 mg/g, as compared to 358.6 mg/g of MCM-41 [75]. The frequently used method for the synthesis of HMSNs includes the 'core-templating method'. In this approach, many soft/hard templates are used to form the core followed by coating with desired substance at different concentrations to obtain a shell around the substrate with a desired thickness. Subsequently, the core template can be eliminated by calcination or treatment with a suitable solvent leaving behind the shell with a hollow core [77]. She et al. synthesized HMSNs using eudragit S-100 and Triton X-100 as the core-shell template [78]. HMSNs using SiO_2@CTAB-SiO_2 nanoparticles as templates were synthesized by selective etching process [79]. Ghasemi et al. synthesized HMSNs using poly tert-butyl acrylate (PtBA) nanospheres as core-forming hard templates in the presence of CTAB as soft templates [80].

Many hard/soft templates like vesicles, polymeric micelles [81,82], gold [83] or silica nanoparticles were used to construct templates [84,85]. Lin and collaborators proposed a new technique for the synthesis of MSNs using water-in-oil microemulsion as a template. The advantages of this method were the uniformly sized particles obtained compared to other methods. Also, the microemulsion is said to be thermodynamically stable [86].

As the commonly used sol-gel process is a laborious, time consuming process, many different fast methods were used for the synthesis of MSNs. Ling and Su proposed a low-cost electrochemistry assisted approach to synthesize MSNs in large-scale. The formation of MSNs was accomplished by the production of hydroxide at the stainless steel substrate/solution interface which resulted in the self-assembly of surfactant micelles and the polycondensation of silica precursors [87]. Microwave assisted technique for the synthesis of MSNs could be another low-cost approach for the synthesis of MSNs. Various reports show that MSNs with ordered pore size and arrangement could be rapidly synthesized by this method [88,89]. Another rapid, cost effective method for the fabrication of MSNs is sonochemcial synthesis. The use of photoacoustic cavitations during the process was found to generate ordered MSNs, giving scope for the fine tuning of the process in a shorter duration of time [90,91].

3.3. Raw Materials Used and Factors Affecting the Characteristics of MSNs

The three main elements that form the heart of MSN includes a silica precursor (tetraethyl orthosilicate-TEOS, tetramethyl orthosilicate-TMOS, tetramethoxyvinylsilane- TMVS, sodium meta-silicate and tetrakis(2-hydroxyethyl) orthosilicate- THEOS), a surfactant (non-ionic or cationic surfactant) as a structure directing agent (SDA) and a catalyst. Other additives like cosolvents, compounds to prevent aggregation may also be incorporated based on the requirements. In order to ensure the scale-up of MSNs at reasonable cost, natural perlite materials like pumice rock, rice husk, and renewable biomass could also be explored for the synthesis of MSNs [92,93]. The common chemical constituents explored so far are listed in Table 3.

Table 3. List of commonly used chemicals in the synthesis of MSNs.

Chemical Constituents	Function	References
Cetyltrimethylammonium bromide (CTAB)	Structure directing agent/template	[94,95]
Cetyltrimethylammonium chloride (CTAC)	Structure directing agent/template	[96,97]
Pluronic F123, F127	Surfactant template	[38,98]
Brij-76	Surfactant template	[99,100]
Triton X-100	Surfactant	[101,102]
Tween 20, 40, 60, 80	Surfactant	[103]
Tetraethyl orthosilicate (TEOS)	Inorganic silica source	[94,95]
Tetramethoxy silane (TMOS)	Inorganic silica source	[104,105]
Tetrakis(2-hydroxyethyl) orthosilicate (THEOS)	Inorganic silica source	[106]
Trimethoxyvinylsilane (TMVS)	Inorganic silica source	[107]
Sodium silicate	Inorganic silica source	[108]
Ethanol	Cosolvent to solubilize TEOS	[97,109]
Sodium hydroxide (NaOH)	Base catalyst	[95]
Ammonium hydroxide (NH₄OH)	Base catalyst	[94]
Triethanolamine (TEA)	Base catalyst, complexing agent and growth inhibitor	[96]
Diethanolamine (DEA)	Base catalyst	[96,109]
Disodium hydrogen phosphate-sodium dihydrogen phosphate buffer solution	Reaction medium	[109]
Triisopropylbenzene (TIPB)	Pore-expanding agent	[110,111]
Tetrapropoxysilane (TPOS)	Pore- expanding agent	[111]
Pluronic polymer P103	Pore-expanding agent	[112]

The particle size, pore size and morphology of MSNs can be successfully modulated as required by varying the reaction conditions (relative amounts of alkoxysilane, water, catalyst) and temperature.

3.3.1. Control of Particle Size

Particle size is a very important feature for the biomedical application of MSNs as drug carriers. Hence careful tuning of particle size is essential for effective drug delivery. pH of the reaction medium plays a pivotal role in governing the size of MSNs. The particle size can be effectively controlled by adding suitable additive agents like alcohols, amine, inorganic bases and inorganic salts. These agents alter the hydrolysis and condensation of silica precursor. They accelerate the reaction kinetics thus resulting in particles of smaller size. Moller et al. replaced the often used base catalyst sodium hydroxide (NaOH) and ammonium hydroxide (NH$_4$OH) with triethanolamine (TEA). In addition to conferring a basic pH, it also acts a complexing agent to obtain discrete nanoparticles. When the molar ratio of TEOS: TEA was changed from 1:1 to 1:4, the largest particle size was observed with the ratio 1:4 [97]. Qiao [96] suggested that the initial pH value of the system greatly affects the particle size of MSNs. When they provided Na$_2$HPO$_4$-NaH$_2$PO$_4$ as a source of OH$^-$ ions, particle size was found to increase with an increase in the initial pH of the solution. El-Toni et al. observed that on increasing the concentration of ammonia beyond a certain level, the agglomeration of silica particles takes place due to the increase in the ionic strength of the reaction medium [113]. Bouchoucha et al. also reported the efficiency of TEA in producing well-dispersed nanoparticles [114]. Use of L-lysine as a base catalyst was found to hinder the growth of silica particles, thus resulting in sub-nanometre size particles. This may be due to the electrostatic interaction between the protonated amine groups of L-lysine and a deprotonated hydroxyl group on silica surface further delaying the condensation process [115]. PEG-silane capping on the surface of silica particles was also found to effectively attenuate the particle growth process by steric stabilization. When PEG-silane was added immediately after addition of TMOS, the particle size was found to be 5 nm but when it was added at a delay of 50 min after addition of TMOS, the particle diameter increased to >13 nm [115]. A change from monodisperse to heterogeneous particle size distribution was observed when the amount of silica precursor TEOS was increased, which may be attributed to the secondary condensation reactions taking place due to the presence of excess silica precursor which starts producing new nuclei amongst the already existing silica particles [107,116]. A similar trend of results was obtained by Chiang et al. who found that particle size was found to increase with an increase in the amount of TEOS [117]. An increase in the particle size was observed by using different tetraalkoxysilane with different alkoxy groups (Si(OR)$_4$, R = Me, Et, Pr and Bu). Along with this, the addition of alcohols also influenced the particle size of the MSNs. This may be due to the alteration in the hydrolysis rate [118]. Low concentration of CTAB as surfactant yielded a homogenous spherical particle size distribution. On investigating the effect of CTAB on the particle size, it was observed that transformation from discrete spherical to agglomerates was observed due to variation in the hydrolysis and micellization of CTAB [119]. By tuning the concentration of F127 polymer, the particle size could be controlled. An increase of particle size up to 300 nm was reported with an increase in the triblock copolymer Pluronic F127 concentration. Reports state that a balance between the molar composition of various reactants was necessary to obtain MSNs with desired size and quality [120]. The reaction parameters equally influenced the mean particle size of MSNs. On increasing the temperature of the reaction from 30 to 70 °C, an increase in the particle size from 28.91 nm to 113.22 nm was observed. This may be due to the increase in the rate of reaction leading to polycondensation of the silica monomers resulting in a dense silica structure and a larger size [107].

3.3.2. Control of Pore Size, Pore Volume and Mesostructural Ordering

Depending on the type of surfactant, the pore size of MSNs can be varied. The longer chain length of surfactant results in MSNs with larger pores and those with short chain length gives MSNs with smaller pores [121–124]. The concentration of TEOS influenced the mesostructural ordering of the particles. The higher amount of TEOS showed a disordered mesostructure whereas lesser amount was not sufficient to form a mesoporous structure [117]. The concentration of surfactant CTAB was also found to have a profound impact on the mesostructural arrangement of the particles. A lower concentration of surfactant fails to form micelles and hence the resulting nanoparticles will be template deficient whereas the too high concentration of CTAB may result in a disordered structure [35]. Hence an optimum balance has to be struck between various reagents used. Moreover, mesostructural ordering takes place in dilute aqueous solutions [125]. Addition of N, N-dimethylhexadecylamine (DMHA) behaves as a pore size mediator and thus helps with efficient control of pore size as per requirements [126]. Pore size was also found to have a profound influence on the release rate of the drugs as observed using ibuprofen [127,128]. The selection of surfactant species greatly influences the mesostructural ordering of the nanoparticles and the pore size. Effect of the templating agent due to change in the counterions present in cetyltrimethylammonium was studied. Cetyltrimethylammonium chloride (CTAC) as pore generating template produced MSNs with the wormhole-like arrangement. On changing the counter ion to a much larger tosylate ion (CTATOS), the pore radius was found to increase and the pore morphology changed from wormlike to stellate [129]. Of late, novel strategies have been adopted by scientists to bring about modifications in the properties of the MSNs in order to overcome the drawbacks of the traditional MSNs such as small pore size and poor particle size uniformity. In this regard, Huang et al. [130], synthesized highly monodisperse silica nanoparticles having a large pore size with dendritic morphology using a novel dual templating sol-gel reaction by mixing partially fluorinated short chain anionic fluorocarbon surfactant, Capstone FS-66 and CTAB. An interesting observation was made by them showing that an increase in the amount of Capstone FS-66 incorporated resulted in a change in the morphology. The particle size was larger with a dendritic channel pore structure. As the amount of Capstone is further increased, the morphology transforms into a flower-like large dendritic structure. The same strategy was used by Yu et al., who synthesized dendritic MSNs with particle size of less than 200 nm using imidazolium ionic liquids with different alkyl lengths as cosurfactants and Pluronic F127 as a particle growth inhibitor. They observed that neither the reaction temperature nor the time showed any influence on the particle size of MSNs [131].

3.3.3. Control of Shape

The shape of the MSNs greatly affects the cellular uptake and biodistribution of MSNs. Hence stringent control of the shape of MSNs is important to regulate its excretion and other effects in vivo [132]. A clear picture of the relationship between particle shape and cellular responses was demonstrated in the paper by Huang et al. [133]. Till date, spherical MSNs have been widely explored for their drug delivery potential. However, the non-spherical MSNs are seldom used. By carefully controlling the reaction conditions, non-spherical materials with rod, ellipsoid, film, platelet, sheet and cube shapes could be generated. The molar concentration of surfactant, water, base catalyst and TEOS was found to have an impact on the morphology of the MSNs. Cai et al. generated MSNs with different shapes like spherical, silica rods and micrometre-sized oblate silica by manipulating the concentration of TEOS, NaOH/NH₄OH and CTAB [134]. By regulating the amount of dodecanol as a soft template and the temperature of synthesis, a broad range of silica particles could be realized varying from sphere to shell, rugby, peanut, hollow and yolk shell-like structures. The six different particles fabricated had controlled size, porosity, interior spaces and shell structure. Their results showed that inclusion of dodecanol as a soft template resulted in particles with different morphologies [135]. This indicates that any changes in the micelle structure at the initial stage leads to a change in the particle morphologies. MSNs of various shapes can be obtained with a wide range of aspect-ratio. Rod-shaped MSNs are widely exploited counterparts of spherical MSNs. These can be obtained by varying the reaction parameters in a typical sol-gel reaction. An increase in the amount of catalyst and addition of co-solvent like heptane, change in temperature, varying the molar composition of reactants yield rod-shaped MSNs [133,136,137]. Ellipsoidal shaped MSNs also form a part of drug delivery carrier. Inability to retain its shape due to minimization of surface free energy leading to spherical particles poses a major challenge. These MSNs can be synthesized by the introduction of a co-surfactant [138], the addition of potassium chloride and ethanol [139]. Platelet-shaped MSNs with high pore accessibility can be synthesized by addition of low amounts of ammonium fluoride and heptane [137], the presence of non-ionic block copolymer P104 [140], using a ternary surfactant system of cetyltrimethylammonium bromide–sodium dodecyl sulfate–Pluronic123 [141].

Apart from the silica precursors, certain organosilanes were incorporated, which performed the dual function of shape transformation and surface functionalization. Morphological variants of MSNs could be synthesized by the co-condensation method of incorporation of organosilanes. The particle morphology depends on the type and amount of the organoalkoxysilane precursors introduced [36,142]. Various shapes of MSNs such as spheres, rods and hexagonal tubes could be generated using 3-aminopropyltrimethoxysilane (APTMS), *N*-(2-aminoethyl)-3-aminopropyltrimethoxysilane (AAPTMS), 3-[2-(2-aminoethyl amino) ethylamino] propyltrimethoxysilane (AEPTMS), ureidopropyltrimethoxysilane (UDPTMS), 3-isocyanatopropyltriethoxysilane (ICPTES), 3-cyanopropyltriethoxysilane (CPTES) and allyltrimethoxysilane (ALTMS) as organoalkoxysilanes. The transformation in shape of the MSNs may be attributed to the different types of interaction such as hydrogen bonding, hydrophobic interactions between the organoalkoxysilane and the surfactant template.

4. Drug Loading and Release of Drugs from MSNs

The unique feature of MSNs which makes it a widely exploited carrier for drug delivery is its high loading capacity due to the large pore volume and surface engineering properties both on the external and internal surface for better drug targeting.

4.1. Drug Loading

The drug loading is mainly based on the adsorptive properties of MSNs. Both hydrophilic and hydrophobic cargos can be incorporated into the pores of MSNs. Owing to their large pore volume, MSNs inherently possess greater loading capacity compared to other carriers. Nevertheless, extensive work has been carried out to further enhance the loading of the drugs. Synthesis of HMSNs is one such approach to enhance the loading of MSNs (explained in Section 3.2). She et al. attempted to increase the loading of 5-fluorouracil (5-FU) into hollow MSNs by functionalizing the surface silanol groups with different silanes *viz*, octadecyltrimethoxysilane (OTMS), (3-aminopropyl) triethoxysilane (APTES), 3-cyanopropyltriethoxysilane (CPTES). An improved loading of 28.89% was observed for amine functionalized HMSNs compared to plain HMSNs with 18.34%. This may be via the electrostatic interactions between the negatively charged 5-FU and positively charged amino modified HMSNs. A similar strategy could be used for improving the loading capacity of drugs by electrostatic attractions by varying the type of functionalization [78]. However, a contrasting theory was put forth by Wang et al. whose paper suggested that loading of a drug prior to surface grafting yielded a carrier with high loading as compared to grafting followed by loading of the drug [143,144]. Compared to MSNs, HMSNs proved to be a better carrier in terms of loading capacity due to their hollow cavities. 3–15 times higher loading of drugs was observed in HMSNs when compared to MSNs. In addition, dual loading of drugs was also achieved using the same carrier [74,75,145]. The loading capacity of MSNs could be further enhanced by utilizing polymer gatekeeping for the entrapment of hydrophobic drugs [146]. Consecutive drug loading process which increases the intermolecular interactions can also lead to improved loading of the drugs [147]. An increase in the drug feeding ratio was also found to have a profound influence on the loading capacity of MSNs [145,148]. The pore volume of MSNs is the major factor which dictates the loading of the drug. Hence pore expansion strategy can be adopted to introduce and hold a large amount of cargo. Pore swelling agents such as alkanes/ethanol, triisopropyl benzene (TIPB), trioctylamine (TOA), decane and *N,N*-dimethylhexadecylamine (DMHA) aid pore expansion [129,149,150]. Table 4 gives a comparison of the drug loading capacity of various MSNs.

Table 4. Comparison of loading in MSNs.

Carrier	Drug	Loading (wt %)	References
MCM-41 HMSNs	Ibuprofen	35.9 74.5	[75]
MCM-41 HMSNs	Doxorubicin	48.16 112.12	[74]
HMSNs HMSNs-NH$_2$ HMSNs-COOH HMSNs-CN HMSNs-CH$_3$	5-fluorouracil	18.54 28.89 20.73 22.54 12.13	[78]
MCM-41$_{(C12)}$ MCM-41$_{(C16)}$ SBA-15	Captopril	23.6 34 22.6	[151]
MCM-41 SBA-15 SBA-15 (C8) SBA-15 (C18)	Erythromycin	29 34 13 18	[152]
MCM-41 MCM-41-NH$_2$ SBA-15 SBA-15-NH$_2$	Alendronate	14 37 8 22	[153]
MSN-C0 MSN-C10	Lysozyme	34 42	[149]

HMSNs—Hollow mesoporous silica nanoparticles.

4.2. Release of Drugs from MSNs

The release profile of drugs from MSNs mainly depends on its diffusion from the pores which can be tailored by modifying the surface of the MSNs to suit the biological needs. The decisive factor responsible for controlling the release is the interaction between the surface groups on pores and the drug molecule [154]. It was observed that drug loading followed by surface functionalization with amine groups played a significant role in sustaining the drug release as compared to the systems which were functionalized first and then loaded with the drug. This could be attributed to the loading of the drugs within the pores and the capping with APTES which prevents the drug release. If the surface was first functionalized and then loaded, there are possibilities that the drug will get adsorbed on the surface of MSNs resulting in burst release. The role of APTES concentration in drug release was studied, the results of which revealed that a change in the APTES concentration played a vital role in controlling the drug release from the pores [143]. Aspirin loading and release from the MSNs were studied by post-synthetic grafting as well as co-condensation method. It was observed that co-condensation method showed a greater drug loading compared to the other method. In case of plain MCM-41, weak interaction between aspirin and silanol groups resulted in faster drug release following Fick's diffusion. With amino functionalized MCM-41, the strong interaction between the amine group and aspirin resulted in slow drug release especially for the co-condensed MCM-41 [155]. Echoing similar results, the release of ibuprofen from SBA-15 was found to be greatly influenced by the surface modification. In case of amino-functionalized SBA-15 by one-pot synthesis, complete drug release was observed at the end of 10 h whereas the release from that of post-synthetically modified SBA-15, the release of ibuprofen up to 3 days was observed [156]. Table 5 presents the comparison of release rates of different MSNs.

Table 5. Comparison of release rate of MSNs.

Carrier	Drug	Release Rate	References
MCM-41 (C12) MCM-41 (C16) SBA-15	Captopril	45 wt % within 2 h, total drug release over 16 h 47.47 wt % within 2 h, total drug release >30 h 60 wt % within 0.5 h, total drug release over 16 h	[151]
SBA-15 SBA-15 (C8) SBA-15 (C18)	Erythromycin	60% release within 5 h, total drug release within 14 h	[152]
SBA-15 unmodified (PS0) SBA-15-NH$_2$ by post synthesis (PS2) SBA-15-NH$_2$ by one pot synthesis (OPS2)	Ibuprofen	Complete release in 10 h Initial burst release of 50% in 10 h followed by 100% release in 3 days Complete release in 10 h	[156]
MSN (grafting-loading approach) MSN (loading-grafting approach)	Doxorubicin	40% in 8 h and stagnant release beyond 8 h 10% in first 24 h, sustained beyond 160 h	[143]

5. Applications of MSNs in Drug Delivery

MSNs have been widely utilized for a variety of purposes ranging from its use in medicine, as a catalyst in chemical synthesis, adsorbents to adsorb wastes, toxic substances and also as sensors. One of the advantages of MSNs is the ease with which it can be functionalized based on the requirements for a wide variety of applications to control the release of drugs. Figure 3 shows a pictorial representation depicting the versatility of MSN carrier. Vast research is being conducted in utilizing these carriers for drug delivery. In the following section, the major applications of MSNs for drug delivery are discussed. Table 6 provides a list of few of the diseases for which MSNs have been exploited.

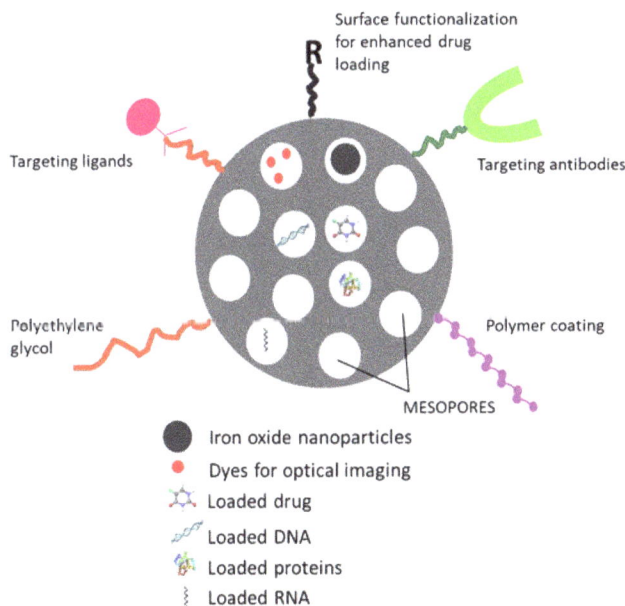

Figure 3. Illustration of versatility of MSN as a carrier in loading variety of drugs.

Table 6. List of some biomedical applications of MSNs.

Category	Drug	Carrier	PS, D_p (nm)	Activity Testing	References
Anticancer	Doxorubicin	Hollow MSNs	120, 2.7	HeLa cells	[157]
	Topotecan	Lipid-coated MSNs	295, 2.3	MCF-7 human breast cancer cells	[158]
	Quercetin	MCM-41	72.9, 2.7	Female athymic nude mice injected with MDA-MB-231 human epithelial breast cancer cells s.c.	[159]
	Curcumin	SLN-silica microcapsules	305, 7.8	Caco-2 cells	[160]
	Paclitaxel	MSNs	100, 2.3	PK studies in peritoneal MIA-PaCa-2 (human pancreatic cancer cell) tumour bearing nude mice	[161]
	5-fluorouracil	MCM-41	135, 2.9	Human colonic HT-29 cells	[162]
	Etoposide	MCM-41-PAA	142.85, 3.69	PC-3 and LNCaP human prostate cancer cells	[163]
	16-hydroxy-cleroda-3,13-dien-16,15-olide (HCD)	Eudragit S100-HCD-Cu-MSN	514, 4.3	Athymic male nude mice injected with C6 Glioma cells s.c.	[164]
Antidepressant	Duloxetine hydrochloride	MSNs	PS not reported, 2.6–7.2	Not reported	[165]
Anti-tuberculosis	Rifampicin	MCM-41	218, 2.4	Not reported	[166]
Anti-inflammatory	Ibuprofen	MSNs	PS not reported, 3.6–4.1	Not reported	[101]
	Ketoprofen	MCM-41 / SBA-15	1500, 3.4 / 970, 6.24	Not reported	[167]
	Budesonide	MCM-41	100, 2.7	Coculture of HT-29 cells and PMA treated human EOL-1 (acute myeloid eosinophilic leukemia) cells	[168]
Antibacterial	Ciprofloxacin	Lipid-coated MSNs	80–100, D_p not reported	*Salmonella typhimurium* administered mice	[169]
	Ciprofloxacin	Arg-MSN	75, 7.2	*Salmonella* infected BALB/c mice	[170]
	Tetracycline	MCM-41	41 and 406, D_p not reported	In vitro against *Escherichia coli*	[171]
Antihypertensive	Captopril	SBA-15	PS not reported, 7.15	Not reported	[172]
	Aliskiren	SBA-15	150, 4.64	Not reported	[172]
	Hydrochlorothiazide, Losartan potassium, Amlodipine besylate, Simvastatin	MCM-41 polypill	60–100, –2.3	Not reported	[173]
Hypoglycemic drugs	Gluconated insulin Rosiglitazone maleate	Alizarin complexone-MSNs	259, 3.9	In vitro monitoring of drug release in human serum	[174]
	16-hydroxycleroda-3,13-dine-16,15-olide (HCD)	MSNs		Diet-induced ICR male diabetic mice	[177]
Osteogenic	Alendronate	MCM-41 / SBA-15	PS not reported, 3.8 / PS not reported, 9.0	Not reported	[153]
	Alendronate	HA-AL-MS-PLGA microspheres	245–258 μm	In vitro on synovium-derived mesenchymal stem cells (MSCs)	[176]
	Dexamethasone	MCM-41	265, D_p not reported	Not reported	[177]
Antioxidant	Morin	MSNs	150, 3	In vitro	[178]

PS—Particle size; D_p—Pore diameter; SLN—Solid lipid nanoparticles; HA-AL-MS-PLGA—Hydroxyapatite-Alendronate-Mesoporous silica-poly(lactic-co-glycolic acid); Arg-MSN—Arginine coated MSN; MCF- Michigan Cancer Foundation; MDA-MB- M.D. Anderson- Metastasis breast cancer; MIA- Melanoma inhibitory activity; PK—Pharmacokinetics; PMA—phorbol myristate acetate ester; PAA—Polyacrylic acid.

5.1. Targeted Antitumor Therapy Using MSNs

The property of surface functionalization of MSNs is widely explored to enhance the site-specific delivery of drugs and avoid side effects. It is a versatile carrier where drugs with different physicochemical properties can be loaded and further functionalized for effective therapy. They can accumulate significantly in the tumour due to the enhanced permeation and retention (EPR) effect [179]. Active targeting aids in maximizing the uptake of actives into the cells. Based on the difference between the normal and tumour cells, suitable receptors overexpressed on tumour cells are selected and ligands specific to those receptors are conjugated on the surface of the MSNs. Specific drug delivery can be achieved by anchoring MSNs with targeting ligands. Folic acid (FA) is a well-known ligand which complements the folate receptors overexpressed on tumour cells. The FA conjugation on the surface of MSNs is brought about by an amide linkage between the carboxyl group of FA and amine group of aminopropyltriethoxysilane (APTES). Ma et al. [180] delivered 5-aminolevulinic acid for photodynamic therapy by conjugating folic acid on the surface of HMSNs against B16F 10 skin cancer cells. The developed formulation was observed to show a high photocytotoxicity to the cancer cells. Similar reports were presented wherein the presence of amine functionalization on the surface aids in the binding of folic acid covalently on the surface of the receptors to ensure selective uptake of doxorubicin (DOX) in breast cancer cells. The apoptosis and cellular uptake studies revealed that FA-MSN-NH_2-DOX showed higher internalization into the cells as compared to MSN-NH_2-DOX [181]. Hyaluronic acid (HA) is another widely explored ligand for targeting CD44 receptors overexpressed on cancer cells. Zhang et al. reported an HA functionalized DOX-MSN which behaved both as enzyme responsive and receptor-mediated delivery system. The increased uptake by colon cancer cells and low in vivo toxicity to the body was proved by in vivo tumour growth inhibition and biodistribution studies. In addition to receptor-mediated uptake, the release of DOX was triggered by hyaluronidase enzyme present in tumour microenvironment [182]. Similar results were reported by Gary-Bobo et al. [183] who fabricated HA-MSNs for photodynamic therapy against colon cancer. The experiments were conducted on HCT-116 colon cancer cell lines which showed the higher efficiency of HA-MSNs owing to their CD44 receptor targeted action as compared to that of plain MSNs. Another novel approach for active targeting of hepatoma cells was reported wherein lactosaminated (Lac) MSNs were designed. These novel delivery systems showed a promising outcome as it had the ability to be endocytosed by asialoglycoprotein (ASGPR) receptors present on the surface of hepatocytes. The findings were supported by the results from cellular uptake studies in ASGPR-positive cells (HepG2 and SMMC7721) wherein Lac-MSNs showed improved cellular uptake when compared to that of plain MSNs. The results also highlighted an interesting point wherein the ligand lactose was recognized only when conjugated with MSNs and not in its free form [184]. Analogues for targeting mannose-6-phosphate receptor overexpressed in cancer cells were grafted onto MSNs to enhance the uptake by tumour cells. These were found to show positive results for the treatment of prostate and colon cancers [185,186]. Arginine-glycine-aspartic acid (RGD) was demonstrated to be selectively engulfed by $\alpha v \beta 3$ and $\alpha v \beta 5$ integrin receptors, which are overexpressed in diverse tumours. The drug-loaded surface engineered RGD-MSNs were thwarted by the normal cells and taken up by the liver cancer cells thus improving the treatment efficacy [187]. In addition to molecular targeting, efforts were also made to club positron-emission tomography (PET) imaging and chemotherapy into a single carrier. Sunitinib as a model anticancer drug was loaded onto the MSNs and surface engineered with cyclo-(Arg-Gly-Asp-D-Tyr-Lys) peptide (cRGDyK) and polyethylene glycol. The efficacy of the receptor uptake was confirmed by flow cytometry studies, PET imaging and histopathological studies. The studies were carried out in U87MG human glioblastoma cells and athymic nude mice were used for in vivo experiments. The tumour uptake of the nanoconjugates was found to be lower in the case of plain HMSNs as compared to that of cRGDyK conjugated HMSNs [188]. Numerous positive outcomes have been demonstrated using a plethora of ligands which are grafted onto the surface of MSNs rendering it target specific. Table 7 lists a few of the ligands which have been explored for cancer drug delivery using MSNs.

Table 7. List of some functionalized MSNs explored for tumour targeting.

Drugs	Application	Targeting Ligand	Receptor	References
5-fluorouracil	Colorectal cancer	Hyaluronic acid	CD44	[189]
5-fluorouracil	Colorectal cancer	EGF	EGF	[190]
Curcumin	Cervical cancer	Chondroitin sulphate	CD44	[191]
Docetaxel	Breast cancer	Folic acid	Folate	[181]
Docetaxel	Hepatoma	Lactose	Asialoglycoprotein	[184]
Doxorubicin	Hepatic cancer	Transferrin	Transferrin	[192]
Doxorubicin	Colon cancer	Aptamer	(EpCAM)	[193]
Photosensitizer merocyanine	Breast cancer	Mannose	Mannose	[194]
Quercetin	Triple negative breast cancer	cRGD peptide	Integrin receptor $\alpha v \beta 3$	[159]
Quercetin	Breast cancer	Folic acid	Folate	[195]
Sunitinib	Glioblastoma	$VEGF_{121}$	VEGF	[196]
Topotecan	Triple-negative breast cancer	cRGD peptide	Integrin receptor $\alpha v \beta 3$	[159]

EGF—Epidermal growth factor; VEGF—Vascular endothelial growth factor; EpCAM—Epithelial cell adhesion molecule.

The surface functionalization of MSNs is not limited to just one ligand. Multiple ligands can be anchored onto the surface of MSNs for receptor targeting. For example, the surface of MSNs loaded with chlorambucil was functionalized with HA and RGD peptide for a synergistic effect. The in vitro cell line studies on human ovarian cancer (SKOV-3) cells showed a significant improvement in the uptake of the MSNs by CD44 and integrin receptors as compared to that of single ligand or plain MSNs [197].

In the recent times, a novel chemotherapeutic strategy utilizing copper impregnated MSNs (Cu-MSNs) have been explored for their potential reactive oxygen species (ROS) mediated apoptosis of cancer cells. Kankala et al. developed a novel Cu-MSN loaded with a catalase inhibitor, 3-amino-1,2,4-triazole (AT) for ROS mediated killing of cancer cells. On uptake by cells and delivery to the endosomal compartment (pH 5.0), the binding between copper and AT breaks off which releases AT to inhibit catalase activity. This in turn, leads to an increase in the ROS production induced by catalysis of copper on MSNs which aids in the cancer cell apoptosis. Positive results were obtained by them when evaluated in HT-29 cells [198]. An effort to overcome the multidrug resistance observed in chemotherapy was made utilizing Cu-MSNs loaded with DOX as model drug. In this system, DOX was conjugated to copper metal through a pH sensitive coordination link susceptible to acidic tumour environment (pH 5.0–6.0). This entire system was further coated with liposomes comprising of cholesterol, D-α-tocopheryl polyethylene glycol 1000 succinate (TPGS), MPEG-2000-DSPE (1,2-Distearoyl-phosphatidylethanolamine-methyl-polyethyleneglycol conjugate-2000), a P-gp inhibitor. Copper ions play a synergistic role in enhancing the intracellular ROS levels which results in killing of cancer cells efficiently. Positive results were obtained by the group when the delivery system was tested in DOX-resistant tumour (MES-SA-DX-5 derived from human uterine sarcoma) and HT-29 cell lines. The antitumor activity of Liposomes-Cu-MSN-DOX was found to be higher when compared to that of pure DOX. The antiproliferative activity of the optimized formulation was found to be profoundly higher in drug resistant cells than the sensitive cells [199].

5.2. MSNs for Anti-Inflammatory Activities

The unique properties of MSNs have been used to accommodate various anti-inflammatory drugs and control their release rate. MCM-41 and SBA-15 are the two widely used silica drug carriers. Ibuprofen was loaded onto multimodal pore channels and the effect on its release was studied. On analysing the release data, it was observed that the release of the drug occurs in three stages *viz*, initial rapid release of the drug adsorbed on the surface of MSNs followed by prolonged release of the drug entrapped in the small pores present in the periphery of the particles having a different pore structural orientation compared to the inner mesopores. The final prolonged release stage occurs by the drug embedded deep in the long length pores of the particles [200]. The bulk of the research

154

work on MSNs for effective delivery of anti-inflammatory drugs has been carried out using ibuprofen as a model drug. Efforts were made to modulate the release rate of the drug by various organic modifications of the surface silanol groups. Surface functionalization was found to alter and also stabilize the drug release rates [127,201]. SBA-15 has also been used to precisely deliver ibuprofen and other anti-inflammatory agents. One such work by Ahmadi et al. demonstrated a change in the release rate of ibuprofen when the surface of the carrier was modified with aminopropyl groups. Plain SBA-15 was not able to sustain the release of the drug due to weak interaction between the surface silanol group and the carboxyl group of ibuprofen. However, on amino functionalization, a relatively prolonged release of the drug was observed due to the strong interaction between the amino groups of silica surface and carboxyl groups of ibuprofen [202]. Other similar studies were carried out to successfully deliver aspirin [155] and indomethacin [203] using MSNs with high drug loading and slow release profile.

5.3. Gated Drug Release/Controlled Drug Delivery

Although the length and the pore structure altered the drug release rate, efforts are constantly underway to achieve smart, zero-release of the drugs by capping the surface of the pores. Controlled and intelligent delivery of drugs to the target site through MSNs is possible due to gated release. The gates of the pores open only in response to certain stimuli like pH, temperature, enzyme, redox and so forth. The principle of gated drug release is very effective when toxic side effects of drugs to other organs are to be avoided [204]. Numerous reports in this regard have been published, a few of which we have discussed in the following section.

5.3.1. pH-Responsive Drug Release

pH is the widely explored stimuli to trigger the drug release as the body has a wide range of pH. MCM-48 particles loaded with prednisolone were coated with succinylated ε-polylysine (SPL) to ensure the pH-dependent release of the drug in the colon region. The in vitro release experiments showed a delay in the release of drug which indicated the successful approach of pH-responsive drug delivery. At acidic pH of the stomach, SPL prevents drug release due to its unionized form whereas, at colonic pH, SPL gets converted to its ionized form facilitating drug diffusion out of the MSNs. The developed nanoparticles could be an alternative for the treatment of diseases of the colon (inflammatory bowel disease and cancer) [205]. The promising outcome of pH-responsive MSNs was observed for tumour-targeted therapy and another disease where the pH of the affected area is slightly acidic than the normal tissues. This pH-responsive drug release can be realized by capping the pores of MSN using acid degradable polymers, polyelectrolytes, some pH-sensitive linkers and so forth. pH sensitive polysaccharide, chitosan was coated onto the MSNs to achieve controlled delivery of curcumin for the treatment of cancer. In vitro drug release studies proved the pH-sensitive nature of chitosan by sustained drug release. The release of curcumin improved when moving from pH 7.4 to pH 5.5. Cell uptake studies in U87MG glioblastoma cancer cell-line showed a decrease in the half maximal inhibitory concentration (IC50) values indicating an improved accumulation of curcumin in cancer cells when encapsulated within chitosan loaded MSNs [206]. Similar studies using chitosan as the pH-triggered cap was carried out by Hu et al. for the release of doxorubicin on MCF-7 breast cancer cells. At acidic pH, the amino groups of chitosan become protonated resulting in swelling of the polymer chains. This opens up the pores of MSNs releasing the drugs [207]. Modulation of doxorubicin via pH-responsive stimuli was also achieved using polymers such as poly(acrylic acid) [208] and polydopamine [209]. Both these reports suggested an enhanced uptake by cancer cells and a sustained release of the drugs. Reports with different polyelectrolytes as pH motifs have shown promising outcomes [208,210]. Tannins as pH motifs were proved by the work of Hu and collaborators. Tannins, by the formation of boronate esters were found to modulate the release of the dye rhodamine at acidic pH [211].

Macromolecular compounds like cyclodextrin (CD) has also been explored for its pH-sensitive property [212]. Tan et al. used a stalk of p-anisidine, loaded the cargo and finally capped the pores with β-CD. The pH sensitivity of the resulting MSNs was evaluated over a pH range of 7.4 to 5.5. A pH-dependent release was observed with a greater release at pH 5.5. When the pH fell below the pKa of the stalk, the interaction between p-anisidine and β-CD reduced thus resulting in the release of the drug. An optimum density of the stalk was the key to control the pH-triggered release. In addition, the effect of both α and β-CD capping on the release of drug was studied. It was observed that the percentage release with α-CD was comparatively lesser that β-CD. This could be due to the different formation constants between CD and p-anisidine stalks [213]. Figure 4 illustrates the release of drug from β-CD capped MSNs in response to stimuli.

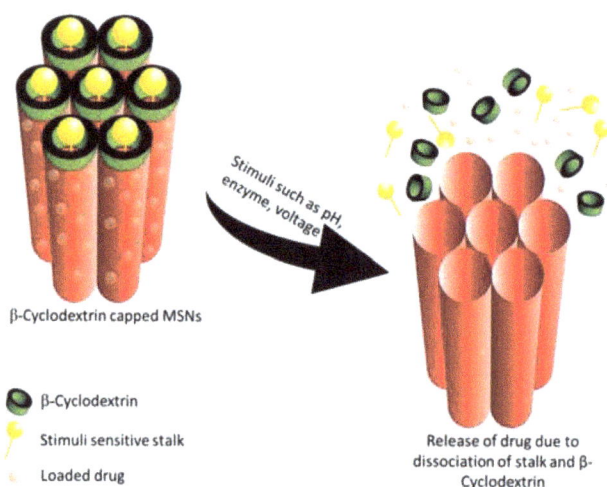

β-Cyclodextrin capped MSNs

- β-Cyclodextrin
- Stimuli sensitive stalk
- Loaded drug

Release of drug due to dissociation of stalk and β-Cyclodextrin

Figure 4. Schematic illustration of the release of drug from β-CD capped MSNs in response to stimuli.

Kuthati et al. devised a strategy to ensure the efficient delivery of antimicrobial agent by modifying the MSN framework via pH sensitive MSNs. Institute of Bioengineering and Nanotechnology-4 (IBN-4) nanoparticles, a type of MSNs was used as a carrier. This was immobilized with silver-indole-3-acetic acid hydrazide (IAAH-Ag) via a pH sensitive hydrazine bond. When exposed to the acidic environment of the site of bacterial infection (pH 5.0), the silver ions are preferentially released up to 12 h to ensure controlled release of the model drug by the cleavage of IAAH-Ag coordination bond. The antibacterial efficacy was investigated on two drug resistant strains of gram negative and gram positive bacteria namely *Escherichia coli* and *Staphylococcus aureus* respectively. In addition to this, the effect of IBN-4-IAAH-Ag NPs on inhibiting the formation of biofilms by four strains of bacteria *viz, Escherichia coli, Bacillus subtilis, Staphylococcus aureus* and *Staphylococcus epidermidis* revealed promising results. The in vitro results were substantiated by in vivo experiments on *Escherichia coli* infected C57BL6 mice. A remarkable reduction in *Escherichia coli* was observed in the formulation treated group of mice. Hence the developed system could be a plausible alternative to the antibiotics used currently [214].

5.3.2. Redox Responsive Drug Release

Redox triggering is another widely used strategy to control the release of cargo from carriers. This technique is being used to deliver anticancer drugs making use of endogenously present reducing agents. Redox cleavable disulfide bonds are often utilized for this kind of drug release. Wang et al. synthesized a disulfide-linked polyethylene glycol (PEG) tethered to MSN for redox responsive drug release. The efficiency of the synthesized MSNs was evaluated by in vitro release studies using Rhodamine B (RhB) as the model drug. Glutathione (GSH) equivalent to intracellular concentration was added to the release media. It was observed that in the absence of GSH, the release of RhB was negligible signifying the efficiency of the cap in blocking the drug release. In addition, the PEG surface modification conferred on the nanoparticles a significant biocompatibility [215]. Dual responsive stalks with β-CD caps were synthesized to control the release of multiple drugs. HMSNs with acetal and ferrocene carboxylic acid units were obtained by selective functionalization. The redox responsiveness of the carrier was confirmed by in vitro experiments using hydrogen peroxide as stimuli. On increasing the concentration of hydrogen peroxide, an increase in the release rate of the drug was observed due to the oxidation of the ferrocenyl moiety. The mechanism behind the release is the strong electrostatic repulsion between β-CD and the oxidized hydrophilic ferrocenyl moiety which results in the dissociation of β-CD caps thus releasing the drug from the pores. The same carrier was also made pH-responsive by introducing an acetal linker to develop a synergistic effect [216].

5.3.3. Temperature Responsive Drug Release

Thermoresponsive MSNs have also been widely been studied as a possible means of controlling drug release. In this context, PEO-b-poly (*N*-isopropylacrylamide) based copolymeric micelles as structure directing agents for the synthesis of functionalized MSNs was developed by Bathfield et al. Ibuprofen as a model drug was loaded into the mesopores using one-pot strategy wherein the drug was incorporated directly into the hybrid material. Ultimately, the structure directing agent in this formulation was the drug-loaded polymer micelles. The drug release profile at 20 and 45 °C revealed a temperature sensitive pattern with a higher drug release at 45 °C than that at 20 °C [217].

5.3.4. Chemical and Enzyme Responsive Drug Release

Several chemicals and enzymes present inherently in the body or produced during diseased conditions have also been explored for the possibility of triggering drug release from the MSNs. Glucose as a chemical has been studied by scientists as a possible trigger to release drugs and has been a boon for diabetes management [218]. In one of the studies, MSNs functionalized with a signal reporter, alizarin complexone (ALC) was developed. Gluconated insulin was then introduced within the pores by benzene-1,4-diboronic acid (BA) mediated esterification reaction. This behaved both as a hypoglycaemic agent as well as pore blocker. In addition, rosiglitazone maleate was also introduced into the pores to form multifunctional MSN. In the presence of glucose, competitive binding between ALC and BA occurs which leads to opening of the pores and release of the drug [174]. Similar work for controlling the drug release using two stimuli that is, glucose and pH was carried out by Tan et al. They fabricated glucosamine-poly(acrylic acid) conjugated MSNs. The pores were capped by the crosslinking of the poly(acrylic acid) chains by the formation of boronate esters. The drug release was governed by pH or the presence of glucose. At mild acidic conditions of pH 6.0 and the presence of 10 mM glucose, the drug release was found to be higher by around 65%. These results suggested that at pH 6.0, combined stimuli showed a sufficiently enhanced release of the drug [219]. Another novel chemical sensitive MSN was with that using thrombin. The MSNs were loaded with an anticoagulant drug (acenocoumarol) and the pores were capped with peptide LVPRGSGGLVPRGSGGLVPRGSK-pentanoic acid (P) which is a substrate for proteolytic α-human thrombin. The results demonstrated that the release of drug was highly specific to the presence of thrombin. Thrombin results in the hydrolysis of the capping peptide releasing the drug [220].

Tailoring the drug release in response to the presence of certain enzymes is another new avenue for modifying the MSN as a carrier. NAD(P)H: quinone oxidoreductase 1 (NQO1) enzyme as stimuli for the release of doxorubicin was demonstrated by Gayam et al. They synthesized MSNs surface functionalized successively with alkyne followed by drug loading. To avoid premature drug release, the mesopores were blocked with rotaxane followed by tethering it to benzoquinone. In the presence of NQO1 enzyme which is upregulated in several tumours, the benzoquinone gets reduced leading to the opening of the pores and the release of doxorubicin. In vivo experiments in nude mice bearing tumour (lung) showed promising results with a significant reduction in tumour volume in the mice treated with MSN-NQO1 compared to those treated with saline and free doxorubicin [221]. Matrix metalloproteinase (MMP-2) triggered drug release for the treatment of liver cancer is another possible line of therapy. Many tumours have shown to overexpress MMP-2, the advantage of which could be explored to target drugs to tumour sites. A two-component that is, a cell penetrating peptide polyarginine and PVGLIG which is a substrate for MMP-2 cleaving based polypeptide was linked with phenylboronic acid-human serum albumin (PBA-HSA) onto the MSNs to render it target specific. Doxorubicin (DOX) was used as the model drug. Human serum albumin was used to cap the pores and phenylboronic acid behaved as the targeting moiety specific to sialic acid overexpressed in liver tumours. The enzyme responsive behaviour of the carrier was studied in vitro where around 73% of the drug released in the presence of MMP-2 as compared to only 15% of release in the absence of MMP-2. In vivo studies in HepG2 cells injected nude mice were performed which revealed encouraging results with DOX-loaded MSN-HSA-PBA showing significant tumour growth inhibition compared to non-functionalized MSN loaded with DOX [222]. An experiment along similar line was performed by Radhakrishnan et al. who explored the use of protamine, a peptide drug as a capping agent to prevent the premature release of diclofenac from MSNs. The protamine cap was found to get hydrolysed in the presence of trypsin enzyme which cleaves the L-arginine residues in protamine thereby releasing the drug. This concept was evaluated by studies on COLO 205 cells. The results showed that about 87% of the drug released within 120 min in COLO 205 cells as compared to 13% in healthy cells. This shows the selective drug release in colon cancer cells as compared to normal cells [223]. Radhakrishnan et al. also demonstrated the use of chondroitin sulphate (CHD) as a gate to the pores of MSNs which would trigger the release of drug in the presence of hyaluronidase enzyme. In addition, CHD also acts as a ligand which gets specifically uptaken by cells overexpressing CD44 receptors. CHD behaves as a cap which prevents the outward diffusion of the drug in the absence of hyaluronidase enzyme [191].

In one of the studies, controlled release of drug was achieved by surface functionalization of MSNs with ferrocenyl moiety β-cyclodextrin complex (Fc-β-CD) to prevent premature release of the drug. The experiments suggested that on stimulation by heme protein (horse-radish peroxidase and hydrogen peroxide) and the production of hydrogen peroxide via the oxidation of glucose by glucose oxidase or +1.5 V stimuli, the ferrocenyl moiety gets dissociated resulting in the opening of the nanovalves and thus releasing the drug. In vitro studies conducted to assess the release property of the carrier revealed that on stimulation with heme protein, a greater amount of drug was released as compared to that with glucose stimulation and without stimuli [224].

5.3.5. External Stimuli for Drug Release

Various other stimuli have also been investigated in modulating the drug delivery from MSNs such as light [225–227], magnetic [227,228], ultrasound [229–231], electroresponsive [224,232] systems. Figure 5 depicts the release of drug from gated MSNs in response to stimuli.

Use of light as an activating mechanism of drug delivery has garnered attention due to its advantages of spatial and temporal control of release of drugs. Febvay et al. [225] combined the advantages of light triggering with a high loading of MSNs in their study to enable the delivery of a model molecule, a fluorescent dye–Alexa546–which is impermeable to the cytosolic compartment. The MSNs were prepared using secondary surfactant pluronic F127 and further tagged with biotin or streptavidin. Following endocytosis, the LN-229 cells (human glioma, ATCC) were exposed to green excitation light for 3 to 120 s which resulted in the dye being released into the cytosol. This could be attributed to the cell membrane damage induced by the light irradiation. Liu et al. [226] explored the potential of deeper tissue penetration potential of near infrared (NIR) radiations to control the release of the drugs. They developed MSNs with gold nanorods forming the inner core and phase changing molecule, 1-tetradecanol as gatekeepers. DOX was chosen as the model drug molecule. These nanoparticles were further functionalized with folate moieties to target KB cells. The system was able to release DOX due to heating induced by near IR radiation generated by a gold nanorod core. The successful release of the drug on IR radiation was ascertained by first subjecting it to external heating which did not show any release at 37 °C. On NIR irradiation of 802 nm for 10 min, the temperature increased to 45 °C which resulted in the release of DOX which may be attributed to the change in the fluid state of tetradecanol molecules above T_m. In vitro studies on KB cells showed preferential uptake by the cell owing to the surface functionalization. The combined effect of phototherapy (NIR irradiation), chemotherapy (DOX) and targeted therapy resulted in remarkable killing of cancer cells. Hence the developed nanoparticulate system could be efficiently used for multimodal therapy. Li et al. [227] worked on similar lines where they explored the potential of MSNs as multimodal carriers using MRI monitored magnetic targeting and NIR mediated phototherapy. In their work, they developed iron oxide (Fe_3O_4) nanoparticles coated with trisoctahedral gold (Au) shell which were loaded with DOX. These were further coated with silica shell capped with oligonucleotides. Au shell here acted as NIR responsive material whereas Fe_3O_4 facilitated magnetically triggered release of drug. The controlled release property of the carrier was confirmed via in vitro studies on HeLa cell lines which showed DOX release upon NIR irradiation at 808 nm and magnetic attraction for a brief period of 2 h. These results were further supported by in vivo studies on nude mice. HeLa cells were transplanted to the nude mice for the development of tumour after which the nanoparticles were injected. On exposure to magnetic attraction for 30 min and laser exposure at 3 W/cm^2 for 30 min, a complete disappearance of tumour was observed after 14 days. These findings suggest the plausible use of these carriers to enable efficient combination therapy options for tumours.

Another novel strategy to induce visible light irradiated delivery of drugs using MSNs as drug carriers was put forth by Kuthati et al. They developed a silver nanoparticle (SNPs) decorated copper impregnated MSNs (Cu-MSNs) to aid in the photodynamic inactivation of antibiotic resistant *Escherichia coli*. Curcumin (Cur), a phototherapeutic agent was loaded into the MSNs. They explored the plasmonic resonance coupling between curcumin and silver nanoparticles to enhance the transfer of silver nanoparticle to photosensitizer to effectively kill gram negative *Escherichia coli*. They hypothesized that curcumin would produce large amounts of ROS under light irradiation which will enhance the release of silver ions. SNP+Cur behaves as a positively charged nanocomposite which improves the binding ability of Cur to the bacterial membrane. The antibacterial efficacy against *Escherichia coli* was studied by constant illumination using LED array at 470 nm at a fluence of 72 J/cm^2. The study yielded promising results revealing that Cur-Cu-MSN-SNP efficiently killed bacteria in light conditions with very mild toxicity in dark conditions. The successful eradication of bacterial cells may be attributed to three factors, namely, improved solubility and local concentration of Cur loaded into MSNs, improved binding of positively charged nanoparticle to bacterial membrane, enhanced ROS production due to Cu-MSN-SNPs. Similar strategy can be used for the development of wide variety of photobactericidal systems [233].

The release of drugs from MSNs can also be triggered via magnetic attraction. Baeza et al. [228] reported the synthesis of a hybrid polymer which responded to both thermal and magnetic stimuli. They incorporated superparamagnetic iron-oxide nanocrystals into the mesopores which was capable of providing a sufficient heating capacity for hypothermia cancer therapy. To enable thermoresponsive release of the drug molecule, poly(N-isopropylacrylamide) was tethered to the surface of MSNs. Fluorescein and soybean trypsin inhibitor type II was loaded into the pores of the MSNs to model the release property. In response to an alternating magnetic field of 24 kA/m and 100 kHz inside a thermostatic chamber maintained at 20 °C, a higher release of fluorescein was observed which may be due to the heat energy and enlargement of the pores leading to greater release of the drugs.

Among the non-invasive routes to enhance the spatio-temporal delivery of drugs, ultrasound is slowly gaining popularity owing to its advantages of lower cost, absence of ionizing radiations and ease of tissue penetration regulation by tuning the frequency of the cycles and exposure time. They are capable of inducing thermal/mechanical effects which can trigger the release of the drugs. Several efforts are underway to utilize this technology for the therapy of diseases especially cancer. Paris et al. formulated an ultrasound responsive MSNs capped with the copolymer, poly(2-(2-methoxyethoxy) ethyl methacrylate-co-2-tetrahydropyranyl methacrylate), with two functional ends and a monomer ratio 90:10 (MEO$_2$MA:THPMA). They utilized fluorescein as the model molecule to monitor the developed system. Ultrasound irradiation resulted in the cleavage of the hydrophobic tetrahydropyranyl moiety of the cap leading to a change in its conformation allowing the drug to be released. They studied this concept further by surface functionalization of the MSNs with biotin and RGD peptide to enable selective uptake by tumour cells (HeLa cell lines). DOX was loaded as the cargo within the mesopores. They successfully proved the efficiency of the developed nanoparticulate system in enhancing the efficiency of the DOX in killing cancer cells [229,231]. Studies on similar line was reported by Kim et al. [230] using ibuprofen as a model drug which were loaded into MSNs and covered with poly(dimethylsiloxane) as the implantable body. On exposure to ultrasound of 28 kHz with a power of 1.5 W/cm^2, an increase in the diffusion of ibuprofen was observed. In addition, negligible damage was observed to the polymer material on subjecting it to ultrasound frequency. These results suggest the possible use of this stimulus in enabling controlled release of drug to the diseased sites.

Another interesting approach to non-invasive drug therapy could be the use of a mild electric field that aids in controlling the release of the cargo by activating certain mechanisms, *viz*, electrochemical reduction-oxidation and movement of a charged molecule. Xiao et al. [224] developed a novel controlled release MSNs sensitive to enzyme or voltage. These were functionalized with ferrocene and further loaded with rhodamine and capped with β-cyclodextrin (β-CD). Voltage ranging from 0.5 V to 1.5 V was applied to trigger the release of the cargo from the pores. Both the enzyme and voltage triggered release was based on the presence of ferrocenyl (Fc) and β-CD valve. The release is based on the conversion of Fc to Fc$^+$ which dissociates from the surface of the pores under a standard potential of +0.32 V. They observed that at a higher voltage, the release rate was higher and vice versa. Wang et al. [232] also utilized the potential of ferrocene functionalized β-CD as nanovalves to modulate the drug release from MSNs. They loaded two drugs that is, gemcitabine and doxorubicin and evaluated the potential of ferrocene in controlling the drug release. On applying a voltage of +1.5 V, a controlled release of 23% of gemcitabine was observed over 15 min. Thereafter −1.5 V was applied, which ceased the release of the drug. Hence, this approach can be effectively used for controlling the drug release from MSNs and thus avoiding side effects.

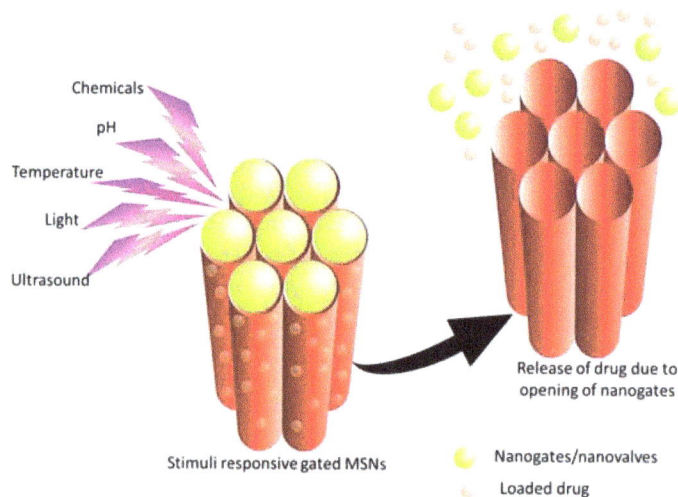

Figure 5. Schematic illustration of the release of drug from gated MSNs in response to stimuli.

5.4. MSNs for Improvement of Solubility of Drugs

MSNs owing to their modifiable surface chemistry can act as carriers for poorly soluble drugs and tackle their solubility issues [234]. Bukara et al. [235] proved this potential of MSNs by loading the poorly soluble drug fenofibrate and assessing them in healthy human volunteers. The volunteers were monitored for a period of 96 h post dosing and their plasma samples were collected and assessed for the pharmacologically active metabolite fenofibric acid. A significant increase in C_{max} with a point estimate of 177% and a reduction in t_{max} were observed for fenofibrate formulation following single oral administration. No serious adverse events were reported and none of the volunteers discontinued the study. This demonstrates that the MSNs could also be used as a possible alternative to other carriers to improve the solubility and bioavailability of drugs. Enhanced oral bioavailability of telmisartan (TEL) was achieved by loading it into MSNs. Based on the results obtained by the study on beagle dogs, Zhang et al. set forth a basis to use MSNs as a drug carrier for poorly soluble drugs. In vitro cellular uptake studies showed that TEL-MSN showed an enhanced uptake in Caco-2 cells resulting in accumulation in the cell membrane as compared to TEL-mesoporous silica microparticles. The uptake mechanism of these MSNs occurred in three major steps: first, binding of MSNs to intestinal cell membrane followed by nonspecific cellular uptake and merging with endosomes and finally, release from endosomes and enters the cytoplasm. In vivo absorption studies of TEL-MSN in beagle dogs revealed a 1.29 times increase in $AUC_{0\rightarrow72h}$ as compared to that of marketed tablet and MSN [236]. Thomas et al. synthesized MSNs loaded with BSC-II antiepileptic drugs, carbamazepine (CBZ), oxcarbazepine (OXC) and rufinamide (RFN). The dissolution profile of the drugs in phosphate buffer, showed faster release for CBZ and OXC whereas RFN showed a slower release of drugs after an initial burst release. The profile resembled a first order release mechanism related to the drug diffusion process. This could be widely exploited for the improvement in drug absorption and bioavailability of poorly soluble drugs by further proving this concept via in vivo studies [237].

5.5. MSNs in Biomedical Imaging and Theranostic Purpose

The versatile features of MSNs such as ability to incorporate wide variety and large number of compounds within them, their stability and controllable size, makes it an ideal platform for biomedical imaging and theranostic applications. Many of the fluorophores face certain drawbacks such as poor solubility and stability especially those for near infrared (NIR) imaging. These compounds can be incorporated within the MSNs to improve their photophysical and photochemical properties. Various literatures have suggested the successful utilization of this carrier for imaging and theranostic purposes.

MSNs can be widely used for optical imaging, magnetic resonance imaging (MRI), positron emission tomography (PET). Optical imaging is a technique wherein the specific probes are excited by incident light usually in the visible or near infrared regions, thus emitting light at a lower energy. MRI is a powerful in vivo imaging technique which gives a three dimensional anatomical picture of the region of interest with a high resolution.

Most often, the dyes are incorporated within the mesopores which gives sufficient stability and protection from the external environment. Sreejith et al. developed a novel hybrid material constituting squaraine loaded MSNs which were further coated with thin sheets of graphene oxide. Squaraine dyes possess significant photophysical properties in the NIR region. In order to ascertain their bioimaging ability, in vitro studies were carried out on HeLa cell lines which showed positive results. The developed hybrid formulation was successful in protecting the dye as well as preventing its leakage from the system showing a potential platform for bioimaging [238]. Moreover, these MSNs can also be tagged with surface active moieties which can be preferentially directed to abnormal tissues for diagnostic and therapeutic purposes. Nakamura et al. reported the synthesis of multimodal MSNs possessing features of imaging as well as drug delivery. The carrier was loaded with ^{19}F, a MRI contrast reagent. These nanoparticles were further labeled with fluorescent dyes and tethered with folic acid to ensure adequate uptake by tumour cells. The developed nanoparticles demonstrated positive results in vitro exhibiting sufficient cellular uptake by folate expressing cancer cells which was observed via ^{19}F MRI and fluorescence microscopy [239]. Jun et al. reported the use of silica nanoparticles embedded with quantum dots (QDs) and constituting a core-shell of CdSe@ZnS for bioimaging purposes (Si@QDs@Si NPs). They observed that the system showed superior fluorescence as compared to single quantum dots when studied in HeLa cells. The same was confirmed via in vivo testing wherein the mice were injected with Si@QDs@Si NPs mixed with HeLa cells. The nanoparticles exhibited enhanced fluorescence and hence can be effectively used for bioimaging which requires minute cell tracking with high sensitivity [240]. Helle et al. explored the potential of cyanine 7-doped silica nanoparticles for lymph node mapping using NIR imaging. They were able to map the lymph nodes for the diagnosis of possible metastatic and draining nodes. In addition, the developed platform were found to be excreted via hepatobiliary route and was found to be safe when tested in mice up to a period of three months showing an efficient hepatobiliary excretion [241].

5.6. MSNs for Bone Tissue Engineering and Repair

MSNs have found a special place in the field of tissue engineering. Most of the research in this area revolves around bone tissue differentiation and osteogenesis. The surface silanol groups present on MSNs react with the body fluids to generate carbonated apatite which can further lead to bone generation. In addition to this, the MSNs can be loaded with osteogenic agents to augment the bone tissue engineering process [242,243]. For instance, bone morphogenetic protein-2 (BMP2) derived peptide functionalized dexamethasone loaded MSNs were formulated to evaluate its efficacy for the osteogenic differentiation. The evaluation was carried out using cell line studies to study the endocytosis and uptake of the functionalized MSNs. The ectopic bone formation was studied in vivo, the results of which indicated that the BMP2-pep functionalized MSNs held great promise in bone repair. The addition of dexamethasone synergized the bone differentiation effect [177]. Similar results were reported by Luo et al. for bone forming peptide incorporated MSNs [244]. Incorporation of bioactive glasses into mesoporous silica is another interesting application of MSN in bone repair. Increased bone tissue regeneration was observed with these materials containing SiO_2-CaO-P_2O_5 as composition. Readers are directed to references [245,246] for a detailed review of these materials.

6. Biodistribution and Biocompatibility of MSNs

The safety and toxicity of nanoparticles are a cause of major concern owing to their high surface-to-volume ratio compared to its counterparts. The biocompatibility of any carrier is a prerequisite property for any pharmaceutical product to ascertain that these products do not accumulate in the body over a period of time causing untoward effects.

Many of the formulations containing conventional nanocarriers have been approved by US FDA (Table 1). Biomaterials such as lipids and polymers constitute these conventional nanocarriers. Due to its inherent biodegradability and biocompatibility, these nanocarriers have been constantly exploited for further research to enhance its biomedical applicability. Liposomes are one such carrier which comprises of phospholipid bilayer within which both hydrophobic and hydrophilic drug can be encapsulated. Liposomes have proven to be capable of being used for site specific drug targeting in a variety of diseases [247,248]. These carriers have been found to be safe which may be attributed to the biocompatible nature of phospholipids used [249]. Another nanocarrier that shares a similar importance to that of liposomes is the polymeric nanocarrier. In this regard, poly(lactic-co-glycolic acid) (PLGA) is one of the renowned polymer-based carriers. This is a part of an FDA approved device [249,250]. Although these encouraging results have been obtained regarding their safety for human use, there are certain drawbacks such as stability related issues, lack of control over drug release and difficulty in overcoming certain biological barriers associated with these carriers. Nevertheless, these are still the most widely explored carriers due to their non-toxic property.

Inorganic nanocarriers with robust characteristics, MSNs, although has shown positive in vitro results, studies are still being carried out extensively due to the age-old toxicity-related issues of silicon dioxide, especially silicosis. Efforts are underway in identifying the major routes of toxicity of silica in both its crystalline as well as amorphous forms. In this section, we have focused on the current data available on the biodistribution and biocompatibility of MSNs. Control over the size, shape, pore order and surface chemistry is crucial in deciding the fate of MSNs.

6.1. Effect of Surface Chemistry, Shape, and Size of MSNs

As per the reports, the major pathway of toxicity associated with silica is due to its surface chemistry (silanol groups) which can interact with the membrane components leading to the lysis of the cells and leaking of the cellular components [251,252]. Mesoporous silica exhibited lower hemolytic effect compared to non-porous silica. This could be attributed to the lower density of silanol groups on the surface of mesoporous structures [94]. Surface properties of MSNs also have a great impact on the biodistribution and biocompatibility of MSNs. Altering the surface features by functionalization with polyethylene glycol (PEG) helps the MSNs to escape from being captured by liver, spleen and lung tissues. This could be attributed to the longer circulation time of PEG-MSNs [253]. Yu et al. studied the impact of pore size, shape and surface features of silica nanoparticles on the cellular toxicity. The cellular toxicity was evaluated on macrophages (RAW 264.7) and cancer epithelial (A549) cells. Post 72 h exposure, they observed that A549 cells were resistant to the nanoparticles even at the concentration of 500 µg/mL. However, at a concentration of 1000 µg/mL, observable toxicity was seen. The IC50 value for the nanoparticles when tested on macrophages was found to be between 50 and 100 µg/mL. The cellular level of association was determined using inductively coupled plasma mass spectrometry (ICP-MS). Interestingly; it was observed that amino modified MSNs showed a higher level of cellular association which is contradictory to literature which report that increase in surface silanol groups are responsible for higher cellular association [251,252]. The plausible explanation for this higher interaction between amino MSNs and cells could be that a particular surface threshold exists beyond which cell interaction is facilitated. The observations from the above study suggest that toxicity depends on the type of cells, concentration of nanoparticles treated and pore size and surface charge of nanoparticles [254].

An interesting experiment to identify the effect of the spatial arrangement of MSN surface amine groups on its interaction pattern with cells was performed by Townson et al. MSNs with the same size, porosity and charge were modified with suitable reagents (trimethoxysilylpropyl modified polyethyleneimine, 2-[methoxy(polyethyleneoxy)propyl]trimethoxysilane, *N*-trimethoxysilylpropyl-*N*,*N*,*N*-trimethyl ammonium chloride) resulting in PEG-PEI and PEG-NMe$_3$$^+$ MSNs to ensure exposed polyamines and distributed, obstructed amine groups respectively. Both in vitro and in vivo experiments were performed to determine the toxicity effects. The synthesized nanoparticles were subjected to cytotoxicity studies on a wide range of cell lines such as A549 (human lung carcinoma), A431 (human epithelial cancer), Hep3B (human hepatocellular carcinoma) and human hepatocytes. PEG-PEI MSNs were found to bind to all the cells whereas PEG-NMe$_3$$^+$ MSNs showed limited binding. To confirm these results and to ascertain if the same effects will be observed in a biological system as well, 50 µg was injected into the veins of ex vivo chick embryos which helped in real-time imaging of particles. The results showed a similar trend as that observed in in vitro studies. PEG-PEI MSNs were found to bind endothelial cells and stationary and circulating white blood cells (WBCs) whereas PEG-NMe$_3$$^+$ MSNs remained in circulation for >6 h. In order to verify the importance of amine groups in binding, the MSNs were subjected to acetylation thereby shielding the amine groups. This reduces the binding affinity of the MSNs. From the study, it was concluded that exposure to charged particles and its effect on the formation of protein corona in vivo should also be considered when designing MSNs for biomedical applications [255].

The biodegradation and toxicity of MSNs also depend on the shape of the MSNs. The effect of shape on in vivo toxicity of MSNs after oral administration was studied by Li et al. for MSNs with different aspect ratios of 1, 1.75 and 5. These MSNs were administered at a dose of 40 mg/kg. Two hours post administration, a significant number of MSNs were observed in the liver and spleen. The number of spherical nanoparticles showed a marked increase in the liver compared to its rod-shaped counterparts. It was observed that MSNs showed a rapid excretion from the body via faeces while some of the unchanged MSNs or their degradation products could be absorbed and later excreted via urine. The in vitro results of degradation showed that spherical nanoparticles showed rapid degradation while long rods have slow degradation rate, especially in intestinal fluid. These results suggest that degradation of MSNs depends on the shape and biological environment. No abnormalities were observed in liver, spleen, lung and heart. However, spherical nanoparticles induced renal tubular necrosis and haemorrhage which may be due to the degradation products. Contrasting results were obtained for MSNs administered via an intravenous route where no major abnormality in kidney was detected [132,256]. However, there is a lack of clear picture of the degradation pathway and pharmacokinetics of MSNs. With this regard, efforts were made by Zhao et al. to study the pharmacokinetics and biodistribution of different shapes of MSNs namely, long rod, short rod and spherical particles following oral administration. The retention of the nanoparticles in the gastrointestinal tract was determined by ex vivo optical imaging method. In vitro cytotoxicity study revealed that all the three nanoparticles were nearly non-toxic in nature which can be attributed to the conversion of nanoparticles to non-toxic silicate ions. To predict the biodistribution of the nanoparticles, Si content in different organs was determined by inductively coupled plasma optical emission spectrometry (ICP-OES). On examining the Si content in different organs, Zhao et al. also arrived at the same conclusion as that by Li [256], that majority of the MSNs accumulate in the liver. The synthesized MSNs did not show any visible histopathological changes when compared with that of the control indicating that the particles did not produce any gastrointestinal toxicity or inflammation [257].

Size of the nanoparticles also has a profound influence on the biodistribution and excretion of MSNs. MSNs with a varying particle size from 80 to 360 nm was prepared and their biodistribution was assessed in ICR mice. An increase in particle size led to an increase in its accumulation in the liver and spleen following intravenous (i.v.) administration. However, no pathological abnormalities were observed at the end of 1 month. Smaller sized MSNs undergo slower degradation as it can escape the degradation by liver and spleen [253]. Different types of MSNs (MCM-41, SBA-15) were injected subcutaneously (s.c.) and intraperitoneally (i.p.) to mice. Intraperitoneal injection resulted in the death of animals which may be attributed to the rapid systemic distribution following i.p. injection as compared to s.c. [258]. Acute and sub-acute toxicity profiling of fluorescent mesoporous silica nanoparticles (FMSNs) were performed in female nude mice. 1 mg/mouse/day was administered via the intravenous route. No observable toxicity was seen in the animals. Long-term toxicity study following intraperitoneal injection of FMSNs at a dose of 1 mg/mouse/day twice per week for 2 months was conducted to assess the long-term effects of MSNs. The histopathological examination of body tissues, haematological parameters displayed no apparent changes compared to control. In addition, the FMSNs also showed an enhanced tumour uptake property resulting in a reduction in tumour volume [259]. Single dose toxicity studies by Tang et al. revealed that the nanoparticles exhibited a size-dependent toxicity [260]. Zhang et al. synthesized DOX-loaded MSNs functionalized with folic acid of varying sizes of 48, 72 and 100 nm and investigated the effect of particle size on its in vivo distribution in MDA-MB-231 tumour-bearing Balb/c mice. The animals were sacrificed at the end of 24, 48 and 72 h post injection and their organs were harvested. The amount of Si content in each of the organs was determined by inductively coupled plasma mass spectrometry (ICP-MS). It was observed that MSNs with size of 48 nm showed the highest accumulation in the tumour tissues. The results suggest that particle size and surface modification alters the biodistribution of MSNs [261].

The data generated from various literatures suggest that careful control of particle size and shape is the determinant factor in ascertaining the biodistribution and toxicity of MSNs. In addition, the safety and toxicity of MSNs also depend on the dosage of the MSNs administered at which no observable biological effects are detected.

Recently, Shen et al. [262] reported that the novel 3D-dendritic MSNs synthesized by them showed a rapid biodegradation in simulated body fluid within 24 h as compared to two weeks for that of plain MSNs reported earlier. In yet another effort to prepare biodegradable MSNs, He et al. [263] synthesized a novel pH responsive mesoporous silica–calcium phosphate (MSN-CAP) hybrid nanoparticles. The MSNs were doped with calcium phosphate during synthesis process which yielded pH responsive MSNs. The in vitro degradation behaviour of MSN-CAP was observed in simulated fluids. The results showed that the complete degradation of the nanoparticles took place in 24 h. Both these novel MSNs could be an alternative prospect for clinical use. However, their in vivo degradation behaviour has to be ascertained.

6.2. In Vivo Safety and Toxicity of MSNs

Determining the safety and biocompatibility of MSNs is crucial owing to its variable characteristics. Over the last few years, the number of literature on the study of the safety of MSNs has drastically increased. The toxicity of the carriers depends on its various characteristics and the conclusions derived from the studies were found to vary. Nevertheless, most of the reports showed that the MSNs get preferentially accumulated in the liver and spleen following administration.

Liu and collaborators made an attempt to study the single and repeated dose toxicity of HMSNs following intravenous administration in mice. LD_{50} of HMSNs was found to be higher than 1000 mg/kg. In single dose toxicity studies, mice were injected with HMSNs at a low dose and high dose. At the higher dose of 1280 mg/kg, mice did not survive. In contrast, the groups treated with low dose HMSNs did not show any behavioural changes nor any haematology or pathological changes. To carry out the detailed repeated dose toxicity studies, intravenous administration of HMSNs were given to mice continuously for 14 days and observed for a month. During the 1 month observation period, no mortality was observed. Moreover, no remarkable changes in pathology or blood parameters were observed. In order to assess the fate of the nanoparticles, HMSNs were injected intravenously at a dose of 80 mg/kg. Following administration, the majority of the nanoparticles were found to localize in the liver and spleen. Analysis of the silicon content using ICP-OES revealed that highest amount of silica was present in the spleen and liver which gradually reduced over a period of 4 weeks [264].

In order to assess the fate of MSNs after different administration routes, Fu and collaborators tested MSNs with a particle size of 110 nm in ICR mice. Following administration via hypodermic, intramuscular and intravenous injection as well as oral administration, the in vivo distribution of fluorescent-tagged MSNs was tracked. It was observed that of all the exposure routes, the oral route was found to be well tolerated even when the dose was increased to 5000 mg/kg and intravenous route seemed to have the least threshold. MSNs administered via intravenous route were found to preferentially accumulate in the liver and spleen at the end of 24 h and 7 days whereas those administered by other routes did not show any fluorescence in these organs. It was observed that a portion of the MSNs administered via intramuscular and hypodermic route could cross different biological barriers with a slow absorption rate. The major routes of excretion of MSNs were found to be via urine and faeces with the highest values after oral administration as compared to other routes. No histopathological changes were observed in liver, spleen, kidney and lung at the end of 24 h and 7 days by different exposure routes. Nonetheless, a low degree of inflammation was seen in the mice which were treated with MSNs via the hypodermic and intramuscular route. The results suggested that MSNs were found to be safe and well tolerated when administered by oral and intravenous routes [265]. For an extensive review on the biocompatibility of MSNs and silica NPs, the readers are directed to references [260,266,267].

6.3. MSNs v/s Silica Nanoparticles

Different forms of silica *viz*, fumed silica, porous silica and non-porous silica can be used as drug carriers. These carriers have shown encouraging results in preclinical studies. However, to translate these materials to the bedside, a clear understanding of the fate and the inherent toxicity of these carriers in vivo is essential. Silica nanoparticles used for biomedical applications are usually amorphous in nature belonging to either porous or non-porous category. The rapid clearance of amorphous silica from the lung compared to the crystalline forms is responsible for its lower toxicity potential [268]. MSNs are found to dissolve rapidly when it is sufficiently below the saturation levels. As per the reports of Martin [269], silica dissolves in the body fluids which subsequently gets absorbed or excreted as silicic acid in the urine. The silica nanoparticles undergo degradation to silicic acid which is non-toxic via three different processes *viz*, hydration, hydrolysis and ion-exchange. This process of degradation was found to depend on the degradation medium and the concentration of nanoparticles. Various strategies have been explored which can manipulate the degradation kinetics of silica nanoparticles. Some of the approaches are noncovalent doping of organic moieties to accelerate the hydrolytic degradation, covalent binding of organically bridged silsesquioxanes- based NPs, and incorporation of cleavable organically bridged silsesquioxanes into silica NPs to enhance the degradation by the biological trigger. The degradation of MSNs is much more complicated than other silica NPs owing to its varying matrix. This is attributed to the difference in the rate and degree of condensation of silica matrices between the various sol-gel procedures of MSN synthesis. As per the review by Croissant et al., partially condensed MSNs degrade in a few days, well condensed MSNs tend to degrade in weeks and calcined MSNs takes months for its degradation [270].

In order to assess the impact of porous structures on the in vivo immunotoxicity, Lee et al. performed repeated-dose toxicity studies on BALB/c mice. MSNs and colloidal silica NPs were injected intraperitoneally into mice for 4 weeks. At the end of the study period, the animals were sacrificed and organs were harvested to study the effects of the particles. The animals treated with MSNs showed an increase in the relative weight of liver and spleen and an increased response to lymphocyte mitogens, concanavalin A (Con A) or lipopolysaccharide (LPS). In addition, a decrease in the $CD4^+/CD8^-$ and $CD4^-/CD8^+$ phenotypes and an increase in the levels of $CD4^+/CD8^-$ and $CD4^+/CD8^+$ were recorded. Elevated IgG/IgM levels were also observed in the MSN treated animals. The results indicate that MSNs showed a greater extent of damage than colloidal silica NPs [271]. However, a careful study of the toxicity is needed to establish the safety of MSNs.

6.4. Biocompatibility of MSNs in Humans

The biocompatibility of silica nanoparticles has long been a topic of controversy as studies conducted by researchers have yielded variable results. Nevertheless, the Food and Drug Administration (FDA) approval of hybrid silica nanoparticles for bioimaging marks an event of utmost importance. These particles were found to be ~7 nm in size within which fluorescent dye, Cy5 was incorporated. These particles were labelled with ^{124}I and surface functionalized with peptide cyclo-(Arg-Gly-Asp-Tyr) (cRGDY) to selectively target integrin-expressing tumours. C dots were synthesized in such a way that they had limited reticuloendothelial system (RES) uptake and promote renal excretion. Preliminary experiments on in vivo safety by Choi et al. (Cornell University) revealed that these fluorescent silica nanoparticles were safe and did not show any toxicity in mice. These particles were also found to be an effective bioimaging probe for cancer imaging [21,22]. Burns et al. carried out in vivo biodistribution studies of the developed C dots in nude mice wherein nanoparticles were injected intravenously. The particles were found to show rapid renal clearance within 45 min of injection and majority of these particles accumulated in the liver. To further modify the clearance, the particles were coated with methoxy-terminated poly(ethylene glycol) chains. By careful manipulation of the surface features of C dots, they can be used for wide variety of biomedical applications including imaging and therapy [22]. Based on the encouraging results of pre-clinical studies, these nanoparticles received approval from the FDA as an Investigational New Drug (IND) to conduct the human clinical trial, phase I. The first human clinical trials suggested its safety for human use. A pilot clinical trial was conducted in five metastatic melanoma patients to assess the pharmacokinetic (PK) profile of C dots following a single injection dose. The PK profiles, renal excretion, metabolic profile assessment in patients suggested that the particles were well tolerated, preferentially accumulated in the tumour site and were found to be safe for human use [272,273].

A study wherein the potential of ordered mesoporous silica nanoparticles (OMS) in enhancing the bioavailability of fenofibrate in man was conducted by Bukara and collaborators which can be considered as another breakthrough step acting as a trigger in evoking interest among the researchers for the use of MSNs for biomedical applications. Promising results obtained by them in their preclinical studies [274] prompted them to complement those results with clinical studies. Fenofibrate was loaded into OMS and these were subsequently enclosed within capsules. The study was carried out with 12 volunteers who were administered a single dose of fenofibrate OMS and the marketed formulation of fenofibrate, Lipanthyl®. Safety assessment was performed by periodic monitoring of the vital signs, 12-lead electrocardiogram (ECG) and blood biochemical parameters in the subjects. The PK profile revealed an increase in the rate and extent of absorption of fenofibrate when incorporated in OMS as compared to the marketed product. In addition, the formulation was found to be well tolerated in the volunteers ensuring the safety of the developed OMS formulation [235].

7. Recent Patents Filed in the Field of MSNs for Biomedical Applications

Ever since its first production, modifications in terms of synthesis aiming to control the particle size and pore volume has led to the filing of several patents on MSNs. Owing to its versatile nature of loading therapeutic agents, both hydrophilic and hydrophobic, patents filed on MSNs mainly include investigating them for biomedical applications, biosensors, imaging and as adsorbents. In the following section, we have laid emphasis on reviewing the recent patents related to the biomedical applications of MSNs.

A novel approach of coating the MSNs with lipids coined as 'protocells' has received significant attention in the fabrication of drug delivery systems. These combine the advantages of liposomes (low toxicity, long circulation times) with the advantages of MSNs (tunable size, shape and loading capacity) (Figure 6). Numerous studies have shown positive results, a few of which are touched upon here.

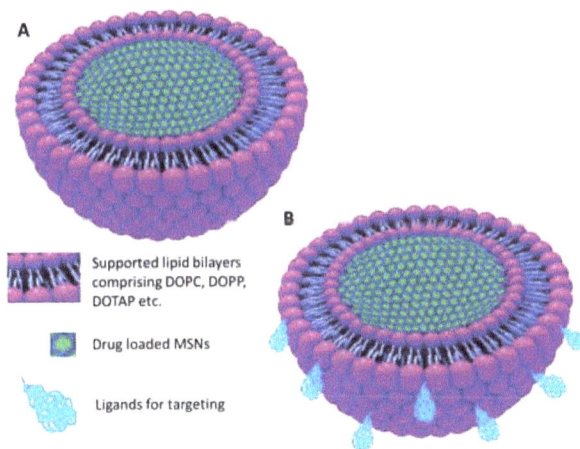

Figure 6. Representation of (**A**) Non-targeted protocell and (**B**) Targeted protocell.

A protocell of MSN encapsulated within lipid bilayer was designed by Ashley and collaborators wherein, MSNs were prepared by aerosol-assisted evaporation-induced self-assembly (EISA) procedure. The MSNs were encapsulated within supported lipid bilayers. The lipid bilayer components (cholesterol and phospholipids) were covalently attached to the glycidoxypropylsilane or APTES functionalized MSNs. Levofloxacin was loaded into the pores of the MSNs. The lipid bilayers were composed of either 1,2-dioleoyl-sn-glycero-3-phosphocholine (DOPC), 1,2-dioleoyl-sn-glycero-3-phosphoethanolamine (DOPE) or 1,2-distearoyl-sn-glycero-3-phosphocholine (DSPC). The protocells were rendered target specific by anchoring peptides (e.g., RGD peptide comprising of Arg-Gly-Asp) onto its surface. The protocells were PEGylated with polyethylene glycol to enhance its circulation time in the body. The pore size of the MSNs ranged from 1 nm to 75 nm. A high drug loading of about 20–55 wt % of the protocell was obtained for individual antibiotics. Fcy targeted protocells were found to show enhanced uptake by THP-1 cells resulting in the effective killing of intracellular organism *F. tularensis*. Only 2 wt % levofloxacin loaded protocell was also found to be cytotoxic as compared to that of free levofloxacin. Biodistribution studies in Balb/c mice showed that Fcy targeted protocells were distributed in various organs of potential *F. tularensis* infection such as lung, liver, spleen and lymph nodes. The results revealed that the biodistribution like many other nanoparticles depends on their size and size distribution. Based on literature reports and approximation of previous work on other antibiotics, the inventors also claimed that oral administration of protocells was far more effective than inhalation therapy for respiratory tularemia. However, these protocells have to be filled in capsules coated with a suitable polymer to prevent its degradation from the gastric environment. The application of protocells could also be extended to incorporate various other antibiotics, macromolecules such as DNA and histone packaged plasmid into the protocells to enhance its penetration into the nucleus of a cell and deposit its contents [275].

Jeffrey and collaborators fabricated MSNs which were functionalized with targeting ligands specific to white blood cells or arterial, venous or capillary vessels. These targeting ligands were either Fc gamma from IgG, human complement C3, ephrin B2 and SP94 peptide. These MSNs were further encapsulated within lipid bi- or multi-layers to form protocells. Polyethyleneglycol-polyethyleneimine (PEG-PEI) was tethered to the surface of MSNs to enhance the colloidal stability of the formulation. The MSNs were around 50 nm in size and positively charged. This helps to bind itself to endothelial cells, serum proteins and white blood cells. To elucidate the binding of these MSNs, they were injected into veins of ex vivo chick embryos. PEI-PEG-MSNs were found to be bound to endothelial cells as well as stationary and circulating white blood cells following injection [276].

Similar use of protocells was extended and reported for multicomponent delivery of drugs DOX, 5-fluorouracil and cisplatin to cancer cells. The protocells constituted MSNs which were surrounded by lipid bilayers also referred to as 'supported lipid bilayer' (SLB) and further functionalized with targeting ligand SP94 peptides which are overexpressed in liver cancer. These ligands were conjugated on the surface of amino-modified MSNs by a PEG spacer. The lipids chosen were N-[1-(2,3-Dioleoyloxy)propyl]-N,N,N-trimethylammonium methyl-sulfate (DOTAP), 1,2-dioleoyl-sn-glycero-3-phospho-L-serine (DOPS) which functions as a pore sealing agent and thereby restricts the release of the drug. Once internalized by the cells, the SLBs get destabilized by endosome acidification, thus releasing the drug. The protocells could also be tethered with nuclear localization sequence (NLS) to enhance the penetration of the drug into the nucleus of the cells. In vitro cellular uptake of the protocells by Hep3B cells (hepatocellular carcinoma) supported the hypothesis of active targeting by the developed protocells [277].

Toroidal MSNs were synthesized and their potential use as a carrier for the transport of different cargos ranging from small molecules to siRNA, mRNA and plasmids was explored by Brinker and Lin. Both ellipsoidal (eMSN) and toroidal shaped MSNs (tMSNs) were synthesized by varying the reaction procedure and the reactants. 'Torus' shaped MSNs refer to MSN with a central pore and two other pores into which macromolecules can be easily loaded. The internal surface area was found to be in the range of 1.1 to 0.5 cc/g with a payload of 50%. These were functionalized with amino groups and modified with PEG to improve the circulation time. Ligands, Fc gamma from IgG, human complement C3, ephrin B2 and SP94 peptide were tethered onto the MSNs for target specificity. DOPC and DOPP (dioctylphenylphosphonate) lipids can be coated onto the MSNs to seal the pores and also improve the biocompatibility. Cellular uptake studies were performed on a variety of cell lines such as human endothelial cells like EAhy 926, ATCC-CRL-2922 and mouse macrophages ATCC-TIB-71 and Raw 264-7. The successful internalization of the MSNs was proved by the in vivo studies. The developed MSNs can be a possible carrier to load large linear molecules due to its unique structure.

They can also be loaded with a variety of small molecules ranging from anti-cancer, anti-inflammatory, antiviral and so forth [278].

Protocells for the efficient delivery of chemotherapeutic agents for the treatment of hepatocellular carcinoma was formulated. The protocells contained nanoparticles protected by supported lipid bilayers comprising of DOTAP, DOPG (1,2-dioleoyl-sn-glycero-3-phosphoglycerol) or DOPE as lipids. The nanoparticles were loaded with DOX, cisplatin and 5-fluorouracil as model cargo. The surface of the protocells was tethered to a novel binding peptide c-MET. The pores can also be loaded with small interfering RNA, microRNA. The surface of the nanoparticles was modified with amino groups to sustain the drug release. These were coated with liposomes by electrostatically fusing them to nanoporous silica core. The surface was coated with a fusogenic peptide that promotes the endosomal escape of protocells. They can also be coated with nuclear localization sequence to enhance the uptake by the nucleus. The applicability of these protocells can also be extended for the transdermal delivery of the drugs wherein the supported lipid bilayers contained permeation enhancers to enhance the permeability via the stratum corneum [279].

Nel et al. developed phospholipid bilayer coated MSN loaded with gemcitabine (GEM) for the treatment of human pancreatic ductal adenocarcinoma (PDAC). The MSNs were synthesized and loaded with GEM. The lipid membrane was rehydrated with GEM-MSNs which led to the coating and capping of the pores of the MSNs. In addition to this, paclitaxel was dissolved in the organic solvent along with the lipids thus leading to MSNs with two drugs; one in the pores and other embedded in the lipid bilayer. The loading of GEM into the MSNs was found to be around 20% w/w. Transforming growth factor β (TGF-β) inhibitor, LY364947 was adsorbed onto MSNs. These TGF-β inhibitors help in enhancing the permeation of GEM laden MSNs to the tumour sites. This proof-of-concept was established in BxPC3 xenograft mouse models (pancreatic tumour model). The delivery system showed enhanced uptake in tumours showing a significant reduction in tumour volume. To prolong the circulation time, the MSNs were coated with PEI/PEG [280].

Silica nanoparticles loaded with antibiotics and their surface coated with a polymer to prevent premature release of the drug were developed by Avni and collaborators. The formulation was designed such that the cargo will be released only in response to stimuli. In this work, the drug within the nanoparticles will be released only if the substance released by the target cell has the property to degrade the gating molecules. Another application of this invention was in the diagnosis of diseases. Signaling molecule loaded silica nanoparticles were gated with nucleic acid molecules. Outside this particle, another molecule which produces a detectable signal was added. In the presence of a nucleic acid which is complementary to the gating molecule, they both hybridize resulting in the opening of the gates of the nanoparticles. In a similar way, the developed nanoparticles were used for various applications by coating the surface of the particles and making it responsive to stimuli [281].

Pore expanded MSNs with a pore diameter ranging from 1 nm to 100 nm for the loading of bioactive material and mainly protein was developed by Cheolhee. The pore expanding agent used was trimethylbenzene. Also, the surface of the MSNs was functionalized with ligands specific to the protein of interest to enhance the binding of the protein either to the inner or outer surface of the carrier. The ligand includes nickel, nickel-nitrilotriacetic acid (NTA), glutathione, dextrin, biotin or streptavidin. The protein of interest in this work was proteasome. Various other proteins such as bovine serum albumin (BSA), IgG proteins, β-galactosidase, horseradish peroxidase were introduced into the pores to study their effect. The surface of the MSNs was further functionalized with the ligand to enhance the intracellular drug delivery using peptides. The intracellular delivery efficiency of the MSNs was studied using fluorescent tagged MSNs. The MSNs were found to show an increased intracellular delivery of the agents as compared to the free proteins. The internalization mechanism of MSN-proteasome complex was studied in HeLa cell lines. It was observed that the complex exhibited energy-dependent caveolae-mediated and clathrin-mediated endocytosis. This drug delivery carrier could be further extended for the delivery of various other proteins and enzymes such as RNase, kinase, phosphatase, antibodies, miRNA or siRNA [282].

Weng et al. worked on improving the efficacy of a natural molecule, 16-hydroxy-cleroda-3,13-dine-15,16-olide (HCD) for the treatment of cancer. Even though HCD has shown great potential in inducing apoptosis, its use is limited by its poor solubility. HCD was incorporated into copper modified silica nanoparticles. To further prolong the release of the drug from the carrier, these nanoparticles were coated with Eudragit®S100 (Cu-MSN-HCD-S100). The loading of the drug was found to be around 18% of the weight of the carrier which was supported by the reduction in surface area with each coating. In vitro release profile of the drug showed a sustained release with Cu-MSN-HCD-S100 as compared to the uncoated MSNs. The cytotoxic potential of the developed formulation was observed in rat G6 glioma cell lines. These results were supported by in vivo studies in tumour xenograft C6 rat glioma bearing mouse models which showed a reduction in the tumour volume on oral administration of the formulation. The formulation was found to be safe without any major reported toxic effects [283].

Modified MSNs were fabricated by Lee and collaborators to monitor the redox-responsive drug release within the system. To validate this concept, doxorubicin-loaded MSN labeled with coumarin and tethered to cysteine was developed. The release of the drug was blocked by fluorescein isothiocyanate-β-cyclodextrin (FITC-β-CD) which was covalently bound to cysteine. These carriers are designated as redox-responsive fluorescent resonance energy transfer-based MSN drug delivery system (FRET-MSNs). These FRET systems have a unique feature of energy transfer between two fluorophores which is sensitive to changes in the donor (Coumarin-labeled cysteine) to acceptor (FITC-β-CD) separation distance. The change in the FRET signal was used to monitor the drug release. When the donor and acceptor are in proximity to MSN surface, a green emission peak at 520 nm was observed (FRET ON). In the presence of glutathione (GSH) which are overexpressed in cancer cells, the disulfide bonds get cleaved resulting in the opening of FITC-β-CD valve and release of drug which shows an increased blue fluorescence at 450 nm corresponding to coumarin (FRET OFF). The pore diameter of these carriers was found to be 2.3 nm with a particle size of around 100 nm. This theory was studied using HeLa cells treated with thioacetic acid (GSH synthesis scavenger) and N-ethylmaleimide (GSH scavenger). In the presence of thioacetic acid, a decrease in cell viability, as well as gradual decrease in FRET signal, was observed. The opposite was true in case of N-ethylmaleimide. Similarly, the same carrier can be used to monitor the release of a wide variety of drugs by suitably modifying the carrier system [284].

A comparatively new avenue of research for the use of MSNs is in the delivery of antibiotic drugs for the treatment of post-operative osteomyelitis and arthroplasty. Polyacrylate based bone cement materials for effective delivery of antibiotics was designed by Shou-Cang and collaborators. A sustained release of 70% of the active principle over a period of 80 days was observed when compared to only 5% release from the currently marketed antibiotic bone cement formulation, Smart-Set GHV.A co-delivery of antibiotics (gentamicin, vancomycin) and anti-inflammatory (indomethacin, ibuprofen) drug was achieved in the current invention. To formulate MSN based bone cement, the drug was loaded into the MSNs and polyacrylate was added to form a mixture to which monomer, methyl methacrylate was added and polymerized to form the bone cement. It was observed that as the content of MSN was increased from 6 wt % to above; an enhanced drug release was observed which was otherwise restricted to <7% as the majority of the drug would be embedded in the bone cement matrix. In the case of MSN, the drug could be released from the matrix via diffusion from the pores. The developed formulation also exhibited low cytotoxicity to mouse fibroblast cells ensuring the safety of the formulation. The compression strength and bending modulus of the bone cement were similar to that of the commercial product. Hence, the current invention can be used as an alternative to treat osteomyelitis, augmentation of the bone crew and bone-implant interface during joint replacement surgery, as bone filler and bone graft substitute [285].

Liu and Lay [286] reported the formulation of stimuli-responsive hollow silica vesicles coated with interpolymer complex for the delivery of bioactive agents. These carriers contained interpolymer complex where the first polymer PEG was immobilized on the surface and the second polymer, poly(methyl methacrylate) (PMMA) was complexed to the first one via hydrogen bond. The principle behind the release of active agent from the pore was related to a pH of the system. At around pH 5, the second polymer will remain complexed to the first one whereas, at pH 7 and above, the interpolymer complex dissociates releasing the drug. The dissociation of the PEG-PMMA complex was due to the deprotonation of PMMA leading to breaking of hydrogen bonds between methyl methacrylate (MMA) and ethylene glycol (EG). This leads to swelling of the complex and dissolving of anionic PMMA. The hollow silica particles were prepared using polystyrene as template and surface modified with amino groups. Calcein blue was loaded as the model cargo to study the behaviour of the delivery system. The ratio of methyl methacrylate: ethylene glycol was in the ratio of 1:3.4. PMMA of varying molecular weights was tried and 6.5 kDa formed a good complex with PEG as it could easily intercalate within the gaps of PEG chains thus providing flexible, smooth PEG-PMMA complex. The developed formulation was evaluated for the proof of concept by in vitro studies. These can be used for delivery of drugs susceptible to gastric pH and can be given via oral route by suitably formulating with additives.

Zink et al. formulated MSNs with its surface modified with mPEG and further coated with a polymer such as a polyethyleneimine (PEI) for the delivery of siRNA and plasmid DNA. Along with this, phosphonate modified MSNs were also synthesized and loaded with drugs. Also, doxorubicin, paclitaxel was loaded into the MSNs. The polymer chain length can effectively control the toxicity of the synthesized MSNs still maintaining the necessary function. To evaluate the toxicity of PEI as a polymer, MSNs were coated with different molecular weights of PEI polymer like 0.6, 1.2, 1.8, 10 and 25 KD. The cytotoxicity potential of the developed formulation was determined in HEPA-1 cells. The results revealed the absence of any toxicity in particles coated with 0.6, 1.2 and 1.8 KD polymers whereas 10 KD polymer showed toxicity at 50 µg/mL whereas 25 KD polymer showed a decline in MTS (3-(4,5-dimethylthiazol-2-yl)-5-(3-carboxymethoxyphenyl)-2-(4-sulfophenyl)-2H-tetrazolium) activity at more than 12.5 µg/mL. In addition to this, paclitaxel was also loaded into the pores to determine the activity of the carrier. The cellular uptake of the paclitaxel-loaded MSNs was determined in PANC-1 and BxPC3 cells (human pancreatic ductal carcinoma). The MSN-PEI-1.2 KD particles exhibited significant cytotoxicity and cellular uptake of paclitaxel whereas MSN-PEI-25 KD showed slight particle related toxicity at a concentration of 25 µg/mL as compared to that of paclitaxel suspension in aqueous media [287].

Liong and collaborators developed MSNs to carry water-insoluble drugs like camptothecin (CPT) and paclitaxel (PCL) for the treatment of pancreatic carcinoma. To render the nanoparticles magnetic in nature for MR imaging, iron oxide nanocrystals were incorporated into the MSNs. They further loaded hydrophobic chemotherapeutic agents into the pores of MSNs. They modified the synthesis of iron oxide nanocrystals by thermal decomposition of iron-oleate complexes which later were merged with cetyltrimethylammonium bromide (CTAB) by the interaction between the hydrophobic tail of CTAB and hydrophobic oleate ligand. The mesoporous silica was formed around the iron oxide nanocrystals at a temperature of 65–80 °C with vigorous stirring to obtain nanoparticles in the range of 100–200 nm. They also successfully utilized the same method with other inorganic nanoparticles like gold and silver in place of iron. The complete removal of surfactant template was brought about by ion exchange method using ammonium nitrate. To avoid agglomeration of the particles, the surface of MSNs was modified with phosphonate groups (that is, trihydroxy silyl propyl methylphosphonate). On loading the drugs into the pores of MSNs, it was observed that only 30 nmol of the drug was loaded onto 1 mg of nanoparticles. To enhance the cellular uptake by cancer cells, the MSNs were functionalized with folic acid moiety. This study was confirmed by cellular uptake studies in pancreatic cell lines (PANC-1, Capan-1 and AsPC-1), colon cancer cell line (SW480) and stomach cancer cell line (MKN-45). Fluorescent MSN clearly indicated the cytotoxic potential of CPT. They also studied the mechanism of cellular uptake in human pancreatic cell line PANC-1 and hepatoma cell line Hepa-1 cells. The results suggested that the uptake of FMSN takes place via temperature and energy dependent manner. This was confirmed by treating the cells with metabolic inhibitors such as sodium azide/sucrose/bafilomycin A, nocodazole/brefeldin A which inhibited the cellular uptake of FMSNs [288].

Sulfasalazine loaded charged MSNs were fabricated by Lee et al. for the effective therapy against diseases of the lower gastrointestinal tract (inflammatory bowel disease, ulcerative colitis, Crohn's disease). The surface of MSNs was functionalized with *N*-trimethoxysilylpropyl-*N,N,N*-trimethylammonium chloride via co-condensation method at varying concentration of 2%, 5%, 8% and 12% *v/v* designated as MSN-TA1, MSN-TA2, MSN-TA3 and MSN-TA4 respectively. Sulfasalazine and a dye named orange II were loaded into the pores of the MSNs. The loading percentage was found to be about 1.7 to 4% in water and DMSO as solvent respectively. The concentration of the dye played a significant role in the adsorption capacity. Higher the concentration of orange II, greater was the adsorption of the dye which suggested diffusion dependent adsorption. However, adsorption was found to be greater with the increased density of TA groups on the surface of MSNs. Similar results were observed with that of sulfasalazine as well. However, the loading efficiency was found to be lesser due to the hydrophobic nature of the drug. pH range of 2–5 was found to be optimum for the loading of the drug as at this pH strong electrostatic attraction was found to be present. The in vitro release profile revealed that MSN-TA4 showed a comparatively slower release of the drug compared to the rest of the modifications and unmodified MSN. Their work indicates that the release and adsorption of the drug onto MSNs could be tailored by tethering TA onto the surface of MSNs [289].

Lin et al. utilized room temperature ionic liquids (RTIL) as a template for the synthesis of MSNs. The organic cation used in this work includes alkylammonium and alkylphosphonium cations and heterocyclic cations like *N*-alkyl pyridinium and *N,N'*-dialkyl imidazolium. These organic cations were treated with suitable anions, such as tetrafluoroborate, hexafluorophosphate, halides such as fluoride, chloride, bromide and iodide to form RTIL. The pores of the MSNs were loaded with antimicrobial agents. These agents could also form part of the cationic group of the RTIL. They suggested that to obtain a delayed release of the drug either the antimicrobial ammonium species can be used as the template of MSN or the pores can be reloaded with the antimicrobial quaternary ammonium salts. To control the release of the drug from the template, the surface of the MSNs can be further coated with a polymer like poly (lactic acid) or any bioadhesive polymer to render the MSNs bioadhesive which can further prolong the drug release. In the present invention, MSNs with different shapes such as spheres, ellipsoids, rods and tubes were synthesized using different tetraalkoxysilanes namely 1-tetradecyl-3-methylimidazolium bromide (C_{14}MIMBr), 1-hexadecyl-3-methylimidazolium bromide (C_{16}MIMBr), 1-octadecyl-3-methylimidazolium bromide (C_{18}MIMBr), 1-tetradecyloxymethyl-3-methylimidazolium chloride (C_{14}OCMIMCl) and cetyl pyridinium bromide (CPBr) respectively. The pores of the MSNs were capped with certain amino acids to alter the drug release. The antibacterial activity of the developed MSNs was determined by disk diffusion assays, minimal inhibitory concentration (MIC), and minimal bactericidal concentration (MBC) against *Escherichia coli* K12. They were also claimed to be effective against fungi. The inventors also developed cetylpyridinium chloride (CPC) containing MSN formulation for the treatment of an oral volatile sulfur compounds (VSC)-prone condition leading to oral malodor problems. The pore surface was blocked with zinc-binding amino acids such as glutamic acid, histidine and aspartic acid groups. In neutral or weakly basic conditions, CPC molecules slowly diffuse out of the pores and suppress the anaerobic protein digestion activities of gram negative bacteria thus preventing VSC formation. The MSN formulation can be administered via oral, topical or parenteral routes depending on the final use. The MSNs can be further formulated using suitable diluents or carriers to convert it into tablets or topical ointments, gels [290].

8. Conclusions

In this review, we have touched upon some exciting research utilizing mesoporous silica nanocarriers as drug delivery systems. Their unique properties of tunable pore size, pore volume, high loading capacity makes them widely exploited nanocarriers. Varying the molar composition of the reactants, type of reactants and the reaction conditions, MSNs with different particle size, shape and pore volume can be obtained. Tailoring the surface properties and pore size of MSNs helps enhance the loading and modify the drug release profile. The major research on MSNs is focused on the use of these in the treatment of cancer wherein variety of ligands can be anchored onto the surface of MSNs due to the ease of functionalization. Moreover, these smart systems can be used to deliver drug at the site of interest by various external and internal stimuli such as pH, temperature, light, chemicals, enzymes, ultrasound and so forth. Review of the patents filed shows that majority of the research focuses on exploring the possible use of protocells (MSNs coated with supported lipid bilayers) for drug and macromolecule delivery. With this kind of systems, it is possible to protect the cargo from the external environment and also achieve 'zero' premature release. However, the pharmacokinetics and biodistribution of these carriers vary depending on its characteristics and the route of administration. Implications associated with long-term use of MSNs remain unanswered. This lacuna holds back the technology platform from stepping to the next level of clinical use.

9. Current and Future Perspectives

Although FDA has approved only a few nanomedicines for treatment and use in the clinics, these novel systems have been successful in laying a huge impact in the field of disease therapy and have the potential to change the conventional treatment or diagnosis. Ever since the first identification of the potential application of MSNs as carriers for drug delivery, exhaustive research is being carried out to prove the importance of this technology in the therapy of multiple diseases. Majority of the work focuses on the use of these carriers for site-specific delivery of chemotherapeutic agents. Nonetheless, regulatory and technical obstacles limit the safe and efficient translation and regulatory approval of these products. Unlike other nanocarriers, the fabrication of MSNs is a simple and cost-effective process. Moreover, these MSNs have an additional scope of being a multifunctional nanocarrier for spatial, temporal placement of drugs and also for theranostic purpose and imaging, and also supports multidrug loading. Remarkable outcomes have been achieved in this regard in both cellular and preclinical studies. However, certain challenges lay ahead in the successful translation of this platform to bedside. Synthesis of MSNs with consistent characteristics and quality can be a major challenge. The industrial transfer of technology mainly depends on scalability and hence the synthesis of MSNs at production scale may be a barrier to its commercialization. There is a need for a better understanding and control of the manufacturing process to ensure reproducibility in the product. In addition, all drugs cannot be loaded in the same concentration and hence the amount of MSN may vary from case to case which may play a role in determining the maximum tolerated dose of MSN. Certain process analytical tools such as custom-built fluorescence correlation spectroscopy (FCS) coupled with size exclusion/gel permeation chromatography (GPC) adopted by Chen et al. [291] would aid in monitoring the particle size and long term stability and thus reduce batch-to-batch variation. While the inherent toxicity issues of most of the inorganic nanoparticles remains a major issue, encouraging reports on the efficacy and biocompatibility of MSNs in animal models shows the tremendous potential of shifting this platform to clinical levels. However, the difference in the physiology of small animals and humans may lead to failure of these carriers in clinical trials. Lack of in-depth understanding of the interaction between MSNs and the biological system needs to be addressed. Comprehensive in vitro screening assays with varying ligands to ensure optimum uptake, stability, specificity and pharmacokinetic profile would be useful in developing a more reliable product for clinical trials especially for anticancer therapy and the same could be extended as a guide to develop more reliable MSN products for other biomedical purposes as well. Recently, a ray of light for the use of silica nanoparticles was seen in the form of FDA's approval to conduct stage I human clinical trial for Cornell dots (C dots). This marked an important step towards the acceptance of silica nanoparticles. Following this, first-in human studies by Bukara and group [235] demonstrated the safety of MSNs. Nevertheless, the potential challenge to the clinical translation of MSN-based drug delivery system lies in the lack of substantial evidence on its chronic toxicity studies, genotoxicity and teratogenic potential, long-term tissue compatibility. Thorough understanding of the degradation mechanism of mesoporous silica in vivo is yet to be established. Efforts are to be made by researchers like us to bridge the gap between

Pharmaceutics **2018**, *10*, 118

the preclinical and clinical use of MSNs to achieve marked progress in this subject. We anticipate that if a careful assessment during the production and in vitro evaluation along with studies to ascertain the biosafety of MSNs is performed, these novel designs can be a vital breakthrough in the future for clinical applications in the diagnosis, imaging and treatment catering to the needs of patients.

Funding: This research received no external funding.

Acknowledgments: The authors would like to acknowledge Manipal Academy of Higher Education (MAHE), Manipal, India for providing financial support and infra-structure to carry out the work.

Conflicts of Interest: The authors declare no conflict of interest.

References

1. Krukemeyer, M.G.; Krenn, V.; Huebner, F.; Wagner, W.; Resch, R. History and Possible Uses of Nanomedicine Based on Nanoparticles and Nanotechnological Progress. *J. Nanomed. Nanotechnol.* **2015**, *6*, 1–7. [CrossRef]
2. Mudshinge, S.R.; Deore, A.B.; Patil, S.; Bhalgat, C.M. Nanoparticles: Emerging carriers for drug delivery. *Saudi Pharm. J.* **2011**, *19*, 129–141. [CrossRef] [PubMed]
3. Kankala, R.K.; Zhang, Y.S.; Wang, S.-B.; Lee, C.-H.; Chen, A.-Z. Supercritical Fluid Technology: An Emphasis on Drug Delivery and Related Biomedical Applications. *Adv. Healthc. Mater.* **2017**, *6*, 1700433. [CrossRef] [PubMed]
4. Kankala, R.K.; Zhu, K.; Sun, X.-N.; Liu, C.-G.; Wang, S.-B.; Chen, A.-Z. Cardiac Tissue Engineering on the Nanoscale. *ACS Biomater. Sci. Eng.* **2018**, *4*, 800–818. [CrossRef]
5. Gong, T.; Xie, J.; Liao, J.; Zhang, T.; Lin, S.; Lin, Y. Nanomaterials and bone regeneration. *Bone Res.* **2015**, *3*, 15029. [CrossRef] [PubMed]
6. Alhariri, M.; Azghani, A.; Omri, A. Liposomal antibiotics for the treatment of infectious diseases. *Expert Opin. Drug Deliv.* **2013**, *10*, 1515–1532. [CrossRef] [PubMed]
7. Deshpande, P.P.; Biswas, S.; Torchilin, V.P. Current trends in the use of liposomes for tumor targeting. *Nanomedicine* **2013**, *8*, 1509–1528. [CrossRef] [PubMed]
8. Puri, A.; Loomis, K.; Smith, B.; Lee, J.-H.; Yavlovich, A.; Heldman, E.; Blumenthal, R. Lipid-based nanoparticles as pharmaceutical drug carriers: From concepts to clinic. *Crit. Rev. Ther. Drug Carr. Syst.* **2009**, *26*, 523–580. [CrossRef]
9. Gad, A.; Kydd, J.; Piel, B.; Rai, P. Targeting Cancer using Polymeric Nanoparticle mediated Combination Chemotherapy. *Int. J. Nanomed. Nanosurg.* **2016**, *2*. [CrossRef]
10. Cheng, C.J.; Tietjen, G.T.; Saucier-Sawyer, J.K.; Saltzman, W.M. A holistic approach to targeting disease with polymeric nanoparticles. *Nat. Rev. Drug Discov.* **2015**, *14*, 239–247. [CrossRef] [PubMed]
11. Han, Y.-H.; Kankala, R.; Wang, S.-B.; Chen, A.-Z. Leveraging Engineering of Indocyanine Green-Encapsulated Polymeric Nanocomposites for Biomedical Applications. *Nanomaterials* **2018**, *8*, 360. [CrossRef] [PubMed]
12. Pandita, D.; Poonia, N.; Kumar, S.; Lather, V.; Madaan, K. Dendrimers in drug delivery and targeting: Drug-dendrimer interactions and toxicity issues. *J. Pharm. Bioallied Sci.* **2014**, *6*, 139–150. [CrossRef] [PubMed]
13. Hiemenz, J.W.; Walsh, T.J. Lipid formulations of amphotericin B: Recent progress and future directions. *Clin. Infect. Dis.* **1996**, *22* (Suppl. 2), S133–S144. [CrossRef] [PubMed]
14. Kaposi's sarcoma: DaunoXome approved. *AIDS Treat. News* **1996**, 3–4.
15. Barenholz, Y. (Chezy) Doxil®—The first FDA-approved nano-drug: Lessons learned. *J. Control. Release* **2012**, *160*, 117–134. [CrossRef] [PubMed]
16. Batist, G.; Barton, J.; Chaikin, P.; Swenson, C.; Welles, L. Myocet (liposome-encapsulated doxorubicin citrate): A new approach in breast cancer therapy. *Expert Opin. Pharm.* **2002**, *3*, 1739–1751. [CrossRef] [PubMed]
17. Junghanns, J.-U.A.H.; Müller, R.H. Nanocrystal technology, drug delivery and clinical applications. *Int. J. Nanomed.* **2008**, *3*, 295–309. [PubMed]
18. Giner-Casares, J.J.; Henriksen-Lacey, M.; Coronado-Puchau, M.; Liz-Marzán, L.M. Inorganic nanoparticles for biomedicine: Where materials scientists meet medical research. *Mater. Today* **2016**, *19*, 19–28. [CrossRef]
19. Kankala, R.K.; Tsai, P.-Y.; Kuthati, Y.; Wei, P.-R.; Liu, C.-L.; Lee, C.-H. Overcoming multidrug resistance through co-delivery of ROS-generating nano-machinery in cancer therapeutics. *J. Mater. Chem. B* **2017**, *5*, 1507–1517. [CrossRef]

20. Kuthati, Y.; Kankala, R.K.; Lee, C.-H. Layered double hydroxide nanoparticles for biomedical applications: Current status and recent prospects. *Appl. Clay Sci.* **2015**, *112–113*, 100–116. [CrossRef]

21. Choi, J.; Burns, A.A.; Williams, R.M.; Zhou, Z.; Flesken-Nikitin, A.; Zipfel, W.R.; Wiesner, U.; Nikitin, A.Y. Core-shell silica nanoparticles as fluorescent labels for nanomedicine. *J. Biomed. Opt.* **2007**, *12*, 64007. [CrossRef] [PubMed]

22. Burns, A.A.; Vider, J.; Ow, H.; Herz, E.; Penate-Medina, O.; Baumgart, M.; Larson, S.M.; Wiesner, U.; Bradbury, M. Fluorescent Silica Nanoparticles with Efficient Urinary Excretion for Nanomedicine. *Nano Lett.* **2009**, *9*, 442–448. [CrossRef] [PubMed]

23. Slowing, I.I.; Trewyn, B.G.; Lin, V.S.-Y. Mesoporous Silica Nanoparticles for Intracellular Delivery of Membrane-Impermeable Proteins. *J. Am. Chem. Soc.* **2007**, *129*, 8845–8849. [CrossRef] [PubMed]

24. Deodhar, G.V.; Adams, M.L.; Trewyn, B.G. Controlled release and intracellular protein delivery from mesoporous silica nanoparticles. *Biotechnol. J.* **2017**, *12*, 1600408. [CrossRef] [PubMed]

25. Cha, W.; Fan, R.; Miao, Y.; Zhou, Y.; Qin, C.; Shan, X.; Wan, X.; Li, J. Mesoporous Silica Nanoparticles as Carriers for Intracellular Delivery of Nucleic Acids and Subsequent Therapeutic Applications. *Molecules* **2017**, *22*, 782. [CrossRef] [PubMed]

26. Tao, C.; Zhu, Y.; Xu, Y.; Zhu, M.; Morita, H.; Hanagata, N. Mesoporous silica nanoparticles for enhancing the delivery efficiency of immunostimulatory DNA drugs. *Dalton Trans.* **2014**, *43*, 5142–5150. [CrossRef] [PubMed]

27. Möller, K.; Müller, K.; Engelke, H.; Bräuchle, C.; Wagner, E.; Bein, T. Highly efficient siRNA delivery from core–shell mesoporous silica nanoparticles with multifunctional polymer caps. *Nanoscale* **2016**, *8*, 4007–4019. [CrossRef] [PubMed]

28. Hanafi-Bojd, M.Y.; Ansari, L.; Malaekeh-Nikouei, B. Codelivery of anticancer drugs and siRNA by mesoporous silica nanoparticles. *Ther. Deliv.* **2016**, *7*, 649–655. [CrossRef] [PubMed]

29. Riikonen, J.; Xu, W.; Lehto, V.-P. Mesoporous systems for poorly soluble drugs—Recent trends. *Int. J. Pharm.* **2018**, *536*, 178–186. [CrossRef] [PubMed]

30. Maleki, A.; Kettiger, H.; Schoubben, A.; Rosenholm, J.M.; Ambrogi, V.; Hamidi, M. Mesoporous silica materials: From physico-chemical properties to enhanced dissolution of poorly water-soluble drugs. *J. Control. Release* **2017**, *262*, 329–347. [CrossRef] [PubMed]

31. Wang, Y.; Zhao, Q.; Han, N.; Bai, L.; Li, J.; Liu, J.; Che, E.; Hu, L.; Zhang, Q.; Jiang, T.; et al. Mesoporous silica nanoparticles in drug delivery and biomedical applications. *Nanomed. Nanotechnol. Biol. Med.* **2015**, *11*, 313–327. [CrossRef] [PubMed]

32. Mamaeva, V.; Sahlgren, C.; Lindén, M. Mesoporous silica nanoparticles in medicine—Recent advances. *Adv. Drug Deliv. Rev.* **2013**, *65*, 689–702. [CrossRef] [PubMed]

33. Tao, Z. Mesoporous silica-based nanodevices for biological applications. *RSC Adv.* **2014**, *4*, 18961–18980. [CrossRef]

34. Huo, Q.; Margolese, D.I.; Stucky, G.D. Stucky Surfactant Control of Phases in the Synthesis of Mesoporous Silica-Based Materials. *Chem. Mater.* **1996**, *8*, 1147–1160. [CrossRef]

35. Beck, J.S.; Vartuli, J.C.; Roth, W.J.; Leonowicz, M.E.; Kresge, C.T.; Schmitt, K.D.; Chu, C.T.W.; Olson, D.H.; Sheppard, E.W.; McCullen, S.B.; et al. A new family of mesoporous molecular sieves prepared with liquid crystal templates. *J. Am. Chem. Soc.* **1992**, *114*, 10834–10843. [CrossRef]

36. Trewyn, B.G.; Slowing, I.I.; Giri, S.; Chen, H.-T.; Lin, V.S.-Y. Synthesis and Functionalization of a Mesoporous Silica Nanoparticle Based on the Sol–Gel Process and Applications in Controlled Release. *Acc. Chem. Res.* **2007**, *40*, 846–853. [CrossRef] [PubMed]

37. Oye, G.; Sjöblom, J.; Stöcker, M. Synthesis, characterization and potential applications of new materials in the mesoporous range. *Adv. Colloid Interface Sci.* **2001**, *89–90*, 439–466. [CrossRef]

38. Zhao, D.; Huo, Q.; Feng, J.; Chmelka, B.F.; Stucky, G.D. Nonionic Triblock and Star Diblock Copolymer and Oligomeric Surfactant Syntheses of Highly Ordered, Hydrothermally Stable, Mesoporous Silica Structures. *J. Am. Chem. Soc.* **1998**, *120*, 6024–6036. [CrossRef]

39. Tozuka, Y.; Wongmekiat, A.; Kimura, K.; Moribe, K.; Yamamura, S.; Yamamoto, K. Effect of Pore Size of FSM-16 on the Entrapment of Flurbiprofen in Mesoporous Structures. *Chem. Pharm. Bull.* **2005**, *53*, 974–977. [CrossRef] [PubMed]

40. Nandiyanto, A.B.D.; Kim, S.-G.; Iskandar, F.; Okuyama, K. Synthesis of spherical mesoporous silica nanoparticles with nanometer-size controllable pores and outer diameters. *Microporous Mesoporous Mater.* **2009**, *120*, 447–453. [CrossRef]

41. Heikkilä, T.; Salonen, J.; Tuura, J.; Hamdy, M.S.; Mul, G.; Kumar, N.; Salmi, T.; Murzin, D.Y.; Laitinen, L.; Kaukonen, A.M.; et al. Mesoporous silica material TUD-1 as a drug delivery system. *Int. J. Pharm.* **2007**, *331*, 133–138. [CrossRef] [PubMed]

42. Kumar, D.; Schumacher, K.; von Hohenesche, C.D.F.; Grun, M.; Unger, K.K. MCM-41, MCM-48 and related mesoporous adsorbents: Their synthesis and characterisation. *Colloids Surf. A Physicochem. Eng. Asp.* **2001**, *187–188*, 109–116. [CrossRef]

43. Wang, S. Ordered mesoporous materials for drug delivery. *Microporous Mesoporous Mater.* **2009**, *117*, 1–9. [CrossRef]

44. Wang, S.; Li, H. Structure directed reversible adsorption of organic dye on mesoporous silica in aqueous solution. *Microporous Mesoporous Mater.* **2006**, *97*, 21–26. [CrossRef]

45. Ukmar, T.; Planinsek, O. Ordered mesoporous silicates as matrices for controlled release of drugs. *Acta Pharm.* **2010**, *60*, 373–385. [CrossRef] [PubMed]

46. Zhao, D.; Zhou, W.; Wan, Y. *Ordered Mesoporous Materials*; Wiley-VCH Verlag GmbH & Co. KGaA: Weinheim, Germany, 2013; ISBN 3527647899.

47. Kim, K.S.; Park, M.; Kim, T.W.; Kim, J.-E.; Papoulis, D.; Komarneni, S.; Choi, J. Adsorbate-dependent uptake behavior of topographically bi-functionalized ordered mesoporous silica materials. *J. Porous Mater.* **2015**, *22*, 1297–1303. [CrossRef]

48. Lu, G.Q.; Zhao, X.S. *Nanoporous Materials: Science and Engineering*; Series on Chemical Engineering; Imperial College Press: London, UK; World Scientific Publishing Co.: Singapore, 2004; Volume 4, ISBN 978-1-86094-210-5.

49. Ge, S.; Geng, W.; He, X.; Zhao, J.; Zhou, B.; Duan, L.; Wu, Y.; Zhang, Q. Effect of framework structure, pore size and surface modification on the adsorption performance of methylene blue and Cu^{2+} in mesoporous silica. *Colloids Surf. A Physicochem. Eng. Asp.* **2018**, *539*, 154–162. [CrossRef]

50. Mayoral, A.; Blanco, R.M.; Diaz, I. Location of enzyme in lipase-SBA-12 hybrid biocatalyst. *J. Mol. Catal. B Enzym.* **2013**, *90*, 23–25. [CrossRef]

51. Galarneau, A.; Cambon, H.; Di Renzo, F.; Ryoo, R.; Choi, M.; Fajula, F. Microporosity and connections between pores in SBA-15 mesostructured silicas as a function of the temperature of synthesis. *New J. Chem.* **2003**, *27*, 73–79. [CrossRef]

52. Lercher, J.A.; Kaliaguine, S.; Gobin, O.C. *SBA-16 Materials Synthesis, Diffusion and Sorption Properties*; Technical University of Munich: Munich, Germany, 2006.

53. Kleitz, F.; Liu, D.; Gopinathan, M.A.; Park, I.-S.; Solovyov, L.A.; Shmakov, A.N.; Ryoo, R. Large Cage Face-Centered-Cubic Fm3m Mesoporous Silica: Synthesis and Structure. *J. Phys. Chem. B* **2003**, *107*, 14296–14300. [CrossRef]

54. Kalbasi, J.R.; Zirakbash, A. Synthesis, characterization and drug release studies of poly(2-hydroxyethyl methacrylate)/KIT-5 nanocomposite as an innovative organic–inorganic hybrid carrier system. *RSC Adv.* **2015**, *5*, 12463–12471. [CrossRef]

55. Jammaer, J.; Aerts, A.; D'Haen, J.; Seo, J.W.; Martens, J.A. Convenient synthesis of ordered mesoporous silica at room temperature and quasi-neutral pH. *J. Mater. Chem.* **2009**, *19*, 8290–8293. [CrossRef]

56. Vialpando, M.; Aerts, A.; Persoons, J.; Martens, J.; Van Den Mooter, G. Evaluation of ordered mesoporous silica as a carrier for poorly soluble drugs: Influence of pressure on the structure and drug release. *J. Pharm. Sci.* **2011**, *100*, 3411–3420. [CrossRef] [PubMed]

57. Stober, W.; Fink, A.; Bohn, E. Controlled growth of monodisperse silica spheres in the micron size range. *J. Colloid Interface Sci.* **1968**, *26*, 62–69. [CrossRef]

58. Grün, M.; Lauer, I.; Unger, K.K. The synthesis of micrometer- and submicrometer-size spheres of ordered mesoporous oxide MCM-41. *Adv. Mater.* **1997**, *9*, 254–257. [CrossRef]

59. Blin, J.L.; Impéror-Clerc, M. Mechanism of self-assembly in the synthesis of silica mesoporous materials: In situ studies by X-ray and neutron scattering. *Chem. Soc. Rev.* **2013**, *42*, 4071–4082. [CrossRef] [PubMed]

60. Gao, C.; Qiu, H.; Zeng, W.; Sakamoto, Y.; Terasaki, O.; Sakamoto, K.; Chen, Q.; Che, S. Formation Mechanism of Anionic Surfactant-Templated Mesoporous Silica. *Chem. Mater.* **2006**, *18*, 3904–3914. [CrossRef]

61. Flodström, K.; Wennerström, H.; Alfredsson, V. Mechanism of Mesoporous Silica Formation. A Time-Resolved NMR and TEM Study of Silica−Block Copolymer Aggregation. *Langmuir* **2004**, *20*, 680–688. [CrossRef] [PubMed]
62. Attard, G.S.; Glyde, J.C.; Göltner, C.G. Liquid-crystalline phases as templates for the synthesis of mesoporous silica. *Nature* **1995**, *378*, 366–368. [CrossRef]
63. Sundblom, A.; Oliveira, C.L.P.; Palmqvist, A.E.C.; Pedersen, J.S. Modeling In Situ Small-Angle X-ray Scattering Measurements Following the Formation of Mesostructured Silica. *J. Phys. Chem. C* **2009**, *113*, 7706–7713. [CrossRef]
64. Hollamby, M.J.; Borisova, D.; Brown, P.; Eastoe, J.; Grillo, I.; Shchukin, D. Growth of Mesoporous Silica Nanoparticles Monitored by Time-Resolved Small-Angle Neutron Scattering. *Langmuir* **2012**, *28*, 4425–4433. [CrossRef] [PubMed]
65. Edler, K.J. Current Understanding of Formation Mechanisms in Surfactant-Templated Materials. *Aust. J. Chem.* **2005**, *58*, 627–643. [CrossRef]
66. Yi, Z.; Dumée, L.F.; Garvey, C.J.; Feng, C.; She, F.; Rookes, J.E.; Mudie, S.; Cahill, D.M.; Kong, L. A New Insight into Growth Mechanism and Kinetics of Mesoporous Silica Nanoparticles by In Situ Small Angle X-ray Scattering. *Langmuir* **2015**, *31*, 8478–8487. [CrossRef] [PubMed]
67. Danks, A.E.; Hall, S.R.; Schnepp, Z. The evolution of "sol–gel" chemistry as a technique for materials synthesis. *Mater. Horiz.* **2016**, *3*, 91–112. [CrossRef]
68. Fowler, C.E.; Khushalani, D.; Lebeau, B.; Mann, S. Nanoscale Materials with Mesostructured Interiors. *Adv. Mater.* **2001**, *13*, 649–652. [CrossRef]
69. Sadasivan, S.; Fowler, C.E.; Khushalani, D.; Mann, S. Nucleation of MCM-41 Nanoparticles by Internal Reorganization of Disordered and Nematic-Like Silica–Surfactant Clusters. *Angew. Chem. Int. Ed.* **2002**, *41*, 2151–2153. [CrossRef]
70. Möller, K.; Kobler, J.; Bein, T. Colloidal suspensions of mercapto-functionalized nanosized mesoporous silica. *J. Mater. Chem.* **2007**, *17*, 624–631. [CrossRef]
71. Brinker, C.J.; Lu, Y.; Sellinger, A.; Fan, H. Evaporation-Induced Self-Assembly: Nanostructures Made Easy. *Adv. Mater.* **1999**, *11*, 579–585. [CrossRef]
72. Fontecave, T.; Boissiere, C.; Baccile, N.; Plou, F.J.; Sanchez, C. Using Evaporation-Induced Self-Assembly for the Direct Drug Templating of Therapeutic Vectors with High Loading Fractions, Tunable Drug Release, and Controlled Degradation. *Chem. Mater.* **2013**, *25*, 4671–4678. [CrossRef]
73. Shi, S.; Chen, F.; Cai, W. Biomedical applications of functionalized hollow mesoporous silica nanoparticles: Focusing on molecular imaging. *Nanomedicine* **2013**, *8*, 2027–2039. [CrossRef] [PubMed]
74. Chen, F.; Hong, H.; Shi, S.; Goel, S.; Valdovinos, H.F.; Hernandez, R.; Theuer, C.P.; Barnhart, T.E.; Cai, W. Engineering of Hollow Mesoporous Silica Nanoparticles for Remarkably Enhanced Tumor Active Targeting Efficacy. *Sci. Rep.* **2015**, *4*, 5080. [CrossRef] [PubMed]
75. Zhu, Y.; Shi, J.; Chen, H.; Shen, W.; Dong, X. A facile method to synthesize novel hollow mesoporous silica spheres and advanced storage property. *Microporous Mesoporous Mater.* **2005**, *84*, 218–222. [CrossRef]
76. Li, Y.; Shi, J.; Hua, Z.; Chen, H.; Ruan, M.; Yan, D. Hollow Spheres of Mesoporous Aluminosilicate with a Three-Dimensional Pore Network and Extraordinarily High Hydrothermal Stability. *Nano Lett.* **2003**, *3*, 609–612. [CrossRef]
77. Lou, X.W.; Archer, L.A.; Yang, Z. Hollow Micro-/Nanostructures: Synthesis and Applications. *Adv. Mater.* **2008**, *20*, 3987–4019. [CrossRef]
78. She, X.; Chen, L.; Li, C.; He, C.; He, L.; Kong, L. Functionalization of Hollow Mesoporous Silica Nanoparticles for Improved 5-FU Loading. *J. Nanomater.* **2015**, *2015*, 1–9. [CrossRef]
79. Liu, J.; Luo, Z.; Zhang, J.; Luo, T.; Zhou, J.; Zhao, X.; Cai, K. Hollow mesoporous silica nanoparticles facilitated drug delivery via cascade pH stimuli in tumor microenvironment for tumor therapy. *Biomaterials* **2016**, *83*, 51–65. [CrossRef] [PubMed]
80. Ghasemi, S.; Farsangi, Z.J.; Beitollahi, A.; Mirkazemi, M.; Rezayat, S.M.; Sarkar, S. Synthesis of hollow mesoporous silica (HMS) nanoparticles as a candidate for sulfasalazine drug loading. *Ceram. Int.* **2017**, *43*, 11225–11232. [CrossRef]
81. Sasidharan, M.; Zenibana, H.; Nandi, M.; Bhaumik, A.; Nakashima, K. Synthesis of mesoporous hollow silica nanospheres using polymeric micelles as template and their application as a drug-delivery carrier. *Dalton Trans.* **2013**, *42*, 13381–13389. [CrossRef] [PubMed]

82. Zhou, X.; Cheng, X.; Feng, W.; Qiu, K.; Chen, L.; Nie, W.; Yin, Z.; Mo, X.; Wang, H.; He, C. Synthesis of hollow mesoporous silica nanoparticles with tunable shell thickness and pore size using amphiphilic block copolymers as core templates. *Dalton Trans.* **2014**, *43*, 11834–11842. [CrossRef] [PubMed]

83. Li, Y.; Li, N.; Pan, W.; Yu, Z.; Yang, L.; Tang, B. Hollow Mesoporous Silica Nanoparticles with Tunable Structures for Controlled Drug Delivery. *ACS Appl. Mater. Interfaces* **2017**, *9*, 2123–2129. [CrossRef] [PubMed]

84. Wang, X.; Feng, J.; Bai, Y.; Zhang, Q.; Yin, Y. Synthesis, Properties, and Applications of Hollow Micro-/Nanostructures. *Chem. Rev.* **2016**, *116*, 10983–11060. [CrossRef] [PubMed]

85. Kong, M.; Tang, J.; Qiao, Q.; Wu, T.; Qi, Y.; Tan, S.; Gao, X.; Zhang, Z. Biodegradable Hollow Mesoporous Silica Nanoparticles for Regulating Tumor Microenvironment and Enhancing Antitumor Efficiency. *Theranostics* **2017**, *7*, 3276–3292. [CrossRef] [PubMed]

86. Lin, Y.-S.; Wu, S.-H.; Tseng, C.-T.; Hung, Y.; Chang, C.; Mou, C.-Y. Synthesis of hollow silica nanospheres with a microemulsion as the template. *Chem. Commun.* **2009**, *0*, 3542–3544. [CrossRef] [PubMed]

87. Ding, L.; Su, B. An electrochemistry assisted approach for fast, low-cost and gram-scale synthesis of mesoporous silica nanoparticles. *RSC Adv.* **2015**, *5*, 65922–65926. [CrossRef]

88. Bian, S.; Gao, K.; Shen, H.; Jiang, X.; Long, Y.; Chen, Y. Organic/inorganic hybrid mesoporous silica membrane rapidly synthesized by a microwave-assisted method and its application in enzyme adsorption and electrocatalysis. *J. Mater. Chem. B* **2013**, *1*, 3267–3276. [CrossRef]

89. Wu, C.-G.; Bein, T. Microwave synthesis of molecular sieve MCM-41. *Chem. Commun.* **1996**, 925–926. [CrossRef]

90. Vetrivel, S.; Chen, C.-T.; Kao, H.-M. The ultrafast sonochemical synthesis of mesoporous silica MCM-41. *New J. Chem.* **2010**, *34*, 2109–2112. [CrossRef]

91. Snoussi, Y.; Bastide, S.; Abderrabba, M.; Chehimi, M.M. Sonochemical synthesis of Fe_3O_4@NH_2-mesoporous silica@Polypyrrole/Pd: A core/double shell nanocomposite for catalytic applications. *Ultrason. Sonochem.* **2018**, *41*, 551–561. [CrossRef] [PubMed]

92. Mourhly, A.; Khachani, M.; Hamidi, A.E.; Kacimi, M.; Halim, M.; Arsalane, S. The Synthesis and Characterization of Low-cost Mesoporous Silica SiO_2 from Local Pumice Rock Regular Paper. *Nanomater. Nanotechnol.* **2015**, *5*. [CrossRef]

93. Akinjokun, A.I.; Ojumu, T.V.; Ogunfowokan, A.O. Biomass, Abundant Resources for Synthesis of Mesoporous Silica Material. In *Microporous and Mesoporous Materials*; InTech: Vienna, Austria, 2016; pp. 105–117.

94. Lin, Y.-S.; Haynes, C.L. Impacts of Mesoporous Silica Nanoparticle Size, Pore Ordering, and Pore Integrity on Hemolytic Activity. *J. Am. Chem. Soc.* **2010**, *132*, 4834–4842. [CrossRef] [PubMed]

95. Williams, S.; Neumann, A.; Bremer, I.; Su, Y.; Dräger, G.; Kasper, C.; Behrens, P. Nanoporous silica nanoparticles as biomaterials: Evaluation of different strategies for the functionalization with polysialic acid by step-by-step cytocompatibility testing. *J. Mater. Sci. Mater. Med.* **2015**, *26*, 125. [CrossRef] [PubMed]

96. Qiao, Z.-A.; Zhang, L.; Guo, M.; Liu, Y.; Huo, Q. Synthesis of Mesoporous Silica Nanoparticles via Controlled Hydrolysis and Condensation of Silicon Alkoxide. *Chem. Mater.* **2009**, *21*, 3823–3829. [CrossRef]

97. Möller, K.; Kobler, J.; Bein, T. Colloidal Suspensions of Nanometer-Sized Mesoporous Silica. *Adv. Funct. Mater.* **2007**, *17*, 605–612. [CrossRef]

98. Feng, P.; Bu, X.; Pine, D.J. Control of Pore Sizes in Mesoporous Silica Templated by Liquid Crystals in Block Copolymer−Cosurfactant−Water Systems. *Langmuir* **2000**, *16*, 5304–5310. [CrossRef]

99. El-Safty, S.A.; Evans, J. Formation of highly ordered mesoporous silica materials adopting lyotropic liquid crystal mesophases. *J. Mater. Chem.* **2002**, *12*, 117–123. [CrossRef]

100. Sayari, A.; Yang, Y. Nonionic oligomeric polymer directed synthesis of highly ordered large pore periodic mesoporous organosilica. *Chem. Commun.* **2002**, *0*, 2582–2583. [CrossRef]

101. Ganesh, M.; Lee, S.G. Synthesis, Characterization and Drug Release Capability of New Cost Effective Mesoporous Silica Nano Particle for Ibuprofen Drug Delivery. *Int. J. Control Autom.* **2013**, *6*, 207–216. [CrossRef]

102. Richer, R. Direct synthesis of functionalized mesoporous silica by non-ionic alkylpolyethyleneoxide surfactant assembly. *Chem. Commun.* **1998**, *0*, 1775–1777. [CrossRef]

103. Prouzet, E.; Cot, F.; Nabias, G.; Larbot, A.; Kooyman, P.; Pinnavaia, T.J. Assembly of Mesoporous Silica Molecular Sieves Based on Nonionic Ethoxylated Sorbitan Esters as Structure Directors. *Chem. Mater.* **1999**, *11*, 1498–1503. [CrossRef]

104. Blin, J.L.; Michaux, F.; Stébé, M.J. Nanostuctured mesoporous materials from different silica sources using fluorinated surfactants as templates. *Colloids Surf. A Physicochem. Eng. Asp.* **2016**, *510*, 104–112. [CrossRef]

105. Brevet, D.; Jouannin, C.; Tourné-Péteilh, C.; Devoisselle, J.-M.; Vioux, A.; Viau, L. Self-encapsulation of a drug-containing ionic liquid into mesoporous silica monoliths or nanoparticles by a sol–gel process. *RSC Adv.* **2016**, *6*, 82916–82923. [CrossRef]

106. Kwon, S.; Singh, R.K.; Perez, R.A.; Abou Neel, E.A.; Kim, H.-W.; Chrzanowski, W. Silica-based mesoporous nanoparticles for controlled drug delivery. *J. Tissue Eng.* **2013**, *4*, 2041731413503357. [CrossRef] [PubMed]

107. Zainal, N.A.; Rizal, S.; Shukor, A.; Azwana, H.; Wab, A.; Razak, K.A. Study on the Effect of Synthesis Parameters of Silica Nanoparticles Entrapped with Rifampicin. *Chem. Eng. Trans.* **2013**, *32*, 2245–2250. [CrossRef]

108. Wang, Y. Synthesis and formation of hierarchical mesoporous silica network in acidic aqueous solutions of sodium silicate and cationic surfactant. *Colloid J.* **2010**, *72*, 737–742. [CrossRef]

109. Das, D.; Yang, Y.; O'Brien, J.S.; Breznan, D.; Nimesh, S.; Bernatchez, S.; Hill, M.; Sayari, A.; Vincent, R.; Kumarathasan, P. Synthesis and Physicochemical Characterization of Mesoporous SiO_2 Nanoparticles. *J. Nanomater.* **2014**, *2014*, 1–12. [CrossRef]

110. Yi, J.; Kruk, M. Pluronic-P123-Templated Synthesis of Silica with Cubic *Ia3d* Structure in the Presence of Micelle Swelling Agent. *Langmuir* **2015**, *31*, 7623–7632. [CrossRef] [PubMed]

111. Yamamoto, E.; Mori, S.; Shimojima, A.; Wada, H.; Kuroda, K. Fabrication of colloidal crystals composed of pore-expanded mesoporous silica nanoparticles prepared by a controlled growth method. *Nanoscale* **2017**, *9*, 2464–2470. [CrossRef] [PubMed]

112. Dunphy, D.R.; Sheth, P.H.; Garcia, F.L.; Brinker, C.J. Enlarged Pore Size in Mesoporous Silica Films Templated by Pluronic F127: Use of Poloxamer Mixtures and Increased Template/SiO_2 Ratios in Materials Synthesized by Evaporation-Induced Self-Assembly. *Chem. Mater.* **2015**, *27*, 75–84. [CrossRef]

113. El-Toni, A.; Ibrahim, M.; Labis, J.; Khan, A.; Alhoshan, M. Optimization of Synthesis Parameters for Mesoporous Shell Formation on Magnetic Nanocores and Their Application as Nanocarriers for Docetaxel Cancer Drug. *Int. J. Mol. Sci.* **2013**, *14*, 11496–11509. [CrossRef] [PubMed]

114. Bouchoucha, M.; Côté, M.-F.; Caudreault, R.C.; Fortin, M.-A.; Kleitz, F. Size-Controlled Functionalized Mesoporous Silica Nanoparticles for Tunable Drug Release and Enhanced Anti-Tumoral Activity. *Chem. Mater.* **2016**, *28*, 4243–4258. [CrossRef]

115. Ma, K.; Werner-Zwanziger, U.; Zwanziger, J.; Wiesner, U. Controlling Growth of Ultrasmall Sub-10 nm Fluorescent Mesoporous Silica Nanoparticles. *Chem. Mater.* **2013**, *25*, 677–691. [CrossRef]

116. Kim, J.W.; Kim, L.U.; Kim, C.K. Size Control of Silica Nanoparticles and Their Surface Treatment for Fabrication of Dental Nanocomposites. *Biomacromolecules* **2007**, *8*, 215–222. [CrossRef] [PubMed]

117. Chiang, Y.-D.; Lian, H.-Y.; Leo, S.-Y.; Wang, S.-G.; Yamauchi, Y.; Wu, K.C.-W. Controlling Particle Size and Structural Properties of Mesoporous Silica Nanoparticles Using the Taguchi Method. *J. Phys. Chem. C* **2011**, *115*, 13158–13165. [CrossRef]

118. Yamada, H.; Urata, C.; Ujiie, H.; Yamauchi, Y.; Kuroda, K. Preparation of aqueous colloidal mesostructured and mesoporous silica nanoparticles with controlled particle size in a very wide range from 20 nm to 700 nm. *Nanoscale* **2013**, *5*, 6145–6153. [CrossRef] [PubMed]

119. Vazquez, N.I.; Gonzalez, Z.; Ferrari, B.; Castro, Y. Synthesis of mesoporous silica nanoparticles by sol–gel as nanocontainer for future drug delivery applications. *Bol. Soc. Esp. Cerám. Vidr.* **2017**, *56*, 139–145. [CrossRef]

120. Wanyika, H.; Gatebe, E.; Kioni, P.; Tang, Z.; Gao, Y. Synthesis and characterization of ordered mesoporous silica nanoparticles with tunable physical properties by varying molar composition of reagents. *Afr. J. Pharm. Pharmacol.* **2011**, *5*, 2402–2410. [CrossRef]

121. Yano, K.; Fukushima, Y. Synthesis of mono-dispersed mesoporous silica spheres with highly ordered hexagonal regularity using conventional alkyltrimethylammonium halide as a surfactant. *J. Mater. Chem.* **2004**, *14*, 1579–1584. [CrossRef]

122. Vallet-Regi, M.; Rámila, A.; del Real, R.P.; Pérez-Pariente, J. A New Property of MCM-41: Drug Delivery System. *Chem. Mater.* **2001**, *13*, 308–311. [CrossRef]

123. Egger, S.M.; Hurley, K.R.; Datt, A.; Swindlehurst, G.; Haynes, C.L. Ultraporous Mesostructured Silica Nanoparticles. *Chem. Mater.* **2015**, *27*, 3193–3196. [CrossRef]

124. Ganguly, A.; Ahmad, T.; Ganguli, A.K. Silica Mesostructures: Control of Pore Size and Surface Area Using a Surfactant-Templated Hydrothermal Process. *Langmuir* **2010**, *26*, 14901–14908. [CrossRef] [PubMed]

125. Palmqvist, A.E.C. Synthesis of ordered mesoporous materials using surfactant liquid crystals or micellar solutions. *Curr. Opin. Colloid Interface Sci.* **2003**, *8*, 145–155. [CrossRef]

126. Gu, J.; Huang, K.; Zhu, X.; Li, Y.; Wei, J.; Zhao, W.; Liu, C.; Shi, J. Sub-150 nm mesoporous silica nanoparticles with tunable pore sizes and well-ordered mesostructure for protein encapsulation. *J. Colloid Interface Sci.* **2013**, *407*, 236–242. [CrossRef] [PubMed]

127. Muñoz, B.; Rámila, A.; Pérez-Pariente, J.; Díaz, I.; Vallet-Regí, M. MCM-41 Organic Modification as Drug Delivery Rate Regulator. *Chem. Mater.* **2002**. [CrossRef]

128. Izquierdo-Barba, I.; Martinez, Á.; Doadrio, A.L.; Pérez-Pariente, J.; Vallet-Regí, M. Release evaluation of drugs from ordered three-dimensional silica structures. *Eur. J. Pharm. Sci.* **2005**, *26*, 365–373. [CrossRef] [PubMed]

129. Möller, K.; Bein, T. Talented Mesoporous Silica Nanoparticles. *Chem. Mater.* **2017**, *29*, 371–388. [CrossRef]

130. Huang, M.; Liu, L.; Wang, S.; Zhu, H.; Wu, D.; Yu, Z.; Zhou, S. Dendritic Mesoporous Silica Nanospheres Synthesized by a Novel Dual-Templating Micelle System for the Preparation of Functional Nanomaterials. *Langmuir* **2017**, *33*, 519–526. [CrossRef] [PubMed]

131. Yu, Y.-J.; Xing, J.-L.; Pang, J.-L.; Jiang, S.-H.; Lam, K.-F.; Yang, T.-Q.; Xue, Q.-S.; Zhang, K.; Wu, P. Facile Synthesis of Size Controllable Dendritic Mesoporous Silica Nanoparticles. *ACS Appl. Mater. Interfaces* **2014**, *6*, 22655–22665. [CrossRef] [PubMed]

132. Huang, X.; Li, L.; Liu, T.; Hao, N.; Liu, H.; Chen, D.; Tang, F. The Shape Effect of Mesoporous Silica Nanoparticles on Biodistribution, Clearance, and Biocompatibility In Vivo. *ACS Nano* **2011**, *5*, 5390–5399. [CrossRef] [PubMed]

133. Huang, X.; Teng, X.; Chen, D.; Tang, F.; He, J. The effect of the shape of mesoporous silica nanoparticles on cellular uptake and cell function. *Biomaterials* **2010**, *31*, 438–448. [CrossRef] [PubMed]

134. Cai, Q.; Luo, Z.-S.; Pang, W.-Q.; Fan, Y.-W.; Chen, X.-H.; Cui, F.-Z. Dilute Solution Routes to Various Controllable Morphologies of MCM-41 Silica with a Basic Medium. *Chem. Mater.* **2001**, *13*, 258–263. [CrossRef]

135. Han, L.; Zhou, Y.; He, T.; Song, G.; Wu, F.; Jiang, F.; Hu, J. One-pot morphology-controlled synthesis of various shaped mesoporous silica nanoparticles. *J. Mater. Sci.* **2013**, *48*, 5718–5726. [CrossRef]

136. Pang, X.; Gao, J.; Tang, F. Controlled preparation of rod- and top-like MCM-41 mesoporous silica through one-step route. *J. Non-Cryst. Solids* **2005**, *351*, 1705–1709. [CrossRef]

137. Björk, E.M.; Söderlind, F.; Odén, M. Tuning the Shape of Mesoporous Silica Particles by Alterations in Parameter Space: From Rods to Platelets. *Langmuir* **2013**, *29*, 13551–13561. [CrossRef] [PubMed]

138. Hao, N.; Li, L.; Tang, F. Facile preparation of ellipsoid-like MCM-41 with parallel channels along the short axis for drug delivery and assembly of Ag nanoparticles for catalysis. *J. Mater. Chem. A* **2014**, *2*, 11565–11568. [CrossRef]

139. Shen, S.; Gu, T.; Mao, D.; Xiao, X.; Yuan, P.; Yu, M.; Xia, L.; Ji, Q.; Meng, L.; Song, W.; et al. Synthesis of Nonspherical Mesoporous Silica Ellipsoids with Tunable Aspect Ratios for Magnetic Assisted Assembly and Gene Delivery. *Chem. Mater.* **2012**, *24*, 230–235. [CrossRef]

140. Cui, X.; Moon, S.-W.; Zin, W.-C. High-yield synthesis of monodispersed SBA-15 equilateral hexagonal platelet with thick wall. *Mater. Lett.* **2006**, *60*, 3857–3860. [CrossRef]

141. Chen, B.-C.; Lin, H.-P.; Chao, M.-C.; Mou, C.-Y.; Tang, C.-Y. Mesoporous Silica Platelets with Perpendicular Nanochannels via a Ternary Surfactant System. *Adv. Mater.* **2004**, *16*, 1657–1661. [CrossRef]

142. Huh, S.; Wiench, J.W.; Yoo, J.-C.; Pruski, M.; Lin, V.S.-Y. Organic Functionalization and Morphology Control of Mesoporous Silicas via a Co-Condensation Synthesis Method. *Chem. Mater.* **2003**, *15*, 4247–4256. [CrossRef]

143. Wang, Y.; Sun, Y.; Wang, J.; Yang, Y.; Li, Y.; Yuan, Y.; Liu, C. Charge-Reversal APTES-Modified Mesoporous Silica Nanoparticles with High Drug Loading and Release Controllability. *ACS Appl. Mater. Interfaces* **2016**, *8*, 17166–17175. [CrossRef] [PubMed]

144. Bouchoucha, M.; Gaudreault, R.C.; Fortin, M.-A.; Kleitz, F. Mesoporous Silica Nanoparticles: Selective Surface Functionalization for Optimal Relaxometric and Drug Loading Performances. *Adv. Funct. Mater.* **2014**, *24*, 5911–5923. [CrossRef]

145. Zhu, Y.; Shi, J.; Shen, W.; Chen, H.; Dong, X.; Ruan, M. Preparation of novel hollow mesoporous silica spheres and their sustained-release property. *Nanotechnology* **2005**, *16*, 2633–2638. [CrossRef]

146. Palanikumar, L.; Kim, H.Y.; Oh, J.Y.; Thomas, A.P.; Choi, E.S.; Jeena, M.T.; Joo, S.H.; Ryu, J.-H. Noncovalent Surface Locking of Mesoporous Silica Nanoparticles for Exceptionally High Hydrophobic Drug Loading and Enhanced Colloidal Stability. *Biomacromolecules* **2015**, *16*, 2701–2714. [CrossRef] [PubMed]

Pharmaceutics **2018**, *10*, 118

147. Vallet-Regí, M.; Balas, F.; Arcos, D. Mesoporous Materials for Drug Delivery. *Angew. Chem. Int. Ed.* **2007**, *46*, 7548–7558. [CrossRef] [PubMed]

148. Palanikumar, L.; Jeena, M.T.; Kim, K.; Yong Oh, J.; Kim, C.; Park, M.-H.; Ryu, J.-H. Spatiotemporally and Sequentially-Controlled Drug Release from Polymer Gatekeeper–Hollow Silica Nanoparticles. *Sci. Rep.* **2017**, *7*, 46540. [CrossRef] [PubMed]

149. Kao, K.-C.; Mou, C.-Y. Pore-expanded mesoporous silica nanoparticles with alkanes/ethanol as pore expanding agent. *Microporous Mesoporous Mater.* **2013**, *169*, 7–15. [CrossRef]

150. Kim, M.-H.; Na, H.-K.; Kim, Y.-K.; Ryoo, S.-R.; Cho, H.S.; Lee, K.E.; Jeon, H.; Ryoo, R.; Min, D.-H. Facile Synthesis of Monodispersed Mesoporous Silica Nanoparticles with Ultralarge Pores and Their Application in Gene Delivery. *ACS Nano* **2011**, *5*, 3568–3576. [CrossRef] [PubMed]

151. Qu, F.; Zhu, G.; Huang, S.; Li, S.; Sun, J.; Zhang, D.; Qiu, S. Controlled release of Captopril by regulating the pore size and morphology of ordered mesoporous silica. *Microporous Mesoporous Mater.* **2006**, *92*, 1–9. [CrossRef]

152. Doadrio, J.C.; Sousa, E.M.B.; Izquierdo-Barba, I.; Doadrio, A.L.; Perez-Pariente, J.; Vallet-Regí, M. Functionalization of mesoporous materials with long alkyl chains as a strategy for controlling drug delivery pattern. *J. Mater. Chem.* **2006**, *16*, 462–466. [CrossRef]

153. Balas, F.; Manzano, M.; Horcajada, P.; Vallet-Regí, M. Confinement and Controlled Release of Bisphosphonates on Ordered Mesoporous Silica-Based Materials. *J. Am. Chem. Soc.* **2006**, *128*, 8116–8117. [CrossRef] [PubMed]

154. Nieto, A.; Colilla, M.; Balas, F.; Vallet-Regí, M. Surface Electrochemistry of Mesoporous Silicas as a Key Factor in the Design of Tailored Delivery Devices. *Langmuir* **2010**, *26*, 5038–5049. [CrossRef] [PubMed]

155. Datt, A.; El-Maazawi, I.; Larsen, S.C. Aspirin Loading and Release from MCM-41 Functionalized with Aminopropyl Groups via Co-condensation or Postsynthesis Modification Methods. *J. Phys. Chem. C* **2012**, *116*, 18358–18366. [CrossRef]

156. Song, S.-W.; Hidajat, K.; Kawi, S. Functionalized SBA-15 Materials as Carriers for Controlled Drug Delivery: Influence of Surface Properties on Matrix−Drug Interactions. *Langmuir* **2005**, *21*, 9568–9575. [CrossRef] [PubMed]

157. Mishra, A.K.; Pandey, H.; Agarwal, V.; Ramteke, P.W.; Pandey, A.C. Nanoengineered mesoporous silica nanoparticles for smart delivery of doxorubicin. *J. Nanopart. Res.* **2014**, *16*, 2515. [CrossRef]

158. Han, N.; Wang, Y.; Bai, J.; Liu, J.; Wang, Y.; Gao, Y.; Jiang, T.; Kang, W.; Wang, S. Facile synthesis of the lipid bilayer coated mesoporous silica nanocomposites and their application in drug delivery. *Microporous Mesoporous Mater.* **2016**, *219*, 209–218. [CrossRef]

159. Murugan, C.; Rayappan, K.; Thangam, R.; Bhanumathi, R.; Shanthi, K.; Vivek, R.; Thirumurugan, R.; Bhattacharyya, A.; Sivasubramanian, S.; Gunasekaran, P.; et al. Combinatorial nanocarrier based drug delivery approach for amalgamation of anti-tumor agents in breast cancer cells: An improved nanomedicine strategy. *Sci. Rep.* **2016**, *6*, 34053. [CrossRef] [PubMed]

160. Kim, S.; Diab, R.; Joubert, O.; Canilho, N.; Pasc, A. Core–shell microcapsules of solid lipid nanoparticles and mesoporous silica for enhanced oral delivery of curcumin. *Colloids Surf. B Biointerfaces* **2016**, *140*, 161–168. [CrossRef] [PubMed]

161. Fu, Q.; Hargrove, D.; Lu, X. Improving paclitaxel pharmacokinetics by using tumor-specific mesoporous silica nanoparticles with intraperitoneal delivery. *Nanomed. Nanotechnol. Biol. Med.* **2016**, *12*, 1951–1959. [CrossRef] [PubMed]

162. Kumar, B.; Kulanthaivel, S.; Mondal, A.; Mishra, S.; Banerjee, B.; Bhaumik, A.; Banerjee, I.; Giri, S. Mesoporous silica nanoparticle based enzyme responsive system for colon specific drug delivery through guar gum capping. *Colloids Surf. B Biointerfaces* **2017**, *150*, 352–361. [CrossRef] [PubMed]

163. Saroj, S.; Rajput, S.J. Tailor-made pH-sensitive polyacrylic acid functionalized mesoporous silica nanoparticles for efficient and controlled delivery of anti-cancer drug Etoposide. *Drug Dev. Ind. Pharm.* **2018**, *44*, 1198–1211. [CrossRef] [PubMed]

164. Thiyagarajan, V.; Lin, S.-X.; Lee, C.-H.; Weng, C.-F. A focal adhesion kinase inhibitor 16-hydroxy-cleroda-3,13-dien-16,15-olide incorporated into enteric-coated nanoparticles for controlled anti-glioma drug delivery. *Colloids Surf. B Biointerfaces* **2016**, *141*, 120–131. [CrossRef] [PubMed]

165. Ganesh, M.; Ubaidulla, U.; Hemalatha, P.; Peng, M.M.; Jang, H.T. Development of Duloxetine Hydrochloride Loaded Mesoporous Silica Nanoparticles: Characterizations and In Vitro Evaluation. *AAPS PharmSciTech* **2015**, *16*, 944–951. [CrossRef] [PubMed]

166. Mohseni, M.; Gilani, K.; Mortazavi, S.A. Preparation and characterization of rifampin loaded mesoporous silica nanoparticles as a potential system for pulmonary drug delivery. *Iran. J. Pharm. Res.* **2015**, *14*, 27–34. [PubMed]

167. El Nabarawi, M.A.; Hassen, D.H.; Taha, A.A. Inclusion and characterization of ketoprofen into different mesoporous silica nanoparticles using three loading methods. *Int. J. Pharm. Pharm. Sci.* **2014**, *6*, 183–191.

168. Yoncheva, K.; Popova, M.; Szegedi, A.; Mihaly, J.; Tzankov, B.; Lambov, N.; Konstantinov, S.; Tzankova, V.; Pessina, F.; Valoti, M. Functionalized mesoporous silica nanoparticles for oral delivery of budesonide. *J. Solid State Chem.* **2014**, *211*, 154–161. [CrossRef]

169. Mudakavi, R.J.; Raichur, A.M.; Chakravortty, D. Lipid coated mesoporous silica nanoparticles as an oral delivery system for targeting and treatment of intravacuolar Salmonella infections. *RSC Adv.* **2014**, *4*, 61160–61166. [CrossRef]

170. Mudakavi, R.J.; Vanamali, S.; Chakravortty, D.; Raichur, A.M. Development of arginine based nanocarriers for targeting and treatment of intracellular *Salmonella*. *RSC Adv.* **2017**, *7*, 7022–7032. [CrossRef]

171. Koneru, B.; Shi, Y.; Wang, Y.-C.; Chavala, S.; Miller, M.; Holbert, B.; Conson, M.; Ni, A.; Di Pasqua, A. Tetracycline-Containing MCM-41 Mesoporous Silica Nanoparticles for the Treatment of *Escherichia coli*. *Molecules* **2015**, *20*, 19690–19698. [CrossRef] [PubMed]

172. Alexa, I.F.; Ignat, M.; Popovici, R.F.; Timpu, D.; Popovici, E. In vitro controlled release of antihypertensive drugs intercalated into unmodified SBA-15 and MgO modified SBA-15 matrices. *Int. J. Pharm.* **2012**, *436*, 111–119. [CrossRef] [PubMed]

173. Doadrio, A.L.; Sánchez-Montero, J.M.; Doadrio, J.C.; Salinas, A.J.; Vallet-Regí, M. Mesoporous silica nanoparticles as a new carrier methodology in the controlled release of the active components in a polypill. *Eur. J. Pharm. Sci.* **2017**, *97*, 1–8. [CrossRef] [PubMed]

174. Zou, Z.; He, D.; Cai, L.; He, X.; Wang, K.; Yang, X.; Li, L.; Li, S.; Su, X. Alizarin Complexone Functionalized Mesoporous Silica Nanoparticles: A Smart System Integrating Glucose-Responsive Double-Drugs Release and Real-Time Monitoring Capabilities. *ACS Appl. Mater. Interfaces* **2016**, *8*, 8358–8366. [CrossRef] [PubMed]

175. Huang, P.-K.; Lin, S.-X.; Tsai, M.-J.; Leong, M.; Lin, S.-R.; Kankala, R.; Lee, C.-H.; Weng, C.-F. Encapsulation of 16-Hydroxycleroda-3,13-Dine-16,15-Olide in Mesoporous Silica Nanoparticles as a Natural Dipeptidyl Peptidase-4 Inhibitor Potentiated Hypoglycemia in Diabetic Mice. *Nanomaterials* **2017**, *7*, 112. [CrossRef] [PubMed]

176. Shi, X.; Wang, Y.; Varshney, R.R.; Ren, L.; Zhang, F.; Wang, D.-A. In-vitro osteogenesis of synovium stem cells induced by controlled release of bisphosphate additives from microspherical mesoporous silica composite. *Biomaterials* **2009**, *30*, 3996–4005. [CrossRef] [PubMed]

177. Zhou, X.; Feng, W.; Qiu, K.; Chen, L.; Wang, W.; Nie, W.; Mo, X.; He, C. BMP-2 Derived Peptide and Dexamethasone Incorporated Mesoporous Silica Nanoparticles for Enhanced Osteogenic Differentiation of Bone Mesenchymal Stem Cells. *ACS Appl. Mater. Interfaces* **2015**, *7*, 15777–15789. [CrossRef] [PubMed]

178. Arriagada, F.; Correa, O.; Günther, G.; Nonell, S.; Mura, F.; Olea-Azar, C.; Morales, J. Morin Flavonoid Adsorbed on Mesoporous Silica, a Novel Antioxidant Nanomaterial. *PLoS ONE* **2016**, *11*, e0164507. [CrossRef] [PubMed]

179. Meng, H.; Xue, M.; Xia, T.; Ji, Z.; Tarn, D.Y.; Zink, J.I.; Nel, A.E. Use of Size and a Copolymer Design Feature To Improve the Biodistribution and the Enhanced Permeability and Retention Effect of Doxorubicin-Loaded Mesoporous Silica Nanoparticles in a Murine Xenograft Tumor Model. *ACS Nano* **2011**, *5*, 4131–4144. [CrossRef] [PubMed]

180. Ma, X.; Qu, Q.; Zhao, Y. Targeted Delivery of 5-Aminolevulinic Acid by Multifunctional Hollow Mesoporous Silica Nanoparticles for Photodynamic Skin Cancer Therapy. *ACS Appl. Mater. Interfaces* **2015**, *7*, 10671–10676. [CrossRef] [PubMed]

181. Khosravian, P.; Shafiee Ardestani, M.; Khoobi, M.; Ostad, S.N.; Dorkoosh, F.A.; Akbari Javar, H.; Amanlou, M. Mesoporous silica nanoparticles functionalized with folic acid/methionine for active targeted delivery of docetaxel. *OncoTargets Ther.* **2016**, *9*, 7315–7330. [CrossRef] [PubMed]

182. Zhang, M.; Xu, C.; Wen, L.; Han, M.K.; Xiao, B.; Zhou, J.; Zhang, Y.; Zhang, Z.; Viennois, E.; Merlin, D. A Hyaluronidase-Responsive Nanoparticle-Based Drug Delivery System for Targeting Colon Cancer Cells. *Cancer Res.* **2016**, *76*, 7208–7218. [CrossRef] [PubMed]

183. Gary-Bobo, M.; Brevet, D.; Benkirane-Jessel, N.; Raehm, L.; Maillard, P.; Garcia, M.; Durand, J.-O. Hyaluronic acid-functionalized mesoporous silica nanoparticles for efficient photodynamic therapy of cancer cells. *Photodiagn. Photodyn. Ther.* **2012**, *9*, 256–260. [CrossRef] [PubMed]

184. Quan, G.; Pan, X.; Wang, Z.; Wu, Q.; Li, G.; Dian, L.; Chen, B.; Wu, C. Lactosaminated mesoporous silica nanoparticles for asialoglycoprotein receptor targeted anticancer drug delivery. *J. Nanobiotechnol.* **2015**, *13*, 7. [CrossRef] [PubMed]

185. Vaillant, O.; El Cheikh, K.; Warther, D.; Brevet, D.; Maynadier, M.; Bouffard, E.; Salgues, F.; Jeanjean, A.; Puche, P.; Mazerolles, C.; et al. Mannose-6-Phosphate Receptor: A Target for Theranostics of Prostate Cancer. *Angew. Chem. Int. Ed.* **2015**, *54*, 5952–5956. [CrossRef] [PubMed]

186. Gary-Bobo, M.; Mir, Y.; Rouxel, C.; Brevet, D.; Basile, I.; Maynadier, M.; Vaillant, O.; Mongin, O.; Blanchard-Desce, M.; Morère, A.; et al. Mannose-Functionalized Mesoporous Silica Nanoparticles for Efficient Two-Photon Photodynamic Therapy of Solid Tumors. *Angew. Chem. Int. Ed.* **2011**, *50*, 11425–11429. [CrossRef] [PubMed]

187. Wu, K.; Liao, Y.-T.; Liu, C.-H.; Yu, J. Liver cancer cells: Targeting and prolonged-release drug carriers consisting of mesoporous silica nanoparticles and alginate microspheres. *Int. J. Nanomed.* **2014**, *9*, 2767–2778. [CrossRef] [PubMed]

188. Chakravarty, R.; Goel, S.; Hong, H.; Chen, F.; Valdovinos, H.F.; Hernandez, R.; Barnhart, T.E.; Cai, W. Hollow mesoporous silica nanoparticles for tumor vasculature targeting and PET image-guided drug delivery. *Nanomedicine* **2015**, *10*, 1233–1246. [CrossRef] [PubMed]

189. Liu, K.; Wang, Z.; Wang, S.; Liu, P.; Qin, Y.; Ma, Y.; Li, X.-C.; Huo, Z.-J. Hyaluronic acid-tagged silica nanoparticles in colon cancer therapy: Therapeutic efficacy evaluation. *Int. J. Nanomed.* **2015**, *10*, 6445–6454. [CrossRef]

190. Chen, L.; She, X.; Wang, T.; He, L.; Shigdar, S.; Duan, W.; Kong, L. Overcoming acquired drug resistance in colorectal cancer cells by targeted delivery of 5-FU with EGF grafted hollow mesoporous silica nanoparticles. *Nanoscale* **2015**, *7*, 14080–14092. [CrossRef] [PubMed]

191. Radhakrishnan, K.; Tripathy, J.; Datey, A.; Chakravortty, D.; Raichur, A.M. Mesoporous silica–chondroitin sulphate hybrid nanoparticles for targeted and bio-responsive drug delivery. *New J. Chem.* **2015**, *39*, 1754–1760. [CrossRef]

192. Chen, X.; Sun, H.; Hu, J.; Han, X.; Liu, H.; Hu, Y. Transferrin gated mesoporous silica nanoparticles for redox-responsive and targeted drug delivery. *Colloids Surf. B Biointerfaces* **2017**, *152*, 77–84. [CrossRef] [PubMed]

193. Xie, X.; Li, F.; Zhang, H.; Lu, Y.; Lian, S.; Lin, H.; Gao, Y.; Jia, L. EpCAM aptamer-functionalized mesoporous silica nanoparticles for efficient colon cancer cell-targeted drug delivery. *Eur. J. Pharm. Sci.* **2016**, *83*, 28–35. [CrossRef] [PubMed]

194. Brevet, D.; Gary-Bobo, M.; Raehm, L.; Richeter, S.; Hocine, O.; Amro, K.; Loock, B.; Couleaud, P.; Frochot, C.; Morère, A.; et al. Mannose-targeted mesoporous silica nanoparticles for photodynamic therapy. *Chem. Commun.* **2009**, 1475–1477. [CrossRef] [PubMed]

195. Sarkar, A.; Ghosh, S.; Chowdhury, S.; Pandey, B.; Sil, P.C. Targeted delivery of quercetin loaded mesoporous silica nanoparticles to the breast cancer cells. *Biochim. Biophys. Acta Gen. Subj.* **2016**, *1860*, 2065–2075. [CrossRef] [PubMed]

196. Goel, S.; Chen, F.; Hong, H.; Valdovinos, H.F.; Hernandez, R.; Shi, S.; Barnhart, T.E.; Cai, W. $VEGF_{121}$-Conjugated Mesoporous Silica Nanoparticle: A Tumor Targeted Drug Delivery System. *ACS Appl. Mater. Interfaces* **2014**, *6*, 21677–21685. [CrossRef] [PubMed]

197. Xu, H.; Wang, Z.; Li, Y.; Guo, Y.; Zhou, H.; Li, Y.; Wu, F.; Zhang, L.; Yang, X.; Lu, B.; et al. Preparation and characterization of a dual-receptor mesoporous silica nanoparticle–hyaluronic acid–RGD peptide targeting drug delivery system. *RSC Adv.* **2016**, *6*, 40427–40435. [CrossRef]

198. Kankala, R.K.; Kuthati, Y.; Liu, C.-L.; Mou, C.-Y.; Lee, C.-H. Killing cancer cells by delivering a nanoreactor for inhibition of catalase and catalytically enhancing intracellular levels of ROS. *RSC Adv.* **2015**, *5*, 86072–86081. [CrossRef]

199. Kankala, R.K.; Liu, C.-G.; Chen, A.-Z.; Wang, S.-B.; Xu, P.-Y.; Mende, L.K.; Liu, C.-L.; Lee, C.-H.; Hu, Y.-F. Overcoming Multidrug Resistance through the Synergistic Effects of Hierarchical pH-Sensitive, ROS-Generating Nanoreactors. *ACS Biomater. Sci. Eng.* **2017**, *3*, 2431–2442. [CrossRef]

200. Jadhav, S.A.; Brunella, V.; Berlier, G.; Ugazio, E.; Scalarone, D. Effect of Multimodal Pore Channels on Cargo Release from Mesoporous Silica Nanoparticles. *J. Nanomater.* **2016**, *2016*, 1–7. [CrossRef]

201. Kamarudin, N.H.N.; Jalil, A.A.; Triwahyono, S.; Salleh, N.F.M.; Karim, A.H.; Mukti, R.R.; Hameed, B.H.; Ahmad, A. Role of 3-aminopropyltriethoxysilane in the preparation of mesoporous silica nanoparticles for ibuprofen delivery: Effect on physicochemical properties. *Microporous Mesoporous Mater.* **2013**, *180*, 235–241. [CrossRef]

202. Ahmadi, E.; Dehghannejad, N.; Hashemikia, S.; Ghasemnejad, M.; Tabebordbar, H. Synthesis and surface modification of mesoporous silica nanoparticles and its application as carriers for sustained drug delivery. *Drug Deliv.* **2014**, *21*, 164–172. [CrossRef] [PubMed]

203. Braz, W.R.; Rocha, N.L.; de Faria, E.H.; Silva, M.L.; Ciuffi, K.J.; Tavares, D.C.; Furtado, R.A.; Rocha, L.A.; Nassar, E.J. Incorporation of anti-inflammatory agent into mesoporous silica. *Nanotechnology* **2016**, *27*, 385103. [CrossRef] [PubMed]

204. Song, Y.; Li, Y.; Xu, Q.; Liu, Z. Mesoporous silica nanoparticles for stimuli-responsive controlled drug delivery: Advances, challenges, and outlook. *Int. J. Nanomed.* **2017**, *12*, 87–110. [CrossRef] [PubMed]

205. Nguyen, C.T.H.; Webb, R.I.; Lambert, L.K.; Strounina, E.; Lee, E.C.; Parat, M.-O.; McGuckin, M.A.; Popat, A.; Cabot, P.J.; Ross, B.P. Bifunctional Succinylated ε-Polylysine-Coated Mesoporous Silica Nanoparticles for pH-Responsive and Intracellular Drug Delivery Targeting the Colon. *ACS Appl. Mater. Interfaces* **2017**, *9*, 9470–9483. [CrossRef] [PubMed]

206. Ahmadi Nasab, N.; Hassani Kumleh, H.; Beygzadeh, M.; Teimourian, S.; Kazemzad, M. Delivery of curcumin by a pH-responsive chitosan mesoporous silica nanoparticles for cancer treatment. *Artif. Cells Nanomed. Biotechnol.* **2017**, 1–7. [CrossRef] [PubMed]

207. Hu, X.; Wang, Y.; Peng, B. Chitosan-Capped Mesoporous Silica Nanoparticles as pH-Responsive Nanocarriers for Controlled Drug Release. *Chem. Asian J.* **2014**, *9*, 319–327. [CrossRef] [PubMed]

208. Yuan, L.; Tang, Q.; Yang, D.; Zhang, J.Z.; Zhang, F.; Hu, J. Preparation of pH-Responsive Mesoporous Silica Nanoparticles and Their Application in Controlled Drug Delivery. *J. Phys. Chem. C* **2011**, *115*, 9926–9932. [CrossRef]

209. Cheng, W.; Nie, J.; Xu, L.; Liang, C.; Peng, Y.; Liu, G.; Wang, T.; Mei, L.; Huang, L.; Zeng, X. pH-Sensitive Delivery Vehicle Based on Folic Acid-Conjugated Polydopamine-Modified Mesoporous Silica Nanoparticles for Targeted Cancer Therapy. *ACS Appl. Mater. Interfaces* **2017**, *9*, 18462–18473. [CrossRef] [PubMed]

210. Zheng, J.; Tian, X.; Sun, Y.; Lu, D.; Yang, W. pH-sensitive poly(glutamic acid) grafted mesoporous silica nanoparticles for drug delivery. *Int. J. Pharm.* **2013**, *450*, 296–303. [CrossRef] [PubMed]

211. Hu, C.; Yu, L.; Zheng, Z.; Wang, J.; Liu, Y.; Jiang, Y.; Tong, G.; Zhou, Y.; Wang, X. Tannin as a gatekeeper of pH-responsive mesoporous silica nanoparticles for drug delivery. *RSC Adv.* **2015**, *5*, 85436–85441. [CrossRef]

212. Park, C.; Oh, K.; Lee, S.C.; Kim, C. Controlled Release of Guest Molecules from Mesoporous Silica Particles Based on a pH-Responsive Polypseudorotaxane Motif. *Angew. Chem. Int. Ed.* **2007**, *46*, 1455–1457. [CrossRef] [PubMed]

213. Bai, L.; Zhao, Q.; Wang, J.; Gao, Y.; Sha, Z.; Di, D.; Han, N.; Wang, Y.; Zhang, J.; Wang, S. Mechanism study on pH-responsive cyclodextrin capped mesoporous silica: Effect of different stalk densities and the type of cyclodextrin. *Nanotechnology* **2015**, *26*, 165704. [CrossRef] [PubMed]

214. Kuthati, Y.; Kankala, R.K.; Lin, S.-X.; Weng, C.-F.; Lee, C.-H. pH-Triggered Controllable Release of Silver–Indole-3 Acetic Acid Complexes from Mesoporous Silica Nanoparticles (IBN-4) for Effectively Killing Malignant Bacteria. *Mol. Pharm.* **2015**, *12*, 2289–2304. [CrossRef] [PubMed]

215. Wang, Y.; Han, N.; Zhao, Q.; Bai, L.; Li, J.; Jiang, T.; Wang, S. Redox-responsive mesoporous silica as carriers for controlled drug delivery: A comparative study based on silica and PEG gatekeepers. *Eur. J. Pharm. Sci.* **2015**, *72*, 12–20. [CrossRef] [PubMed]

216. Zhu, X.; Wang, C.-Q. pH and redox-operated nanovalve for size-selective cargo delivery on hollow mesoporous silica spheres. *J. Colloid Interface Sci.* **2016**, *480*, 39–48. [CrossRef] [PubMed]

217. Bathfield, M.; Reboul, J.; Cacciaguerra, T.; Lacroix-Desmazes, P.; Gérardin, C. Thermosensitive and Drug-Loaded Ordered Mesoporous Silica: A Direct and Effective Synthesis Using PEO-*b*-PNIPAM Block Copolymers. *Chem. Mater.* **2016**, *28*, 3374–3384. [CrossRef]

218. Zhao, Y.; Trewyn, B.G.; Slowing, I.I.; Lin, V.S.-Y. Mesoporous Silica Nanoparticle-Based Double Drug Delivery System for Glucose-Responsive Controlled Release of Insulin and Cyclic AMP. *J. Am. Chem. Soc.* **2009**, *131*, 8398–8400. [CrossRef] [PubMed]

219. Tan, L.; Yang, M.-Y.; Wu, H.-X.; Tang, Z.-W.; Xiao, J.-Y.; Liu, C.-J.; Zhuo, R.-X. Glucose- and pH-Responsive Nanogated Ensemble Based on Polymeric Network Capped Mesoporous Silica. *ACS Appl. Mater. Interfaces* **2015**, *7*, 6310–6316. [CrossRef] [PubMed]

220. Bhat, R.; Ribes, À.; Mas, N.; Aznar, E.; Sancenón, F.; Marcos, M.D.; Murguía, J.R.; Venkataraman, A.; Martínez-Máñez, R. Thrombin-Responsive Gated Silica Mesoporous Nanoparticles as Coagulation Regulators. *Langmuir* **2016**, *32*, 1195–1200. [CrossRef] [PubMed]

221. Gayam, S.R.; Venkatesan, P.; Sung, Y.-M.; Sung, S.-Y.; Hu, S.-H.; Hsu, H.-Y.; Wu, S.-P. An NAD(P)H:quinone oxidoreductase 1 (NQO1) enzyme responsive nanocarrier based on mesoporous silica nanoparticles for tumor targeted drug delivery in vitro and in vivo. *Nanoscale* **2016**, *8*, 12307–12317. [CrossRef] [PubMed]

222. Liu, J.; Zhang, B.; Luo, Z.; Ding, X.; Li, J.; Dai, L.; Zhou, J.; Zhao, X.; Ye, J.; Cai, K. Enzyme responsive mesoporous silica nanoparticles for targeted tumor therapy in vitro and in vivo. *Nanoscale* **2015**, *7*, 3614–3626. [CrossRef] [PubMed]

223. Radhakrishnan, K.; Gupta, S.; Gnanadhas, D.P.; Ramamurthy, P.C.; Chakravortty, D.; Raichur, A.M. Protamine-Capped Mesoporous Silica Nanoparticles for Biologically Triggered Drug Release. *Part. Part. Syst. Charact.* **2014**, *31*, 449–458. [CrossRef]

224. Xiao, Y.; Wang, T.; Cao, Y.; Wang, X.; Zhang, Y.; Liu, Y.; Huo, Q. Enzyme and voltage stimuli-responsive controlled release system based on β-cyclodextrin-capped mesoporous silica nanoparticles. *Dalton Trans.* **2015**, *44*, 4355–4361. [CrossRef] [PubMed]

225. Febvay, S.; Marini, D.M.; Belcher, A.M.; Clapham, D.E. Targeted Cytosolic Delivery of Cell-Impermeable Compounds by Nanoparticle-Mediated, Light-Triggered Endosome Disruption. *Nano Lett.* **2010**, *10*, 2211–2219. [CrossRef] [PubMed]

226. Liu, J.; Detrembleur, C.; De Pauw-Gillet, M.-C.; Mornet, S.; Jérôme, C.; Duguet, E. Gold Nanorods Coated with Mesoporous Silica Shell as Drug Delivery System for Remote Near Infrared Light-Activated Release and Potential Phototherapy. *Small* **2015**, *11*, 2323–2332. [CrossRef] [PubMed]

227. Li, W.-P.; Liao, P.-Y.; Su, C.-H.; Yeh, C.-S. Formation of Oligonucleotide-Gated Silica Shell-Coated Fe_3O_4-Au Core–Shell Nanotrisoctahedra for Magnetically Targeted and Near-Infrared Light-Responsive Theranostic Platform. *J. Am. Chem. Soc.* **2014**, *136*, 10062–10075. [CrossRef] [PubMed]

228. Baeza, A.; Guisasola, E.; Ruiz-Hernández, E.; Vallet-Regí, M. Magnetically Triggered Multidrug Release by Hybrid Mesoporous Silica Nanoparticles. *Chem. Mater.* **2012**, *24*, 517–524. [CrossRef]

229. Paris, J.L.; Cabañas, M.V.; Manzano, M.; Vallet-Regí, M. Polymer-Grafted Mesoporous Silica Nanoparticles as Ultrasound-Responsive Drug Carriers. *ACS Nano* **2015**, *9*, 11023–11033. [CrossRef] [PubMed]

230. Kim, H.-J.; Matsuda, H.; Zhou, H.; Honma, I. Ultrasound-Triggered Smart Drug Release from a Poly(dimethylsiloxane)– Mesoporous Silica Composite. *Adv. Mater.* **2006**, *18*, 3083–3088. [CrossRef]

231. Paris, J.L.; Villaverde, G.; Cabañas, M.V.; Manzano, M.; Vallet-Regí, M. From proof-of-concept material to PEGylated and modularly targeted ultrasound-responsive mesoporous silica nanoparticles. *J. Mater. Chem. B* **2018**, *6*, 2785–2794. [CrossRef]

232. Wang, T.; Sun, G.; Wang, M.; Zhou, B.; Fu, J. Voltage/pH-Driven Mechanized Silica Nanoparticles for the Multimodal Controlled Release of Drugs. *ACS Appl. Mater. Interfaces* **2015**, *7*, 21295–21304. [CrossRef] [PubMed]

233. Kuthati, Y.; Kankala, R.K.; Busa, P.; Lin, S.-X.; Deng, J.-P.; Mou, C.-Y.; Lee, C.-H. Phototherapeutic spectrum expansion through synergistic effect of mesoporous silica trio-nanohybrids against antibiotic-resistant gram-negative bacterium. *J. Photochem. Photobiol. B Biol.* **2017**, *169*, 124–133. [CrossRef] [PubMed]

234. McCarthy, C.A.; Ahern, R.J.; Dontireddy, R.; Ryan, K.B.; Crean, A.M. Mesoporous silica formulation strategies for drug dissolution enhancement: A review. *Expert Opin. Drug Deliv.* **2016**, *13*, 93–108. [CrossRef] [PubMed]

235. Bukara, K.; Schueller, L.; Rosier, J.; Martens, M.A.; Daems, T.; Verheyden, L.; Eelen, S.; Speybroeck, M.V.; Libanati, C.; Martens, J.A.; et al. Ordered mesoporous silica to enhance the bioavailability of poorly water-soluble drugs: Proof of concept in man. *Eur. J. Pharm. Biopharm.* **2016**, *108*, 220–225. [CrossRef] [PubMed]

236. Zhang, Y.; Wang, J.; Bai, X.; Jiang, T.; Zhang, Q.; Wang, S. Mesoporous Silica Nanoparticles for Increasing the Oral Bioavailability and Permeation of Poorly Water Soluble Drugs. *Mol. Pharm.* **2012**, *9*, 505–513. [CrossRef] [PubMed]

237. Thomas, M.J.K.; Slipper, I.; Walunj, A.; Jain, A.; Favretto, M.E.; Kallinteri, P.; Douroumis, D. Inclusion of poorly soluble drugs in highly ordered mesoporous silica nanoparticles. *Int. J. Pharm.* **2010**, *387*, 272–277. [CrossRef] [PubMed]

238. Sreejith, S.; Ma, X.; Zhao, Y. Graphene Oxide Wrapping on Squaraine-Loaded Mesoporous Silica Nanoparticles for Bioimaging. *J. Am. Chem. Soc.* **2012**, *134*, 17346–17349. [CrossRef] [PubMed]

239. Nakamura, T.; Sugihara, F.; Matsushita, H.; Yoshioka, Y.; Mizukami, S.; Kikuchi, K. Mesoporous silica nanoparticles for ^{19}F magnetic resonance imaging, fluorescence imaging, and drug delivery. *Chem. Sci.* **2015**, *6*, 1986–1990. [CrossRef] [PubMed]

240. Jun, B.-H.; Hwang, D.W.; Jung, H.S.; Jang, J.; Kim, H.; Kang, H.; Kang, T.; Kyeong, S.; Lee, H.; Jeong, D.H.; et al. Ultrasensitive, Biocompatible, Quantum-Dot-Embedded Silica Nanoparticles for Bioimaging. *Adv. Funct. Mater.* **2012**, *22*, 1843–1849. [CrossRef]

241. Helle, M.; Rampazzo, E.; Monchanin, M.; Marchal, F.; Guillemin, F.; Bonacchi, S.; Salis, F.; Prodi, L.; Bezdetnaya, L. Surface Chemistry Architecture of Silica Nanoparticles Determine the Efficiency of in Vivo Fluorescence Lymph Node Mapping. *ACS Nano* **2013**, *7*, 8645–8657. [CrossRef] [PubMed]

242. Vallet-Regí, M. Ordered Mesoporous Materials in the Context of Drug Delivery Systems and Bone Tissue Engineering. *Chem. Eur. J.* **2006**, *12*, 5934–5943. [CrossRef] [PubMed]

243. Izquierdo-Barba, I.; Ruiz-González, L.; Doadrio, J.C.; González-Calbet, J.M.; Vallet-Regí, M. Tissue regeneration: A new property of mesoporous materials. *Solid State Sci.* **2005**, *7*, 983–989. [CrossRef]

244. Luo, Z.; Deng, Y.; Zhang, R.; Wang, M.; Bai, Y.; Zhao, Q.; Lyu, Y.; Wei, J.; Wei, S. Peptide-laden mesoporous silica nanoparticles with promoted bioactivity and osteo-differentiation ability for bone tissue engineering. *Colloids Surf. B Biointerfaces* **2015**, *131*, 73–82. [CrossRef] [PubMed]

245. Wu, C.; Chang, J. Mesoporous bioactive glasses: Structure characteristics, drug/growth factor delivery and bone regeneration application. *Interface Focus* **2012**, *2*, 292–306. [CrossRef] [PubMed]

246. López-Noriega, A.; Arcos, D.; Izquierdo-Barba, I.; Sakamoto, Y.; Terasaki, O.; Vallet-Regí, M. Ordered Mesoporous Bioactive Glasses for Bone Tissue Regeneration. *Chem. Mater* **2006**, *18*, 3137–3144. [CrossRef]

247. Bozzuto, G.; Molinari, A. Liposomes as nanomedical devices. *Int. J. Nanomed.* **2015**, *10*, 975–999. [CrossRef] [PubMed]

248. Davis, M.E.; Chen, Z.; Shin, D.M. Nanoparticle therapeutics: An emerging treatment modality for cancer. *Nat. Rev. Drug Discov.* **2008**, *7*, 771–782. [CrossRef] [PubMed]

249. Palazzolo, S.; Bayda, S.; Hadla, M.; Caligiuri, I.; Corona, G.; Toffoli, G.; Rizzolio, F. The Clinical translation of Organic Nanomaterials for Cancer Therapy: A Focus on Polymeric Nanoparticles, Micelles, Liposomes and Exosomes. *Curr. Med. Chem.* **2017**, *24*. [CrossRef] [PubMed]

250. Kamaly, N.; Xiao, Z.; Valencia, P.M.; Radovic-Moreno, A.F.; Farokhzad, O.C. Targeted polymeric therapeutic nanoparticles: Design, development and clinical translation. *Chem. Soc. Rev.* **2012**, *41*, 2971–3010. [CrossRef] [PubMed]

251. Slowing, I.I.; Wu, C.-W.; Vivero-Escoto, J.L.; Lin, V.S.-Y. Mesoporous Silica Nanoparticles for Reducing Hemolytic Activity towards Mammalian Red Blood Cells. *Small* **2009**, *5*, 57–62. [CrossRef] [PubMed]

252. Nash, T.; Allison, A.C.; Harington, J.S. Physico-Chemical Properties of Silica in Relation to its Toxicity. *Nature* **1966**, *210*, 259–261. [CrossRef] [PubMed]

253. He, Q.; Zhang, Z.; Gao, F.; Li, Y.; Shi, J. In vivo Biodistribution and Urinary Excretion of Mesoporous Silica Nanoparticles: Effects of Particle Size and PEGylation. *Small* **2011**, *7*, 271–280. [CrossRef] [PubMed]

254. Yu, T.; Malugin, A.; Ghandehari, H. Impact of Silica Nanoparticle Design on Cellular Toxicity and Hemolytic Activity. *ACS Nano* **2011**, *5*, 5717–5728. [CrossRef] [PubMed]

255. Townson, J.L.; Lin, Y.-S.; Agola, J.O.; Carnes, E.C.; Leong, H.S.; Lewis, J.D.; Haynes, C.L.; Brinker, C.J. Re-examining the Size/Charge Paradigm: Differing in Vivo Characteristics of Size- and Charge-Matched Mesoporous Silica Nanoparticles. *J. Am. Chem. Soc.* **2013**, *135*, 16030–16033. [CrossRef] [PubMed]

256. Li, L.; Liu, T.; Fu, C.; Tan, L.; Meng, X.; Liu, H. Biodistribution, excretion, and toxicity of mesoporous silica nanoparticles after oral administration depend on their shape. *Nanomed. Nanotechnol. Biol. Med.* **2015**, *11*, 1915–1924. [CrossRef] [PubMed]

257. Zhao, Y.; Wang, Y.; Ran, F.; Cui, Y.; Liu, C.; Zhao, Q.; Gao, Y.; Wang, D.; Wang, S. A comparison between sphere and rod nanoparticles regarding their in vivo biological behavior and pharmacokinetics. *Sci. Rep.* **2017**, *7*, 4131. [CrossRef] [PubMed]

258. Hudson, S.P.; Padera, R.F.; Langer, R.; Kohane, D.S. The biocompatibility of mesoporous silicates. *Biomaterials* **2008**, *29*, 4045–4055. [CrossRef] [PubMed]

259. Lu, J.; Liong, M.; Li, Z.; Zink, J.I.; Tamanoi, F. Biocompatibility, biodistribution, and drug-delivery efficiency of mesoporous silica nanoparticles for cancer therapy in animals. *Small* **2010**, *6*, 1794–1805. [CrossRef] [PubMed]

260. Tang, F.; Li, L.; Chen, D. Mesoporous Silica Nanoparticles: Synthesis, Biocompatibility and Drug Delivery. *Adv. Mater.* **2012**, *24*, 1504–1534. [CrossRef] [PubMed]

261. Zhang, Q.; Wang, X.; Li, P.-Z.; Nguyen, K.T.; Wang, X.-J.; Luo, Z.; Zhang, H.; Tan, N.S.; Zhao, Y. Biocompatible, Uniform, and Redispersible Mesoporous Silica Nanoparticles for Cancer-Targeted Drug Delivery In Vivo. *Adv. Funct. Mater.* **2014**, *24*, 2450–2461. [CrossRef]

262. Shen, D.; Yang, J.; Li, X.; Zhou, L.; Zhang, R.; Li, W.; Chen, L.; Wang, R.; Zhang, F.; Zhao, D. Biphase Stratification Approach to Three-Dimensional Dendritic Biodegradable Mesoporous Silica Nanospheres. *Nano Lett.* **2014**, *14*, 923–932. [CrossRef] [PubMed]

263. He, Y.; Zeng, B.; Liang, S.; Long, M.; Xu, H. Synthesis of pH-Responsive Biodegradable Mesoporous Silica–Calcium Phosphate Hybrid Nanoparticles as a High Potential Drug Carrier. *ACS Appl. Mater. Interfaces* **2017**, *9*, 44402–44409. [CrossRef] [PubMed]

264. Liu, T.; Li, L.; Teng, X.; Huang, X.; Liu, H.; Chen, D.; Ren, J.; He, J.; Tang, F. Single and repeated dose toxicity of mesoporous hollow silica nanoparticles in intravenously exposed mice. *Biomaterials* **2011**, *32*, 1657–1668. [CrossRef] [PubMed]

265. Fu, C.; Liu, T.; Li, L.; Liu, H.; Chen, D.; Tang, F. The absorption, distribution, excretion and toxicity of mesoporous silica nanoparticles in mice following different exposure routes. *Biomaterials* **2013**, *34*, 2565–2575. [CrossRef] [PubMed]

266. Chen, Y.; Chen, H.; Shi, J. In Vivo Bio-Safety Evaluations and Diagnostic/Therapeutic Applications of Chemically Designed Mesoporous Silica Nanoparticles. *Adv. Mater.* **2013**, *25*, 3144–3176. [CrossRef] [PubMed]

267. Asefa, T.; Tao, Z. Biocompatibility of Mesoporous Silica Nanoparticles. *Chem. Res. Toxicol.* **2012**, *25*, 2265–2284. [CrossRef] [PubMed]

268. Napierska, D.; Thomassen, L.C.; Lison, D.; Martens, J.A.; Hoet, P.H. The nanosilica hazard: Another variable entity. *Part. Fibre Toxicol.* **2010**, *7*, 39. [CrossRef] [PubMed]

269. Martin, K.R. The chemistry of silica and its potential health benefits. *J. Nutr. Health Aging* **2007**, *11*, 94–97. [PubMed]

270. Croissant, J.G.; Fatieiev, Y.; Khashab, N.M. Degradability and Clearance of Silicon, Organosilica, Silsesquioxane, Silica Mixed Oxide, and Mesoporous Silica Nanoparticles. *Adv. Mater.* **2017**, *29*, 1604634. [CrossRef] [PubMed]

271. Kim, S.-H.; Lee, M.-S.; Kim, D.; Lee, T.K.; Kwon, T.K.; Yun, H.; Khang, S.-H. The comparative immunotoxicity of mesoporous silica nanoparticles and colloidal silica nanoparticles in mice. *Int. J. Nanomed.* **2013**, *8*, 147–158. [CrossRef] [PubMed]

272. Phillips, E.; Penate-Medina, O.; Zanzonico, P.B.; Carvajal, R.D.; Mohan, P.; Ye, Y.; Humm, J.; Gonen, M.; Kalaigian, H.; Schoder, H.; et al. Clinical translation of an ultrasmall inorganic optical-PET imaging nanoparticle probe. *Sci. Transl. Med.* **2014**, *6*, 260ra149. [CrossRef] [PubMed]

273. Benezra, M.; Penate-Medina, O.; Zanzonico, P.B.; Schaer, D.; Ow, H.; Burns, A.; DeStanchina, E.; Longo, V.; Herz, E.; Iyer, S.; et al. Multimodal silica nanoparticles are effective cancer-targeted probes in a model of human melanoma. *J. Clin. Investig.* **2011**, *121*, 2768–2780. [CrossRef] [PubMed]

274. Bukara, K.; Schueller, L.; Rosier, J.; Daems, T.; Verheyden, L.; Eelen, S.; Martens, J.A.; Van den Mooter, G.; Bugarski, B.; Kiekens, F. In Vivo Performance of Fenofibrate Formulated With Ordered Mesoporous Silica Versus 2-Marketed Formulations: A Comparative Bioavailability Study in Beagle Dogs. *J. Pharm. Sci.* **2016**, *105*, 2381–2385. [CrossRef] [PubMed]

275. Ashley, C.E.; Carnes, E.C.; Wu, T.; Felton, L.A.; Sasaki, D.Y. Antibiotic Protocells and Related Pharmaceutical Formulations and Methods of Treatment. U.S. Patent 20170165375A1, 15 June 2017. Available online: https://www.google.com/patents/US20170165375 (accessed on 7 November 2017).

276. Brinker, C.J.; Townson, J.; Lin, Y.-S.; Durfee, P.N. Core and Surface Modification of Mesoporous Silica Nanoparticles to Achieve Cell Specific Targeting In Vivo. U.S. Patent 20160287717A1, 6 October 2016. Available online: https://www.google.com/patents/US20160287717 (accessed on 7 November 2017).

277. Brinker, C.J.; Ashley, C.E.; Jiang, X.; Liu, J.; Peabody, D.S.; Wharton, W.R.; Carnes, E.; Chackerian, B.; Willman, C.L. Protocells and Their Use for Targeted Delivery of Multicomponent Cargos to Cancer Cells. U.S. Patent 8992984B1, 31 March 2015. Available online: https://www.google.com/patents/US8992984 (accessed on 7 November 2017).

278. Brinker, J.C.; Lin, Y. Torroidal Mesoporous Silica Nanoparticles (TMSNPS) and Related Protocells. U.S. Patent 20160338954A1, 24 November 2016. Available online: http://www.freepatentsonline.com/y2016/0338954.html (accessed on 7 November 2017).

279. Ashley, C.E.; Brinker, C.J.; Carnes, E.C.; Fekrazad, M.H.; Felton, L.A.; Negrete, O.; Padilla, D.P.; Wilkinson, B.S.; Wilkinson, D.C.; Willman, C.L. Porous Nanoparticle-Supported Lipid Bilayers (Protocells) for Targeted Delivery Including Transdermal Delivery of Cargo and Methods Thereof. U.S. Patent EP2765997A4, 24 June 2015. Available online: https://www.google.co.in/patents/EP2765997A4?cl=esCached (accessed on 7 November 2017).

280. Nel, A.E.; Zink, J.I.; Meng, H. Lipid Bilayer Coated Mesoporous Silica Nanoparticles with a High Loading Capacity for One or More Anticancer Agents. U.S. Patent 20160008283A1, 14 January 2016. Available online: https://www.google.com/patents/US20160008283?cl=en (accessed on 7 November 2017).

281. Oktem, H.A.; Ozalp, V.C.; Hernandez, F.J.; Hernandez, L.I. Applications and Tools Based on Silica Particles Coated with Biological or Synthetic Molecules. U.S. Patent 20170172935A1, 22 June 2017. Available online: https://www.google.com/patents/US20170172935 (accessed on 7 November 2017).

282. Won, C. Composition for Delivering Bioactive Material or Protein, and Use Thereof. U.S. Patent 20170172923A1, 22 June 2017. Available online: https://www.google.com/patents/US20170172923 (accessed on 7 November 2017).

283. Weng, C.-F.; Chia, Y.-C.; Lee, C.-H.; Varadharajan, T. HCD Formulation for Cancer Treatment. U.S. Patent 20160243236A1, 25 August 2016. Available online: https://www.google.com/patents/US20160243236 (accessed on 7 November 2017).

284. Lee, K.; Lai, J.; Shah, B. FRET-Based Mesoporous Silica Nanoparticles for Real-Time Monitoring of Drug Release. U.S. Patent 9408918B1, 9 August 2016. Available online: http://www.freepatentsonline.com/9408918.html (accessed on 7 November 2017).

285. Shou-Cang, S.; Kiong, N.W.; Chia, L.; Tan, R. Nanostructured Material Formulated with Bone Cement for Effective Antibiotic Delivery. U.S. Patent 9155814B2, 13 October 2015. Available online: https://www.google.com/patents/US9155814 (accessed on 7 November 2017).

286. Liu, Y.; Lay, C.L. Stimuli-Responsive Interpolymer Complex Coated Hollow Silica Vesicles. U.S. Patent 20150182468A1, 2 July 2015. Available online: https://www.google.com/patents/US20150182468 (accessed on 7 November 2017).

287. Zink, J.I.; Nel, A.E.; Xia, T.; Ji, Z.; Meng, H.; Li, Z.; Liong, M.; Xue, M.; Tarn, D.Y. Cationic Polymer Coated Mesoporous Silica Nanoparticles and Uses Thereof. U.S. Patent 20120207795A1, 16 August 2012.

288. Liong, M.; Lu, J.; Tamanoi, F.; Zink, J.I.; Nel, A. Mesoporous Silica Nanoparticles for Biomedical Applications. U.S. Patent 20100255103A1, 7 October 2010. Available online: https://www.google.ch/patents/US20100255103 (accessed on 7 November 2017).

289. Lee, C.-H.; Lo, L.-W.; Yang, C.-S.; Mou, C.-Y. Charged Mesoporous Silica Nanoparticle-Based Drug Delivery System for Controlled Release and Enhanced Bioavailability. U.S. Patent 20100104650A1, 29 April 2010. Available online: https://www.google.com/patents/US20100104650 (accessed on 7 November 2017).

290. Lin, V.; Trewyn, B.; Huh, S.; Whitman, C. Antimicrobial Mesoporous Silica Nanoparticles. U.S. Patent 20060018966A1, 26 January 2006. Available online: https://www.google.com/patents/US20060018966 (accessed on 7 November 2017).

291. Chen, F.; Ma, K.; Benezra, M.; Zhang, L.; Cheal, S.M.; Phillips, E.; Yoo, B.; Pauliah, M.; Overholtzer, M.; Zanzonico, P.; et al. Cancer-Targeting Ultrasmall Silica Nanoparticles for Clinical Translation: Physicochemical Structure and Biological Property Correlations. *Chem. Mater.* **2017**, *29*, 8766–8779. [CrossRef] [PubMed]

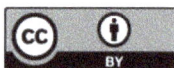

MDPI

St. Alban-Anlage 66

4052 Basel

Switzerland

Tel. +41 61 683 77 34

Fax +41 61 302 89 18

www.mdpi.com

Pharmaceutics Editorial Office

E-mail: pharmaceutics@mdpi.com

www.mdpi.com/journal/pharmaceutics

www.ingramcontent.com/pod-product-compliance
Lightning Source LLC
Chambersburg PA
CBHW051852210326
41597CB00033B/5871